MR

New Perspectives
on Down Syndrome

New Perspectives on Down Syndrome

edited by

Siegfried M. Pueschel, M.D., Ph.D., M.P.H.
Director
Child Development Center
Rhode Island Hospital
Providence

Carol Tingey, Ph.D.
Associate Professor
Department of Psychology
Utah State University
Logan

John E. Rynders, Ph.D.
Professor
Department of Educational Psychology
Special Education Programs
University of Minnesota
Minneapolis

Allen C. Crocker, M.D.
Director
Developmental Evaluation Clinic
Children's Hospital
Boston

and

Diane M. Crutcher
Executive Director
National Down Syndrome Congress
Chicago

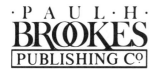
·P·A·U·L·H·
BROOKES
PUBLISHING CO.

Baltimore · London

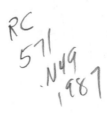

Paul H. Brookes Publishing Co.
Post Office Box 10624
Baltimore, Maryland 21285–0624

Typeset by The Composing Room, Grand Rapids, Michigan.
Manufactured in the United States of America by
The Maple Press Company, York, Pennsylvania.

This project has been funded at least in part with federal funds from the U.S. Department of Education under contract number 300-85-0071. The content of this publication does not necessarily reflect the views or policies of the U.S. Department of Education nor does mention of trade names, commercial products, or organizations imply endorsement by the U.S. Government.

Permission to reprint the following quotation is gratefully acknowledged:
Page 298: Quotation from Featherstone, H. (1980). *A difference in the family* (pp. 77–78). New York: Basic Books. Reprinted by permission.

The illustration by Martha Perske appearing on page 19 is reprinted with permission from: Perske, R., & Perske, M. (1980). *New life in the neighborhood.* Nashville: Abingdon Press.
The illustrations by Martha Perske appearing on pages 145, 269, and 333 are reprinted with permission from: Perske, R., & Perske, M. (1981). *Hope for the families: New directions for parents of persons with retardation or other disabilities.* Nashville: Abingdon Press.

Library of Congress Cataloging-in-Publication Data

New perspectives on Down syndrome.

    Papers from the Down Syndrome State-of-the-Art Conference, held in Boston, Mass., Apr. 23–25, 1985.
    Bibliography: p.
    Includes index.
    1. Down's syndrome—Congresses. I. Pueschel, Siegfried M. II. Down Syndrome State-of-the-Art Conference (1985 : Boston, Mass.)
RC571.N49   1987   618.92′858842   86-12993
ISBN 0-933716-69-9

Contents

✦✦✦

v

Contributors

G. Thomas Bellamy, Ph.D.
Professor and Director
Specialized Training Program
College of Education
University of Oregon
Eugene, OR 97403-1211

Diane Bricker, Ph.D.
University of Oregon
Center on Human Development
901 East 18th Street
Eugene, OR 97403

Paige Calvin
399 Marrett Road
Lexington, MA 02173

Claire D. Canning, B.A.
35 Narragansett Avenue
Pawtucket, RI 02861

Allen C. Crocker, M.D.
Director
Developmental Evaluation Clinic
The Children's Hospital
300 Longwood Avenue
Boston, MA 02115

Diane M. Crutcher
Executive Director
National Down Syndrome Congress
1800 Dempster Street
Park Ridge, IL 60068-1146

Michael R. Cummings, Ph.D.
Department of Biological Sciences
University of Illinois at Chicago
Institute for the Study of Developmental
  Disabilities
1640 West Roosevelt Road
Chicago, IL 60608

Mercedes B. Ducayen, M.S.
Research Worker
Center for Reproductive Sciences of the
  International Institute for the Study of
  Human Reproduction
College of Physicians and Surgeons
Columbia University
630 West 168th Street
New York, NY 10032

Chris DeRoest
Instructor
Teaching Research Division
Oregon State System of Higher
  Education
345 North Monmouth Avenue
Monmouth, OR 97361

Jean Edwards, D.S.W.
Professor, Special Education
Box 751
Portland State University
Portland, OR 97207

Charles J. Epstein, M.D.
Division of Medical Genetics
Department of Pediatrics
Box 6106, 650-M
University of California–San Francisco
San Francisco, CA 94143

Jye-Siung Fang, Ph.D.
Assistant Professor of Obstetrics and
  Gynecology
Center for Reproductive Sciences of the
  International Institute for the Study of
  Human Reproduction
College of Physicians and Surgeons
Columbia University
630 West 168th Street
New York, NY 10032

Douglas Fenderson, Ph.D.
University of Minnesota
Medical School
Minneapolis, MN 55455

H.D. Bud Fredericks, Ed.D.
Research Professor
Teaching Research Division
Oregon State System of Higher
 Education
345 North Monmouth Avenue
Monmouth, OR 97361

Sharon Graw
Eleanor Roosevelt Institute for Cancer
 Research
1899 Gaylord Street
Denver, CO 80206

James Gusella, Ph.D.
Director of Neurogenetics Laboratory
Genetics Unit
Harvard Medical School
Massachusetts General Hospital
Fruit Street, Research 3
Boston, Massachusetts 02114

Marci Hanson, Ph.D.
Professor
Department of Special Education
San Francisco State University
1600 Holloway Avenue
San Francisco, CA 94132

Lewis Holmes, M.D.
Embryology, Teratology Unit
Massachusetts General Hospital
Boston, MA 02114

DeAnna Horstmeier, Ph.D.
Project Coordinator, G.A.P.S.
Advocacy and Protective Services, Inc.
986 West Goodale Boulevard
Columbus, OH 43212

Carl A. Huether, Ph.D.
Department of Biological Sciences
University of Cincinnati
Cincinnati, OH 45221

Georgiana Jagiello, M.D., D.Sc.
Virgil Damon Professor of Obstetrics
 and Gynecology and of Human
 Genetics and Development
Director, Center for Reproductive
 Sciences of the International Institute
 for the Study of Human Reproduction
College of Physicians and Surgeons
Columbia University
630 West 168th Street
New York, NY 10032

Orv C. Karan, Ph.D.
Director, Clinical Service and Training
Research and Training Center in
 Community Integration of the
 Mentally Retarded
Waisman Center on Mental Retardation
 and Human Development
University of Wisconsin–Madison
1500 Highland Avenue
Madison, WI 53706

Catherine Berger Knight, Ph.D.
Waisman Center on Mental Retardation
 and Human Development
1500 Highland Avenue
University of Wisconsin–Madison
Madison, WI 53706

David Kurnit, M.D., Ph.D.
The Children's Hospital
Genetics Division
300 Longwood Avenue
Boston, MA 02115

Jon F. Miller, Ph.D.
Department of Communicative
 Disorders
and
Waisman Center on Mental Retardation
 and Human Development
University of Wisconsin–Madison
1500 Highland Avenue
Madison, WI 53706

John Mushlitz, Jr., B.S.
Instructor
Teaching Research Division
Oregon State System of Higher
 Education
345 North Monmouth Avenue
Monmouth, OR 97361

Rachael L. Neve, Ph.D.
The Children's Hospital
Genetics Division
300 Longwood Avenue
Boston, MA 02115

Thomas J. O'Neill
National Down Syndrome Congress
1800 Dempster Street
Park Ridge, IL 60068-1146

David Patterson, Ph.D.
President
Eleanor Roosevelt Cancer Research
    Institute
1899 Gaylord Street
Denver, CO 80206

Donna Pauls
Administrative Assistant
Education, Rehabilitation and
    Augmentative Communications Unit
Waisman Center on Mental Retardation
    and Human Development
University of Wisconsin–Madison
1500 Highland Avenue
Madison, WI 53706

Robert Perske
159 Hollow Tree Ridge Road
Darien, CT 06820

Siegfried M. Pueschel, M.D., Ph.D., M.P.H.
Director, Child Development Center
Rhode Island Hospital
593 Eddy Street
Providence, RI 02902

John E. Rynders, Ph.D.
Professor
Special Education Programs
University of Minnesota
249 Burton Hall
Minneapolis, MN 55455

Miriam Schweber, Ph.D.
School of Medicine
Boston University
80 East Concord Street
Boston, MA 02118

Denis W. Stoddard, Ph.D.
Comprehensive Training and
    Development Institute, Inc.
Third Floor
51 North High Street
Columbus, OH 43215

Jean Ann Summers, B.S.G.
Acting Director
Lawrence University Affiliated Facility
University of Kansas
Lawrence, KS 66045

Weng Kong Sung, Ph.D.
Associate Research Scientist
Center for Reproductive Sciences of the
    International Institute for the Study of
    Human Reproduction
College of Physicians and Surgeons
Columbia University
630 West 168th Street
New York, NY 10032

Horace C. Thuline, M.D.
Head, Genetic Services Section
Division of Health
Department of Social and Health
    Services
State of Washington
1704 NE 150th Street
Seattle, WA 98155

Carol Tingey, Ph.D., F.A.A.M.D.
Associate Professor
Department of Psychology
Early Intervention Research Institute
Developmental Center for Handicapped
    Persons
College of Education
Utah State University
Logan, UT 84322-6850

Ann P. Turnbull, Ed.D.
Professor, Department of Special
    Education
and
Acting Associate Director
Bureau of Child Research
University of Kansas
223 Haworth Hall
Lawrence, KS 66045

Paul Watkins
Senior Scientist
Integrated Genetics
31 New York Avenue
Framingham, MA 01701

Madeleine C. Will
Assistant Secretary
Office of Special Education and
    Rehabilitative Services
U.S. Department of Education
Room 3006—Switzer
330 C Street, S.W.
Washington, DC 20202

Barbara Wilcox, Ph.D.
Associate Professor
Special Education and Rehabilitation
University of Oregon
Eugene, OR 97403

Jean M. Zadig, Ph.D.
The Children's Hospital
300 Longwood Avenue
Boston, MA 02115

Foreword

Turning Possibilities
into Realities

✦✦✦

As you open this book, I think it is particularly exciting to find among these pages the work of professionals from the fields of biomedicine, education, psychosocial studies, and community living who have come together to coordinate efforts to reaffirm the humanity and potential of individuals with Down syndrome. Each of us, to some extent, is involved with questions of ultimate worth, with defining the indices that measure the quality of life—but we are involved in different ways. Some time ago, I read about a marvelous exchange between Robert R. Wilson, then-head of the Fermilab Accelerator Project, which developed a high-speed proton accelerator to produce nuclear energy, and a senator during a hearing. It goes like this: Appearing before a congressional committee, Wilson was being pressed for a justification for Fermilab. "Is there anything connected with the hopes of this accelerator that in any way involves the security of this country?" asked the senator. "No sir, I do not believe so," said Wilson. "It has no value in that respect?" pursued the senator. Wilson replied, "It has only to do with the respect with which we regard each other, the dignity of men, our love of culture. It has to do with, are we good painters, good sculptors, great poets? I mean all the things we really venerate and honor in our country and are patriotic about. It has nothing to do with defending our country except to make it worth defending." President Ronald Reagan expressed it well, in announcing our country's endorsement of and participation in the International Decade of the Disabled. He said: "The disabled want what all of us want: the opportunity to contribute to our communities, to use our creativity, and to go as far as our God-given talents will take us."

I have heard from many parents and professionals who fear that, as handicapped students near the end of their formal education, they often lack the necessary socialization skills to succeed in the world of work. In one instance, professionals tried work-study programs and found that the skills for doing the job were present, but that the young man was doing very poorly in dealing with supervisors and co-workers. The reason was that he had not learned appropriate socialization skills. With the help of professionals who act as job coaches and personal advocates, many handicapped individuals, in-

cluding those with mental impairments, such as Down syndrome, are learning
necessary socialization skills while engaging in meaningful employment in
supported work programs.

I would like to share something of the dream and vision that I have been
developing during my tenure as the Assistant Secretary for the Office of
Special Education and Rehabilitative Services (OSERS). But more than
dreams and visions, the elements are there, the possibilities have been demonstrated. To turn them into everyday realities is the real challenge. The supported work initiative of my office is addressing that challenge. It is an
intensive effort to assist states with the implementation of their supported
employment programs as an alternative to the day activity services that now
include many individuals with severe disabilities. The development of viable
supported employment programs is slowly replacing institutionalization and
day activity programs as the method of choice in dealing with individuals with
disabilities. As we envision it, supported employment combines the ongoing
support typically provided in day activity programs with paid work opportunities. Such supported employment programs could occur in a variety of
settings: in dispersed individual placements in a community, with publicly
funded support staff rotating among sites; or in a mobile crew working in
neighborhood settings; or in group placements, with many individuals hired
as a team, supervised directly by a job coach.

Supported employment is defined by four characteristics that together
distinguish it from both vocational rehabilitation services and traditional
methods of providing day activity services.

1. *Service recipients.* Supported employment is designed for individuals
   who are served in day activity programs because they appear to lack the
   potential for unassisted competitive employment and consequently are
   not served by the vocational rehabilitation system.
2. *Ongoing support.* Supported employment involves the continuing provision of training, supervision, and support services that would be available
   in a traditional day activity program. Unlike vocational rehabilitation
   programs, however, supported employment is not designed to lead to
   unassisted competitive work.
3. *Employment focus.* Supported employment is designed to produce the
   same benefits for disabled persons that other people receive from work.
   Employment quality can be measured by: income level, quality of working life, security, mobility, advancement opportunity, and so forth. In
   contrast, outcome measures currently used in day activity programs
   reflect mastery of skills and behaviors that are thought to be prerequisite
   to obtaining employment and receiving employment benefits.
4. *Flexibility in support strategies.* Supported employment incorporates a
   variety of techniques to assist individuals in obtaining and performing

work. For example, support could involve assistance to a service agency that provided training and supervision at an individual's worksite; support to an employer to offset the excess costs of equipping, training, and supervising a severely disabled individual; and salary supplements to a co-worker who provided regular assistance in performance of personal care activities while at work.

The central part of the OSERS supported work demonstration is a one-time, time-limited, grant, contract, or cooperative agreement program that provides funds to help states convert traditional day activity programs to alternative supported employment methods. In order for supported employment programs to be effective, we need people who are trained to develop jobs, match individual strengths to work tasks, communicate with employers, plan transportation, and handle complex interactions with Social Security, education, and related programs. Job coaches or trainer advocates will be needed to work closely with difficult-to-place workers until they learn to function at an acceptable performance rate (i.e., in bench work, electronic assembly, or other entry-level positions). As needed, job coaches should perform the work themselves to assure employers that the job will be done correctly, and to act as role models for the employees.

Job coaches will also learn what is involved in monitoring the employees' progress on the job, getting regular written feedback from employers and co-workers, utilizing behavioral data, and implementing communication with the employees' families. They will learn what is involved in helping an employee keep a job. Social skills also play a major role in an individual's ability to succeed in the workforce. The job coaches play a pivotal role in the development and enhancement of social skills which may be lacking in some severely disabled individuals at the time of their entry into supported employment programs.

Intensive, individualized and ongoing training tends to be expensive. But we contend that supported employment programs are less expensive in the long run than total public support. Most trainees become at least partially self-supporting subsequent to their involvement in the program. Although supported employment programs for severely handicapped youth and adults make up only a tiny fraction of the programs available, they do provide a powerful demonstration that, with assistance, even individuals with the most severe physical and mental handicaps can move from welfare programs to employment programs.

This nation is experiencing a new declaration of independence for persons with disabilities, with 4 million students enrolled in special education programs. That is more than the total population of the United States at the time of our Declaration of Independence over 200 years ago. When the United States became an independent nation, we were motivated by idealism. Ameri-

cans dared to believe in their abilities. Today, many people are too preoc-
cupied with supposed limitations. In the area of rehabilitation—and other
aspects of our lives—too little is expected. And we get exactly what we
expect.

As professionals and parents, we must not expect too little. I challenge
and encourage all members of the allied and divergent professions represented
in this book to look for ways to unify toward our common goal—the improvement and expansion of education, employment, independent living, and social opportunities for children, youth, and adults with Down syndrome.
Through our support and vigilance, we can assure that state and local jurisdic-
tions provide adequate educational and employment services for their disabled
citizens. All disabled individuals need the opportunities to become self-sustaining or potentially self-sustaining adults in the communities in which they
live. Collectively, we can make these opportunities possible.

Madeleine C. Will
Assistant Secretary
Office of Special Education and Rehabilitative Services

REFERENCES

Reagan, R. (1983, November 28). *Weekly compilation of presidential documents.*
Washington, DC: U.S. Government Printing Office.

Foreword

These Things
Are Most Important

✦✦✦

Hello. My name is Paige Calvin. I have done a lot of things in my life. These things are most important to me—my family, my friends, and my work. I am a student in the LAB program at Lexington High School. I like to go to work. I have a job after school. I am becoming more involved. I go to school on my own. I go out to swim and out to dinner or to the movies with my friends. This summer, I am a staff member at Camp Calumet. I have been camping for 5 years. Someday I want to be independent, live with my friends, and go to work every day. Here are some pictures at my work. I hope you can help to find jobs for people with Down syndrome like me.

Paige Calvin
Age 20

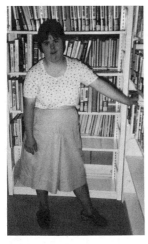

I am at the library. I file slips by numbers.

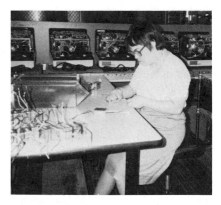

Here I am at Honeywell on the sixth floor. I put transformers on the wires.

Foreword

The Person Comes First

✦✦✦

I would like to tell you about someone I know. He's not real tall; he's got an award-winning smile and a great sense of humor; in fact, he's a real kidder. He's an excellent swimmer; he can manage an olympic-size pool quite well. He's a very pleasant guy and when you consider the fact that he is known as chronically ill to the medical community, you marvel at his ability to remain so pleasant—taking it all in stride. He goes to school, really does quite well; he achieves a great deal of satisfaction within that setting. He's got a very pleasant personality. I've even seen people meet him, be a little uncomfortable, and then be put at ease by him. He's got a certain wisdom and understanding of the world, and his dad, well, his dad is real proud of him. If you're in doubt, just ask me!

You see, I am introducing you to my son, Joshua. Josh is 7 years old. He's diligent to the task, a unique kid, a hard worker and, yes, Josh has Down syndrome. I mention the Down syndrome last because Josh is a person first. Josh is not a "Down's"; he's not "a Down syndrome child"; but rather he's an individual who happens to have Down syndrome. He's not a category or a diagnosis. He is a person before he is anything else.

That is so important for all of us to keep in mind as we deal with families that are touched by Down syndrome. As a parent of a child with Down syndrome, I have a lot of concerns about the many physical problems that my son experiences. I have concerns about the educational services that are sometimes available and sometimes not. I certainly have concerns about Josh's future: Will he have the opportunity for the socialization that he needs? Will there be needed community living and employment opportunities for him? Will he be afforded the opportunities to which he is entitled and that he has the right to receive?

If we all work together, our goals will be met. The opportunities can become realities and everyone's rights will be protected. None of us can do this alone. We need each other. I pledge to you the cooperation of the National Down Syndrome Congress. We look forward to a continuing relationship with our friends from government and our friends from the professional community. We look forward to a continuing spirit of shared hope for the future.

In the past several years, we have seen infant stimulation become the norm; we have seen Public Law 94-142 enacted; we have seen the Child Abuse Amendments become law; we have seen the birth and growth of services for the mentally retarded and developmentally disabled. We now need to continue working and making sure that these accomplishments progress and remain true to task. So, too, we need to expand our horizons and set new goals. We need to continue working and ensure that we'll never stop looking for the answers that will someday help us unravel the many mysteries surrounding Down syndrome. Today, the opportunity is at hand—to provide a brighter future for all individuals with Down syndrome through learning and sharing.

Thomas J. O'Neill
President
National Down Syndrome Congress

Preface

✦✦✦

In 1982, the idea of a state-of-the-art conference relevant to life span issues surrounding Down syndrome was conceived by Madeleine C. Will, Assistant Secretary of the Office of Special Education and Rehabilitative Services, along with some members of the National Institute of Handicapped Research (NIHR) as well as the leadership of the National Down Syndrome Congress. Behind the initiation of planning discussions was a concept representing pride and acknowledgment in the accomplishments thus far achieved for individuals with Down syndrome and, concurrently, dissatisfaction in some areas of services, attitudes, and research. Primary authorizing legislation of NIHR has mandated a comprehensive research rehabilitation plan that must lead to an interagency committee on disability research representing the approximately 32 federal agencies conducting research in various aspects of disabilities and rehabilitation.

The Down Syndrome State-of-the-Art Conference (April 23–25, 1985, Parker House Hotel, Boston, Massachusetts) helped fulfill NIHR's mandates by sharpening issues and providing "cutting edge" information and research findings from a biomedical, educational, psychosocial, and community living perspective. The format of this program was created to ensure that all disciplines presented would leave the conference with a more accurate, well-rounded perception of Down syndrome and the people affected by it. Our intent was to expose participants representing a range of fields to individuals with Down syndrome and their families, looking at prospects and problems from all angles.

The material contained in this book represents major topical presentations plus allied comments from peer reviewers. All chapters and the accompanying responses have been revised and updated for publication. This book is not intended to be totally comprehensive, but rather addresses many of the most pertinent aspects of life span issues surrounding Down syndrome as well as offering research recommendations.

We hope that the goals of Madeleine Will, NIHR, conference initiators, and the planning commitee have been met. Furthermore, it is our hope that this book can be used as a stepping stone for identification of where we are and where we need to go in order to maximize the abilities of persons with Down syndrome as we approach the 21st century.

Diane M. Crutcher
Executive Director
National Down Syndrome Congress

Acknowledgments

✦✦✦

The National Down Syndrome Congress gratefully acknowledges the ongoing support of the National Institute of Handicapped Research (NIHR) in bringing this book and the Down Syndrome State-of-the-Art Conference to fruition. We especially thank Madeleine Will, Assistant Secretary of the Office of Special Education and Rehabilitative Services, for initiating the concept and trusting a national parent group to accomplish the goal successfully. Further, we thank our project officer, Naomi Karp; Dr. Douglas Fenderson, former director of NIHR; and the members of the planning committee (see Appendix) for their constant insight, availability, and assistance. Finally, we extend our deepest appreciation to the conference presenters, reactors, moderators, and conferees who spent 2½ days learning and sharing about the *total* person with Down syndrome as well as the families touched by it.

People with Down syndrome will benefit greatly from the knowledge that has been shared. It is the hope of the planning committee and those connected with this book and the conference that this knowledge will facilitate continued interest—in order to apply and implement what is now known for the benefit of all those touched by Down syndrome.

History of Down Syndrome
The Need for a New Perspective

John E. Rynders

✦✦✦

For more than 120 years—ever since J. Langdon Down's historic paper was published in 1866—the realization that persons with Down syndrome *have value and give value* has grown, although sometimes with serious setbacks, in the public consciousness. The purpose of this chapter is to look at those years through "value-colored glasses." (A synopsis of the events to be covered is shown in Table 1.[1])

THE FIRST FORMAL DESCRIPTION OF DOWN SYNDROME

There are hints in the historical record that an awareness of the condition of Down syndrome existed hundreds, perhaps even thousands of years ago. Images in old paintings and ancient stone carvings suggest that this might be so (Milton & Gonzalo, 1974; Zellweger, 1968). But there can be no doubt that a paper by J. Langdon Down in 1866 stands as a landmark document in the written history of Down syndrome.

Down, in attempting to classify the various forms of "feeblemindedness" that he had observed, probably influenced by Charles Darwin's thoughts on evolution, concluded that individuals with mental disabilities belonged to various ethnic classifications, including the "Ethiopian and Malay varieties." His description of persons he felt belonged to the "Mongolian family" is of particular interest.

This work was supported in part by Contract #300-82-0363 from Special Education Programs, U.S Department of Education, awarded to the University of Minnesota. The material does not necessarily reflect the policy of the U.S. Department of Education, and no official endorsement should be inferred.

[1]In deciding which events to include in this review, a simple selection procedure was employed: The author outlined a proposed total set of events and sent it to the other four editors of this book for their inclusion-exclusion critique. What is included represents a consensus across editors that the events chosen provide a reasonably comprehensive portrayal of significant occurrences from the historical record on Down syndrome and mental retardation.

1

Table 1. Historical events: Down syndrome since 1866

Date	Event
1866	J. Langdon Down provides the first formal description of Down syndrome.
1896	Smith attempts to treat Down syndrome with a drug (thyroid hormone extract) for the first time.
1920	The "Eugenics Scare" leads to a massive state residential institution construction program. Many of those institutionalized were persons with Down syndrome.
1940s–1950s	World War II heightens awareness that the human rights of vulnerable people must be established and protected.
1959	Lejeune and his associates discover that Down syndrome is a chromosomal disorder.
1960s–1970s	Deinstitutionalization begins on a national scale, prompted by litigation. Head Start helps to spawn early education efforts for children with Down syndrome.
1973	The Down's Syndrome Congress (now the National Down Syndrome Congress) is formed.
1970s–1980s	Passage of major social, educational, and vocational legislation, such as PL 94-142 (Education for All Handicapped Children Act) and Sections 503 and 504 of PL 93-112 (Rehabilitation Act of 1973).
1982	The case of Baby Doe leads to a new application of Section 504 of the Rehabilitation Act of 1973, establishing the right of newborn children with Down syndrome to customary medical care.

The great Mongolian family has numerous representatives, and it is to this division, I wish, in this paper, to call special attention. A very large number of congenital idiots [not a derogatory term at that time] are typical Mongols. So marked is this, that when placed side by side, it is difficult to believe that the specimens [people] compared are not children of the same parents. The number of idiots [mentally retarded persons] who arrange themselves around the Mongolian type is so great, and they present such a close resemblance to one another in mental power, that I shall describe an idiot member of this racial division, selected from the large number that have fallen under my observation.

The hair is not black, as the real Mongol, but of a brownish colour, straight and scanty. The face is flat and broad, and destitute of prominence. The cheeks are roundish, and extended laterally. The eyes are obliquely placed, and the internal canthi more than normally distant from one another. . . . The lips are large and thick with transverse fissures. The tongue is long, thick, and is much roughened. The nose is small. The skin has a slight dirty yellowish tinge, and is deficient in elasticity, giving the appearance of being too large for the body.

The boy's aspect is such that it is difficult to realize that he is the child of Europeans, but so frequently are these characters presented, that there can be no doubt that these ethnic features are the result of degeneration. (Down, 1866, pp. 260–261)

In light of the era of racial elitism in which he lived, it is remarkable that Down did not portray the developmental prospects of persons with Down syndrome as devoid of hope. To the contrary, near the end of his historic article in *Clinical Lectures and Reports* (1866), he wrote: "They are cases which very much repay judicious treatment. . . . The improvement which training effects in them is greatly in excess of what would be predicated if one did not know the characteristics of the type" (pp. 261–262).

Unfortunately, views leading to the devaluing of persons with Down syndrome have occurred several times since 1866. For example, in 1924, Crookshank concluded that persons with Down syndrome represented a regression to a nonhuman species (i.e., to an orangutan). In 1968, Joseph Fletcher, a well-known theologian, in attempting to comfort a bereaved parent (Mr. Bard) who, after an emotional struggle, had concluded that he must institutionalize his child with Down syndrome, wrote:

> People in the Bards' situation have no reason to feel guilty about putting a Down's syndrome baby away, whether it's "put away" in the sense of hidden in a sanitarium or in a more responsible lethal sense. It is sad, yes. Dreadful. But it carries no guilt. True guilt arises only from an offense against a person, and a *Down's is not a person* [emphasis added]. (Bard & Fletcher, 1968)[2]

As recently as 1970, the *Encyclopaedia Britannica* listed the condition of Down syndrome under the heading, "Monster." (The 1974 edition shows it under the appropriate heading of "Down's syndrome.")

THE FIRST "THERAPEUTIC" DRUG TREATMENT FOR DOWN SYNDROME

In addition to hypothesizing that "mongolism" was a manifestation of ethnic degeneracy, Down (1866) also suggested that the degeneracy stemmed from tuberculosis in the parents. Thus, the search for a biomedical "cure" began in 1866 and has been pursued actively from that date onward.

Many drug treatments have been attempted to improve the functioning ability of persons with Down syndrome. This chapter offers only a few illustrative examples of this interesting body of work, drawing most of the material from a 1982 review by Horrobin and Pueschel (see Table 2). They concluded that, based on the evidence available, there is no drug treatment that significantly improves the overall functioning of children with Down syndrome.

THE "EUGENICS SCARE" AND THE INSTITUTIONALIZATION MOVEMENT

The movement to build large, state-operated, residential institutions for persons with mental retardation did not begin with the "Eugenics Scare" in 1920. It received impetus in part, it appears, from the thoughts of Johann

---

[2]See Chapter 10, by Robert Perske, for a more detailed account of this incident, and the events that followed.

Table 2. History of drug treatments for Down syndrome: Selected examples

Treatment	Rationale for use	Current status of treatment
Thyroid hormone extract	Benda (1960) and Smith (1896) advocated its use based on their work.	Koch, Share and Gralicker (1965) did not find any significant differences between treated and untreated children with Down syndrome in a contolled study. Administration of thyroid hormone does not benefit children with Down syndrome unless there is laboratory documentation of concurrent hypothyroidism (Horrobin & Pueschel, 1982).
Pituitary extract	Benda (1960) and Goldstein (1954, 1956a) suggested its use on the premise that panhypopituitarism is a contributing factor in Down syndrome.	Berg, Kirman, Stern, and Mittwoch (1961), Diamond and Moon (1961), and Freeman (1970) found that pituitary extract given to children with Down syndrome did not improve their intellectual and social functioning.
Glutamic acid and its derivatives	Some workers have reported good results with this therapy (Gadson, 1951; Goldstein, 1956a; Kugelmass, 1959).	Astin and Ross (1960) and Lombard, Gilbert, and Donofrio (1955) reported no significant improvement after glutamic acid administration to persons with Down syndrome.
Vitamins	Vitamin E (Saxl, 1972) and vitamin B_6 (Coleman, 1973) have been tried in an attempt to improve functioning (e.g., intelligence).	Coleman (1980) studied the effect of pyridoxine administration in a controlled trial and reported no significant improvement in intellectual functioning of children with Down syndrome in the treatment group.
Various combinations of vitamins, hormones, enzymes, minerals, and other substances	Enthusiastic claims of success for such combinations have been made (Haubold, 1967; Turkel, 1975).	White and Kaplitz (1964), who treated children with Down syndrome according to Haubold's instruction, did not find any significant improvement. Bumbalo, Morelewicz,

(continued)

Table 2. *(continued)*

Treatment	Rationale for use	Current status of treatment
		and Berens (1964) investigated the effect of Turkel's "U-series" on children with Down syndrome in a double-blind study; except for improvement in socialization, they did not find any other effect from this treatment approach.
Sicca cell therapy	Lyophylized material prepared from embryonic animal organs is injected, assuming that this biological material will stimulate the growth and function of the corresponding tissue in the human body (Mommsen, 1961; Schmid, 1976a,b).	Black, Kato, and Walker (1966), in a double-blind study, found no evidence that sicca cell treatment improved children's development; Bardon (1964) did not find a significant difference between experimental and control groups. Reports from the German medical literature (Bierich, 1975; Bremer, 1975; Hitzig, 1975; Schulte, 1975) provided evidence that sicca cell injection is not effective in children with Down syndrome.
		Concerns exist now that there may be danger per transmittal of fatal slow virus infection by animal cell therapy (Crocker, personal communication, 1985).
Dehydroepiandrosterone	DeMoragas (1958) used this treatment, claiming that both appearance and development of children with Down syndrome could be influenced favorably through its use.	Studies by Diamond and Moon (1961) did not corroborate DeMoragas's claim.
Dimethyl sulfoxide	Chilean investigators have claimed improvement of intellectual functioning following the administration of dimethyl sulfoxide (Aspillage, Morizon, & Avendano, 1975).	In 1973, a short-term study with dimethyl sulfoxide was carried out in Oregon to assess the effects of this treatment on academic achievement. This investigation did not

(continued)

Table 2. *(continued)*

Treatment	Rationale for use	Current status of treatment
		produce a significant positive change in children with Down syndrome (Gabourie, Becker, & Bateman, 1975).
Tryptophan compounds	Bazelon et al. (1967), employing this treatment, noted improvement in muscle tone, less tongue protrusion, and better activity level in infants with Down syndrome who had been administered 5-hydroxytryptophan (5-HTP).	Coleman (1973), using a double-blind study design, did not find any significant difference between experimental and control group children, nor did Partington, MacDonald, and Tu (1971), Pueschel, Reed, Cronk, and Goldstein (1980), or Weise, Koch, Shaw, and Rosenfeld (1974).

Guggenbühl, who, in 1836, founded a small community (a colony of cottages) on a mountainside in Switzerland (see Kanner, 1967, for a description of this effort). Guggenbühl's intent was to cure cretinism (a generic term often used in the 1800s to refer to many types of mental disabilities, including Down syndrome and genuine cretinism). Unfortunately, Guggenbühl's idyllic plan for creating an intimate community to "protect people with mental disabilities from society," was seized upon in the late 1800s and early 1900s as a way to "protect society from people with mental disabilities." Ironically, because of irrational fears about persons with mental retardation, "cottages" on state institution grounds often took form in huge dormitories that became "human warehouses"; the "colony" idea, also adopted by designers of institutions, lost its originally intended form as a community of persons with common needs, becoming instead a geographically isolated, fenced-in set of facilities that were often operated in a highly regimented manner.

The "Eugenics Scare" was premised on the erroneous notion that mental retardation (at least the form often termed cultural-familial retardation) is inherited. It was thus believed that society's gene pool would be ruined by persons with mental retardation, who were believed to be sexually promiscuous and would, therefore, breed rampantly and indiscriminately. This fueled a worldwide frenzy to build large institutions. Sounding the alarm, Goddard, a former superintendent of Vineland Training School, a large residential institution in the eastern United States, wrote, in 1912:

"Feeblemindedness is hereditary and transmitted as surely as any other character. We cannot successfully cope with these conditions until we recognize feeblemindedness and its hereditary nature, recognize it early, and take care of it. In considering the question of care, *segregation through colonization* [emphasis added] seems in the present state of our knowledge to be the ideal and perfectly satisfactory method." (Kanner, 1967, p. 132)

Goddard's ideas, accepted virtually without challenge in the early 1900s, led to the passage of permissive sterilization laws and the promotion of a policy favoring lifelong institutional segregation for persons with mental retardation. Persons with Down syndrome became one of the largest subpopulations within these residential facilities. It would take the atrocities against the "unfit" that occurred during World War II, coupled with evidence that institutionalized children with Down syndrome did not compare favorably with home-reared children with Down syndrome in terms of their development (Stedman & Eichorn, 1964) to begin to alter the acceptance of institutions.

WORLD WAR II AND ITS AFTERMATH
HEIGHTENS AWARENESS OF HUMAN AND CIVIL RIGHTS

The Nazi ideology of World War II gave rise to the Holocaust, undoubtedly the ultimate devaluing event of all time: more than 6 million Jews, thousands of persons with mental illness and mental disability (including many with Down syndrome), and other persons considered to be "inadequate" were exterminated. When the war ended, advocates of human rights in democratic societies, seeing the horrible consequences of unbridled prejudice, looked to strengthening human and civil rights legislation in their countries. Litigation resulted in stronger laws to protect the rights of ethnic and racial minority groups, and struck down school districts' authority to exclude school children with handicaps from a public education.

DOWN SYNDROME DISCOVERED
TO BE A CHROMOSOMAL DISORDER

Until 1956, textbooks on human development and medical genetics reported that humans normally have 48 chromosomes. In the mid 1950s, novel cytogenetic techniques (nonhardening fixatives, colchicine treatment, and hypotonic shock) allowed researchers to visualize chromosomes in metaphase preparations as never seen before. Thus, in 1956, Tjio and Levan were able to demonstrate clearly that there were 46 chromosomes in normal human cells. Then, in 1958, Lejeune, a French geneticist, found an additional chromosome in the cells of a child with Down syndrome. Lejeune and his co-workers studied two more individuals before reporting that persons with Down syndrome have a supernumerary chromosome in the G group (Lejeune, Gautier, & Turpin, 1959). Shortly thereafter, other investigators found that some persons with Down syndrome have translocations (Polani, Briggs, Ford, Clarke, & Berg, 1960) and mosaicism (Clarke, Edwards, & Smallpiece, 1961).

DEINSTITUTIONALIZATION

The mood of the 1970s was very conducive to the deinstitutionalization movement. As Schulz and Turnbull (1983) noted, the push to establish rights for persons with handicaps was consistent with the public's increased sensitivity to establishing equal rights for other groups, such as blacks, Native Americans, and women. In this change-oriented atmosphere, parents and professionals had expanding opportunities to move children with Down syndrome from large state institutions to community settings. A key opportunity for opening regular education programs to children with Down syndrome did not come until the landmark 1972 case of *Pennsylvania Association for Retarded Children v. Commonwealth of Pennsylvania,* known as the PARC case. The judge ruled that every child, regardless of mental ability, has a right to a free, appropriate public program of education, and that placement in a regular public school class is preferable to placement in a special public school class.

Following the PARC case, right-to-education class action suits were brought in almost every state, with similar results. It was not long until the "waves" created in those cases "brought down the walls" of large state institutions, eventually carrying children with Down syndrome from the institutions and special schools into group homes and regular public schools at an ever-increasing rate.

But not all segments of the population were prepared to capitalize on new opportunities. Educational environments were often particularly unprepared for students with Down syndrome, especially when it came to holding appropriate expectations of their educability. A quotation from an article published in *Psychology Today* illustrates this problem. In a 1975 issue of that magazine, a physician in charge of the reproductive genetics unit in an eastern university hospital was quoted as saying "You show me just one mongoloid that has an educable IQ. . . . I've never seen even one who is educable in my experience with over 800 mongols" (Restak, 1975, p. 92).

Disturbed by that statement, Rynders, Spiker, and Horrobin (1978) reviewed the professional literature to see what evidence of educability existed in studies involving persons with Down syndrome. A computerized search yielded more than 650 references, of which 105 contained data pertinent to the question of educability. The first thing the search revealed was that studies reporting educability data were often marred by serious methodological insufficiencies, appearing to have been conducted as if the authors of the studies believed that the condition has such a powerful genotypic impact that it is not important to provide information about children's age, rearing history, or even their gender. For instance, in 63 of the 105 studies that were reviewed, 60% did not provide data on whether the persons with Down syndrome in the studies were male or female. The absence of such basic developmental data across the 63 studies was certainly not paralleled in literature devoted to research on nonhandicapped children. In any case, after a careful sifting of the 105 studies, several instances were found in which children with Down syndrome manifested educable behaviors in terms of intellectual, academic, or other types of achievements. Hence, the physician's perception, as quoted in that 1975 issue of *Psychology Today,* appears to be too pessimistic.

HEAD START AND THE EARLY EDUCATION MOVEMENT

Spawned by President Lyndon Johnson's War on Poverty, Head Start was designed to prevent mental retardation from occurring in young high-risk children (e.g., black children living in slum areas). Gradually, Head Start–type programs began to serve young children with at-risk conditions (e.g., children with serious brain damage, congenital hearing and vision impairment, and children with Down syndrome).

During the late 60s, new laws such as PL 90-538, the Handicapped Children's Early Education Act Program (HCEEP), generated funding for an array of research and demonstration projects specifically for infants and preschool children with handicaps. By then, it was becoming obvious that "quick-fix" Head Start Programs, such as summer-only programs, could not produce the sustained, whole-family, lifelong achievements that were desired.

In a 1985 review (Rynders & Stealey) that identified eight current early education studies involving children with Down syndrome, each of which had acceptably strong experimental rigor, it was shown, consistent with Hanson's review in this book, (see Chapter 6), that early education is usually effective for young children with Down syndrome (seven out of eight studies showed significant differences favoring the experimental group or condition). However-er, in the Rynders and Stealey (1985) review, as in the Rynders et al. (1978) review, most studies on Down syndrome that were examined did not report, and perhaps did not collect, routine developmental data about child characteristics. For example, five of the eight early education studies in the 1985 review provide no data confirming the chromosome presence of Down syndrome; even fewer indicated the subgroup of the syndrome to which a karyotype belonged; and only two of the eight described children in terms of gender. Ignoring such basic developmental data implies the continuing existence of the devaluing stereotype that "a Downs, is a Downs, is a Downs."

DOWN'S SYNDROME CONGRESS ESTABLISHED

During the 1940s and 1950s, parents of children with mental disabilities, including Down syndrome, formed parent-professional groups such as the National Association for Retarded Children (now the Association for Retarded Citizens of the United States). In the 1970s, parents of children with Down syndrome began to organize across the country. In 1973, the Down's Syndrome Congress was formed, following a national meeting of parents of children with Down syndrome, held in Anaheim, California in October, 1972. Eleven years later, the membership voted to drop the possessive from "Down's" (because Down did not "own" the condition) and, due to its growing national status, decided to become the National Down Syndrome Congress (NDSC).

NDSC accomplishments since that time include:

1. Successfully lobbying that Down syndrome become one of the priorities of the National Genetics Disease Act
2. Organizing 13 consecutive national conventions and co-sponsoring three international conventions on Down syndrome
3. Helping to bring about the 1984 presidential proclamation on Down syndrome, and the 1985 Public Law designating October as National Down Syndrome Month
4. Promoting legislative awareness concerning "Baby Doe" issues
5. Fostering public awareness of the value of persons with Down syndrome through TV and other media
6. Publishing literature on Down syndrome, including a journal, the *Down Syndrome News,* as well as several books and booklets.
7. Coordinating a nationwide parent group network and offering parent group leadership seminars annually
8. Initiating a national conference focusing on the adolescent/adult with Down syndrome and a national conference on fostering appropriate behavior
9. Convening a state-of-the-art conference on Down syndrome, with federal support

MAJOR SOCIAL, EDUCATIONAL, AND VOCATIONAL LEGISLATION PASSED

Created by President John F. Kennedy's "national plan to combat mental retardation," the President's Panel on Mental Retardation, in 1963, established several important long-term goals. In the 1970s, Congress began to convert many of the goals of the 1960s into legislation. The resulting public laws of the 1970s and 1980s have had a significant impact on guaranteeing the right of individuals with Down syndrome to substantial social, educational, and vocational opportunities; indeed, they might be considered a "Bill of Rights" for persons with handicaps.

Educational Issues

PL 94-142, the Education for All Handicapped Children Act of 1975, is the most important of the group of laws. Prior to 1975, parents of school-age children with Down syndrome could not require public school officials in most states to provide an education (even a segregated education) for their children. Instead, they were totally reliant on the goodwill of school officials to accept their children, a situation that often forced them into a supplicant role. With PL 94-142, however, the U.S. Congress not only provided parents of children with Down syndrome a guarantee of a free public education for their children in the least restrictive, appropriate environment, but also mandated the writing of educational objectives and the right to due process hearings.

How successful has PL 94-142 been? It has been highly successful in guaranteeing a free public education for children with Down syndrome; the legal process assures that. But it is not yet totally clear what a least restrictive, appropriate environment contains or should contain. Part of the problem is that educational researchers have not been able to fully validate several major assumptions about the effectiveness of educating children with disabilities in the mainstream.

One of the assumptions undergirding the mainstreaming movement has been that students with disabilities such as Down syndrome profit from interacting with nonhandicapped students. However, there is a problem in approaching mainstreaming in an overly simplistic manner. Simply arranging for handicapped and nonhandicapped students to be in physical proximity with one another does *not* ensure that positive interactions and interpersonal attraction will result. In fact, there is evidence that nonhandicapped students when integrated casually sometimes have feelings of rejection toward handicapped peers (Goodman, Gottlieb, & Harrison, 1972; Iano et al., 1974). This is particularly true when an educational situation is created without deliberate planning for positive child-to-child interactions. In fact, rejection or acceptance of students with Down syndrome by nonhandicapped peers depends extensively on the way in which learning goals and rewards are structured by the teacher. Within any group learning situation, a teacher can structure interactions for cooperation, competition, or individualization (Johnson and Johnson, 1975). Evidence is accumulating that properly structured cooperative experiences result in a greater liking of and a greater number of positive interactions with handicapped students by nonhandicapped peers (Ballard, Corman, Gottlieb, and Kaufman, 1977; Cooper, Johnson, Johnson, and Wilderson, 1980; Johnson, Rynders, Johnson, Schmidt, and Haider, 1979; Martino and Johnson, 1979; Rynders, Johnson, Johnson, & Schmidt, 1980).

A second consideration in advocating for a greater number of positive heterogeneous interaction opportunities in regular schools is that school officials might be reluctant to have students with Down syndrome in a regular public school where "the three Rs" are emphasized. A low expectation for school-age children with Down syndrome, perhaps a carry-over from the one described earlier for infants (Restak, 1975), poses serious difficulties for parents beyond the early education period. Sadly, few specific attempts have been made to promote academic achievement in school-age children with Down syndrome. In other words, advocacy "ammunition" is in short supply. Fortunately, a few researchers have provided evidence that children with Down syndrome, given sound instruction, can learn basic and sometimes relatively sophisticated academic skills, such as functional arithmetic (Dalton, Rubino, & Hislop, 1973) and functional reading (Brown et al., 1972). (For a description of secondary education curricula for individuals with Down syndrome, see Chapter 8 in this book.) It should also be noted that the child with Down syndrome needs a balanced curriculum, including physicial education, art, music, home economics, and industrial arts, as well as academic instruction.

Beyond the School Years

Several pieces of federal legislation have opened up local community mainstreaming opportunities for persons with Down syndrome. For example, the Rehabilitation Act of 1973 (PL 93-112), Sections 503 and 504, prescribed far-reaching civil rights protections for persons with handicaps. Hiring, access to facilities, retention, and testing practices have all come under federal scrutiny and have led to enhanced independent living opportunities.

Furthermore, Medicaid waiver legislation (in the Omnibus Budget Reconciliation Act of 1981) authorized a case-based plan for expenditure of funds in promoting a community care plan for individuals with handicaps. One of the best features of this Medicaid legislation was that it maximized family and community options rather than emphasizing institutionalization.

Such laws help to promote the productivity of adults with Down syndrome, so that they can remain in the community. In addition, there is an increasing body of literature showing that adults with Down syndrome respond well to proper training in vocational tasks, even some relatively complex tasks such as bicycle brake assembly (Gold, 1973; personal communication, 1980). Moreover, they can, again, with proper training, considerably improve their communication abilities (Talkington & Hall, 1970) and independent living skills (Corcoran, 1979). Caution needs to be observed in reviewing this literature, however, since the results are often more clinical than experimental. Nonetheless, 120 years after J. Langdon Down said,

"They are cases that very much repay judicious treatment..." (1866, p. 261), it is beginning to be appreciated that the developmental potential of persons with Down syndrome is far greater than previously imagined.

BABY DOE AND THE AFTERMATH

In 1982, Baby Doe, a newborn child with Down syndrome, was nearing death due to starvation because his parents refused to allow routine surgery to correct an incomplete esophagus. As death approached, several organizations representing citizens with disabilities, including the National Down Syndrome Congress, sought feverishly to find legal means to save his life. Moreover, a number of parents, some of whom already had a child with Down syndrome, offered to adopt him. However, all advocacy efforts were to no avail.

Following Baby Doe's death, a lawyer representing the child's parents said, "There would have been horrific trauma—trauma to the child who would never have enjoyed a quality of life of any sort, trauma to the family, trauma to society . . .." (cited in Will, 1982). In his column, reacting to the lawyer's statement, George Will wrote, "The task of convincing communities to provide services and human sympathy for the retarded is difficult enough without incoherent lawyers laying down the law about whose life does and does not have 'meaning.' "

To understand meaning (and value) more fully, consider the words of a young woman with Down syndrome, who testified before a Wisconsin subcommittee hearing on the topic of abortion:

> I am 21 years old. I was born a Down syndrome. That means I have a disability. My parents told me about it when I was around ten years old. There are a lot of things I can do. I can swim. I can read. I can make friends. I can listen to my records. I can watch television. I can make my own lunch. I can go to see a movie. I can take the bus by myself to Chicago and to work. I can count money. I can sing like a bird. I can brush my teeth. I can do latch hook rugs. I can cook dinner. I can think. I can pray. I can square dance. I can play drums. I know what is right. I know what is wrong. I can write letters. I can scuba dive. I can paint pictures. I work at Madison Opportunity Center. I live at a group home with my friends. . . . (McGee, 1982, p. 120)

The words *I can* are of historic importance. They emphasize the need for a new societal perspective, one which shows that individuals with Down syndrome *have value* and *give value*.

REFERENCES

Aspillage, M. J., Morizon, G., & Avendano, I. (1975). Dimethyl sulfoxide therapy in severe retardation in mongoloid children. *Annals of the New York Academy of Science, 243,* 421–431.

Astin, A. W., & Ross, S. (1960). Glutamic acid and human intelligence. *Psychological Bulletin, 57*, 429–434.

Ballard, M., Corman, L., Gottlieb, J., & Kaufman, M. (1977). Improving the social status of mainstreamed retarded children. *Journal of Educational Psychology, 69*, 605–611.

Bard, B., & Fletcher, J. (1968). A right to die. *The Atlantic Monthly, 3*, 59–64.

Bardon, L. M. (1964). Sicca cell treatment in mongolism. *Lancet, 2*, 234–235.

Bazelon, M., Paine, R. S., Cowie, V. A., Hunt, P., Houck, J. C., & Manhanad, D. (1967). Reversal of hypotonia in infants with Down's syndrome by administration of 5-hydroxytryptophan. *Lancet, 1*, 1130.

Benda, C. E. (1960). *The child with mongolism.* New York: Grune & Stratton.

Benda, C. E. (1969). *Down's syndrome: Mongolism and its management.* New York: Grune & Stratton.

Berg, J. M., Kirman, B. H., Stern, J., & Mittwoch, U. (1961). Treatment of mongolism. *Journal of Mental Science, 107*, 475–480.

Bierich, J. R. (1975). Stellungnahme zur Frage der Indikation der Frischbzw. Sicca-Zelltherapie beim Mongolismus aud padiatrischendokrinologischer Sicht [Discussion concerning the indication of fresh- and sicca cell therapy in mongolism from a pediatric-endocrine point of view]. *Mschr. Kinderheilk, 123*, 671–674.

Black, D. B., Kato, J. G., & Walker, G. W. H. (1966). A study of improvement in mentally retarded children accruing from sicca cell therapy. *American Journal on Mental Deficiency, 70*, 499–508.

Bremer, J. H. (1975). Stellungnahme zur Zelltherapie bei Kindern unter besonderer Berucksichtigung padiatrisch-metabolischer Fragen [Discussion of cell therapy in children in relation to pediatric-metabolic issues]. *Mschr. Kinderheik, 123*, 674–675.

Brown, L., Jones, S., Troccolo, E., Heiser, C., et al. (1972). Teaching functional reading to young trainable students: Toward longitudinal objectives. *Journal of Special Education, 3*, 237–246.

Bumbalo, T. S., Morelewicz, H. V., & Berens, D. L. (1964). Treatment of Down's syndrome with the "U" series of drugs. *Journal of the American Medical Association, 5*, 187.

Clarke, C. M., Edwards, J. H., & Smallpiece, V. (1961). 21 trisomy/normal mosaicism in an intelligent child with mongoloid characters. *Lancet, 1*, 1028.

Coleman, M. (1973). *Serotonin in Down's syndrome.* New York: Elsevier/North Holland.

Cooper, L., Johnson, D. W., Johnson, R., & Wilderson, F. (1980). Effects of cooperative, competitive, and individualistic experiences on interpersonal attraction among heterogeneous peers. *Journal of Social Psychology, 111*, 243–252.

Corcoran, E. L. (1979). Campus life for retarded citizens. *Education Unlimited, 1*, 22–24.

Cornwell, A. C., & Birch, H. G. (1969). Psychological and social development in home-reared children with Down's syndrome (mongolism). *American Journal of Mental Deficiency, 74*, 341–350.

Crookshank, F. (1924). *The mongol in our midst.* London: Kegan Paul, Trench and Trubner Ltd.

Dalton, A., Rubino, C., & Hislop, M. (1973). Some effects of token rewards on school achievement of children with Down's syndrome. *Journal of Applied Behavior Analysis, 6*, 251–259.

DeMoragas, J. (1958). Treatment of mongolism with dehydroepiandrosterone. *Rev. Esp. de Ped, 14*, 545.

Diamond, E. F., & Moon, M. S. (1961). Neuromuscular development in mongoloid children. *American Journal of Mental Deficiency, 66,* 218.

Down, J. L. H. (1866). Observations on an ethnic classification of idiots. *London Hospital, Clinical Lectures and Reports, 3,* 259–262.

Encyclopaedia Britannica. (1970). Monster (p. 794–795). Chicago: William Benton.

Encyclopaedia Britannica. (1974). Down's syndrome. Chicago: William Benton.

Freeman, R. (1970). Psychopharmacology and the retarded child. In F. Menolascino (Ed.), *Psychiatric approaches to mental retardation.* New York: Basic Books.

Gabourie, J., Becker, J. W., & Bateman, B. (1975). Oral dimethyl sulfoxide in mental retardation. Part I. Preliminary behavioral and psychometric data. In S. W. Jacobs & R. Herschler (Eds.), Biological actions of dimethyl sulfoxide. *Annals of the New York Academy of Science, 243,* 1–508.

Gadson, E. J. (1951). Glutamic acid and mental deficiency. *American Journal of Mental Deficiency, 55,* 521–528.

Goddard, H. (1914). *Feeble-mindedness, its causes and consequences.* New York: Macmillan.

Gold, M. (1973). Research on the vocational habilitation of the retarded: The present, the future. In N. R. Ellis (Ed.), *International review of research in mental retardation* (Vol. 6). New York: Academic Press.

Goldstein, H. (1954). Treatment of mongolism and nonmongoloid mental retardation in children. *Archives of Pediatrics, 71,* 77–89.

Goldstein, H. (1956a). Treatment of congenital acromicria syndrome in children. *Archives of Pediatrics, 13,* 153.

Goldstein, H. (1956b). Sicca cell therapy in children. *Archives of Pediatrics, 73,* 234.

Goodman, H., Gottlieb, J., & Harrison, R. (1972). Social acceptance of EMR's integrated into a nongraded elementary school. *American Journal of Mental Deficiency, 76,* 412–417.

Haubold, H. (1967). Beeinflussung des phenotyps mongoloider kinder durch eine Fruheinsetzende Dauerbehandlung [Impact on the phenotype of mongoloid children through early initiated, continued therapy]. *Anesth. Med., 13,* 3.

Hitzig, W. H. (1975). Stellungnahme zur Frischzellenbebandlung bei Kindern unter besonderer Berucksichtigung des Down-syndromes und andersartiger cerebraler Schadigungen [Discussion concerning cell therapy in children with special reference to Down syndrome and other cerebral insults]. *Mschr. Kinderheilk, 123,* 676–678.

Horrobin, J., & Pueschel, S. (1982). Medical care and management. In S. Pueschel and J. Rynders (Eds.), *Down syndrome: Advances in biomedicine and the behavioral sciences* (pp. 269–303). Cambridge, MA: Ware Press.

Iano, R., Ayers, D., Heller, H., McGettigan, J., & Walker, V. (1974). Sociometric status of retarded children in an integrated program. *Exceptional Children, 40,* 267–271.

Johnson, D. W., & Johnson, R. (1975). *Learning together and alone: Cooperation, competition, and individualization.* Englewood Cliffs, NJ: Prentice-Hall.

Johnson, R., Rynders, J., Johnson, D. W., Schmidt, B., & Haider, S. (1979). Producing positive interaction between handicapped and nonhandicapped teenagers through cooperative goal structuring: Implications for mainstreaming. *American Educational Research Journal, 16,* 161–168.

Kanner, L. (1967). *A history of the care and study of the mentally retarded.* Springfield, IL: Charles C Thomas.

Koch, R., Share, J., & Graliker, B. (1965). The effects of cytomel on young children with Down's syndrome (mongolism): A double-blind longitudinal study. *Journal of Pediatrics, 66,* 776.

Kugelmass, I. N. (1959). Chemical therapy of mentally retarded children. *Int. Rec. Med., 172,* 119–136.

Lejeune, J., Gautier, M., & Turpin, R. (1959). Les chromosomes humains en culture de tissus [Human chromosomes in tissue culture]. *C. R. Acad. Sci., 248,* 602–603.

Lombard, J. P., Gilbert, J. G., Donofrio, A. F. (1955). The effects of glutamic acid upon the intelligence, social maturity, and adjustment of a group of mentally retarded children. *American Journal of Mental Deficiency, 60,* 122–132.

Martino, L., & Johnson, D. W. (1979). Cooperative and individualistic experiences among disabled and normal children. *Journal of Social Psychology, 107,* 177–183.

McGee, T. (1982). Testimony in Madison. *Down Syndrome News, 6,* 113–126.

Milton, G., & Gonzalo, R. (1974). Jaguar cult–Down's syndrome—were—jaguar. *Expedition, 16,* 33–37.

Mommsen, H. (1961). Die Zellular-therapie des mongolismus [Cell therapy in mongolism]. *Arztl. Praxis, 13,* 646.

Partington, M. W., MacDonald, M. R., & Tu, J. B. (1971). 5-Hydroxytryptophan (5-HTP) in Down's syndrome. *Developmental Medicine and Child Neurology, 13,* 362–372.

Pennsylvania Association for Retarded Children v. Commonwealth of Pennsylvania, Civil Action No. 71-42 (1971).

Polani, P. E., Briggs, J. H., Ford, C. E., Clarke, C. M., & Berg, J. M. (1960). A mongol girl with 46 chromosomes. *Lancet, 1,* 1028.

Pueschel, S. M., Reed, R. B., Cronk, C. E., & Goldstein, B. I. (1980). The effect of 5-hydroxytryptophan and/or pyridoxin in young children with Down syndrome. *American Journal of Disabled Children, 134,* 838–844.

Restak, R. (1975). Genetic counseling for defective parents: The danger of knowing too much. *Psychology Today, 9,* 21–23, 92–93.

Rynders, J., Johnson, R., Johnson, D. W., & Schmidt, B. (1980). Effects of cooperative goal structuring in producing positive interaction between Down's syndrome and nonhandicapped teenagers: Implications for mainstreaming. *American Journal of Mental Deficiency, 85,* 268–273.

Rynders, J., Spiker, D., & Horrobin, J. (1978). Underestimating the educability of Down's syndrome children: Examination of methodological problems in recent literature. *American Journal of Mental Deficiency, 82,* 440–448.

Rynders, J. E., & Stealey, D. J. (1985). Early education: A strategy for producing a less (least) restrictive environment for young children with severe handicaps. In K. C. Lakin & R.H. Bruininks (Eds.), *Strategies for achieving community integration of developmentally disabled citizens* (pp. 129–158). Baltimore: Paul H. Brookes Publishing Co.

Saxl, O. (1972). New biomedical and gastroenterological findings in Down's syndrome and their importance for its treatment. *Cas. Lek. Cesk., 11,* 281–285.

Schmid, F. (1976a). Das mongolismus-syndrom [Mongolism syndrome]. *Deutsch. Hebammen-Z, 28,* 169–173.

Schmid, F. (1976b). *Das mongolismus-syndrom* [Mongolism syndrome]. Muensterdorf: Hansen and Hansen.

Schulte, F. J. (1975). Stellungnahme zur Behandlung des Down-syndroms, speziell zur Zelltherapie aus neurophysiologisch/neuropadiatrischer sicht [Discussion concerning the treatment of Down syndrome with special reference to cell therapy from a neurophysiologic-neuropediatric point of view]. *Mschr. Kinderheilk, 123,* 671–674.

Schultz, J., & Turnbull, A. (1983). *Mainstreaming handicapped students: Guide for classroom teachers* (2nd ed., p. 59). Boston: Allyn & Bacon.

Smith, T. T. (1896). A peculiarity in the shape of the hand in idiots of the mongol type. *Pediatrics, 2,* 315–320.

Stedman, D., & Eichorn, A. (1964). A comparison of the growth and development of institutionalized and home-reared mongoloids during infancy and early childhood. *American Journal of Mental Deficiency, 69,* 391–401.

Talkington, L. W., & Hall, S. M. (1970). Matrix language program with mongoloids. *American Journal of Mental Deficiency, 75,* 88–91.

Tjio, J. H., & Levan, A. (1956). The chromosome number of man. *Hereditas, 42,* 1–6.

Turkel, H. (1975). Medical amelioration of Down's syndrome incorporating the orthomolecular approach. *Journal of Ortho-Molecular Psychiatry, 4,* 102–115.

Weise, P., Koch, R., Shaw, K. N., & Rosenfeld, M. J. (1974). The use of 5-HTP in the treatment of Down's syndrome. *Pediatrics, 54,* 165.

White, D., & Kaplitz, S. E. (1964). Treatment of Down's syndrome with a vitamin mineral hormone preparation. *International Copenhagen Congress Scientific Study of Mental Retardation, 1,* 224.

Will, G. (1982, April 22). If the baby's not "meaningful," kill it [Editorial]. *Minneapolis Star and Tribune* (reprinted from the Washington Post).

Zellweger, H. (1968). Is Down's syndrome a modern disease? *Lancet, 2,* 458.

SECTION I

BIOMEDICINE

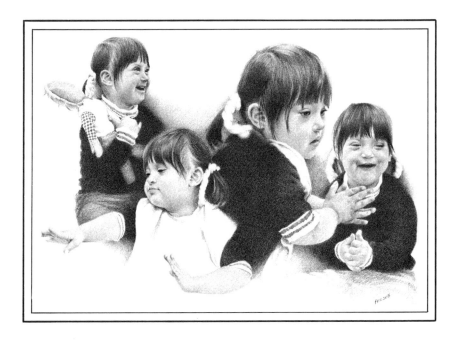

Introduction

Allen C. Crocker

In considering "new perspectives on Down syndrome," it is appropriate to begin with a presentation of new knowledge about the basic circumstances of this human condition. The occurrence of Down syndrome in a person can be viewed as an instance of human variation, with a causation, however presently obscure, and a sequence of effects. There is an understandable desire to learn how these events come to be, for both personal and professional reasons. This search for a scientific anchor in Down syndrome does not diminish one's respect for the special values of the involved individual. Rather, it can provide useful clues for intelligent intervention on the person's behalf and for more accurate continuing assistance. The potential for preventing the chromosomal aberration is another complex and important matter.

Section I explores the current best perceptions about the biological and medical features of Down syndrome. The fundamental premise is that the syndrome derives from an altered configuration of the individual's chromosomes, resulting in a surfeit of one specific element—functionally a "trisomy," three units instead of the normal two, of the 21st chromosome. Chapter 1 analyzes the wide range of hypotheses that have been suggested for the possible etiology of trisomy 21. Chapter 2 works with the reality of the trisomy, and discusses the possible "gene effects" that are demonstrable or theoretical as an outcome to the presence of the additional chromosome 21 material. Chapter 3 goes further, and speculates on mechanisms by which the gene effects might lead to the alterations in development that are seen in the fetus with Down syndrome. Chapter 4 explores recent information on the incidence and worldwide distribution of the phenomenon of trisomy 21. Finally, Chapter 5 records the ways in which the body is affected by Down syndrome and presents guidelines regarding health maintenance for involved individuals.

There are a number of recurrent themes in the chapters of Section I. The 21st chromosome is obviously the central component. The settings in which its "function" is affected before, during, and shortly after conception are of critical importance. The increasing risk for the birth of infants with trisomy 21 as maternal age advances remains the single observation of substance in the epidemiological study of Down syndrome; yet theories of causation must acknowledge human factors that are much more broad. It is probable that there are multiple influences in the story of etiology. Given the actuality of trisomy 21, the equation of gene dosage effects is still a riddle, with the probability existing that strongly unequal roles are contributed by diverse genes. There is an energetic research commitment to the pursuit of identification of the gene activity that is located on the 21st chromosome, a dedication that is vigorously motivated by concerns for the person with Down syndrome.

In these chapters, the reader may be bewildered by the technicality of the language necessary to use in describing the research projects, but interpretative conclusions are offered in each instance. There are simultaneous elements of puzzlement, valuable first-order data, and good prospects for ultimate elucidation. It is hoped that knowing how trisomy 21 originates and how it affects individuals will provide a sound platform for understanding and helping persons with Down syndrome.

Chapter 1

Etiology
of Human Trisomy 21

Georgiana M. Jagiello,
Jye-Siung Fang, Mercedes B. Ducayen,
and Weng Kong Sung

One is struck by the ubiquitous nature of geography, socioeconomic conditions, parental age, and ethnicity pertaining to the occurrence of Down syndrome. Clearly this is not a human problem that is restricted to one population cluster. It is, in another sense, an apparently peculiarly human problem resulting from maldistribution of a chromosome whose uniqueness may have unfortunately deprived one of most ideal domestic or laboratory animal test models. In seeking the etiology of the nondisjunction that results in this maldistribution, the researcher must think in the biological terms that encompass all of these general features. It is a purpose of this chapter to discuss some of the research approaches that have been put forward and tested during the past few decades, and also to provide a brief description of some new directions that one hopes will be more effective in solving this puzzle than the pursuit of earlier hypotheses has been thus far.

In attempting an examination of the characteristics of human trisomy 21, one is inevitably drawn into a consideration of whether the maldistribution of this and other chromosomes is a single effect of a single cause or a symptom of malfunctioning in one or several mechanisms leading to incorrect chromosomal distribution. The categorization of human trisomies as being both dependent on and independent of maternal age suggests that at least two modes of error are operative. Examination of the intricate cascade of events in human oogenesis, which must follow a true course to provide a normal haploid complement in the fertilized ovum, easily reveals many potentially vulnerable stages in which problems can occur, the immediate or delayed effect of which can be maldistribution of chromosomes. Thus the position of this chapter is that several developmental errors may exist, any one or combination of which can produce progeny with trisomy 21.

A related consideration in developing the strategies of investigation into the causes of human trisomy concerns the possibility of nonconjunction as the primary disturbance of chromosome behavior, as opposed to the later phenomenon of nondisjunction. The suggestion of nonconjunction of chromosome 21 was made more than 2 decades ago by Polani, Biggers, Ford, Clark, and Berg (1960). It had not had much experimental support until recently when Speed (1985) noted a high incidence of synaptic errors at pachytene in human fetal oocytes. This provocative finding rekindles interest in the possibility that incorrect pairing, and/or faulty recombination may underlie later chromosome misbehavior, and deserves further testing.

At this time, however, the bulk of epidemiological and experimental evidence definitely points to nondisjunction or failure of separation of chromosomes as the manifest error in trisomy 21. If one considers this from the viewpoint of maternal age and the occurrence of Down syndrome, one finds that the instances of trisomy 21 classified as "maternal age independent" have a peak frequency at age 28.5 years (Bond & Chandley, 1983). These include situations of translocation trisomies, mosaic mothers, or trisomic mothers. "Maternal age dependent" trisomy 21, with a peak frequency at age 43 years (Bond & Chandley, 1983), has emerged from several series of marker studies as being an event most probably occurring as an error at meiosis I of oogenesis in the preovulatory period. This concept forms the linchpin for much of this chapter, which will explore both positive and negative findings in a variety of experiments designed to probe mechanisms that may have gone awry before human ovulation and fertilization.

CLASSIC THEORIES OF NONDISJUNCTION

The five most durable theories for causes of nondisjunction are listed in Table 1. Their survival under experimental assault has been variable. The "production line" hypothesis that Henderson and Edwards expressed in 1968 has been tested extensively (Bodmer, 1961; Jagiello & Fang, 1979; Polani & Jagiello, 1976; Martin, Dill, & Miller, 1976; Speed & Chandley, 1983). The basic tenets of this hypothesis are: 1) oocytes entering meiosis early in gestation have more chiasmata than oocytes switching into meiosis later in gestation and 2) oocyte populations are either ovulated early or late during the reproductive life span; they are vulnerable to nondisjunction if ovulated late because of the reduced number of chiasmata, which leads to inefficiency of interaction with the meiotic spindle. Though data have been produced in cytological studies with several strains of aging female mice (Bodmer, 1961; Jagiello & Fang, 1979; Martin et al., 1976; Polani & Jagiello, 1976; Speed & Chandley, 1983) to support the notion of differences in chiasmata between "early" and "late" oocytes, resultant hyperdiploidy has not been proven unequivocally. In addition, recombination studies (Wallace, MacSwiney, &

Table 1.   Advanced maternal age (over
34 years) hypotheses

1. Production line (fetal)
2. Persistent nucleoli (fetal or adult)
3. Hormonal imbalance (adult)
4. Delayed fertilization (adult)
5. Relaxed selection (adult)

Edwards, 1976) have failed to document a consistent relationship between recombination and maternal age. Thus, the production line hypothesis remains an open question.

The notion of a persistent nucleolus with or without viral involvement (Evans, 1967) implies prophase pairing defects or preovulatory interference with the distribution of acrocentric chromosomes with satellites (Polani et al., 1960). Since data from spontaneous abortion studies (Hassold & Jacobs, 1984) reveal trisomy of nonacrocentric as well as acrocentric chromosomes, the notion of nucleolar persistence and interference cannot be considered satisfactory.

The invocation of hormonal imbalance as producing chromosomal trisomy and Down syndrome was proposed by Rundle, Coppen, and Cowie (1961) and further developed by Crowley, Gulati, Hayden, Lopez, and Dyer (1979). The essential proposition was that the rate of oocyte meiotic resumption in the preovulatory period was hormonally controlled, as was the accompanying phenomenon of chiasma terminalization. The variability of the level and timing of ovarian steroids and gonadotrophins was held to be extensive in older women (and very young women); hence, it was held to be an effector of meiotic behavior. Though hormonal levels in the perimenopausal cycle certainly vary, no evidence for a change in meiotic kinetics between diplotene and metaphase II with increased chiasma terminalization has been produced. Without this, the theory remains speculative.

The "delayed fertilization" concept, developed by German in 1968, had a reasonable basis in work with lower form oocytes and fetal abnormalities with maternal or germ cell aging. However, even if accurate, it would account for only the few *second* meiosis errors of trisomy 21. Such a postovulatory etiology takes the onus away from an abnormality that was structured during early oogenesis and transfers it to the period of fertilization. Consideration of this as the primary point for nondisjunction has not had many advocates, but the idea of delayed fertilization and the more recent one of "relaxed selection" have shifted attention to this time period. (Both concepts are discussed later in this chapter.) The idea of relaxed selection (Ayme & Lippman-Hand, 1982) suggests a declining capability of the aging human uterus to reject trisomic progeny, with a resultant apparent increase in frequency with increasing age. Hook (1983, 1985) recently stated that, thus far, the evidence for substantiating this idea is lacking.

OTHER PUTATIVE ETIOLOGIES OF NONDISJUNCTION

Other potential etiologies for nondisjunction that have been put forth have either had a basis in phenomenology or have been partially derived from experimental data. A few of these propositions are discussed in this section (see Table 2).

The use of oral contraceptives around the day of conception, as opposed to other times or duration of ingestion, may be associated with a trisomic birth. The report of Harlap et al. (1979), resuscitated the possible association of hormones and meiotic control but remained speculative.

X-irradiation, an extensively studied potential hazard, must be viewed at this time as a serious candidate for producing trisomy only when small doses accumulating over a time period are coupled with a long lag period to conception (Alberman, 1972). Though many reports of other paradigms of an association of X-irradiation with trisomy have been published (Uchida, 1979), no solid evidence of etiology in the human population, particularly with advanced maternal age, has been presented.

A recent examination of data relating to potential chemical mutagens and oocyte aneuploidy (Mailhes, Preston & Lavappa, 1985) analyzed 72 published papers dealing with the possibility of the production of aneuploidy in developing female mammalian germ cells. It revealed that only 28 papers

Table 2. Other theoretical etiologies

1. Gonadotrophins
2. Oral contraceptives
3. X-irradiation
4. Radar
5. Chemicals: Cd, Hg, Pb, etc.
6. Vaginal spermicides
7. Cigarettes; alcohol
8. Seasons
9. Viruses
10. Thyroid (other endocrine; e.g., ovarian) autoantibodies
11. Alpha^1-antitrypsin
12. HLA
13. Nondisjunction genes
14. Heterochromatin
15. Structural rearrangements
16. Spindle aging

involving 16 chemicals were found to be experimentally valid for demonstrating hyperploidy induction. The indicted agents included cadmium chloride, cyclophosphamide, triaziquone, and colchicine. The task of demonstrating a capability of such agents for gaining access in threshold amounts to the developing fetal or periovulatory human oocyte at critical developmental stages has complicated the accumulation of proof of their relevance to the etiology of human nondisjunction.

Vaginal spermicides, smoking, alcohol, and seasonal variation all remain unproven culprits, as do the varied theoretical causes of viruses, autoantibodies, human genes for nondisjunction, or large heterochromatin blocks on chromosomes. Putative associations of HLA types and alpha^1-antitrypsin with Down syndrome have not proven to be valid. Interchromosomal effects of structural rearrangements not involving chromosome 21 and aging of the spindle apparatus itself remain provocative and in need of much further investigation. At this point, there is an excess of theories that have been tested and remain either unproven or tentative.

NEW MAMMALIAN MODELS FOR STUDYING NONDISJUNCTION

Three models that may hold promise for attempting to understand the abnormality of the etiology of nondisjunction are discussed in this section. Two are designed to explore the earliest phases of chromosome behavior—pairing of bivalents and genetic exchange. The premise that these fetal events in human oogenesis have a subsequent program of developmental behavior up to and including the periovulatory period is integral. A corollary of this premise, not explicitly included in these two models, is that this program must eventually include the apparatus of distribution: kinetochores (centromeres), centrioles, spindle fibers and associated proteins, and other organelles of movement. The third model focuses on the much later period between human fertilization and implantation.

Disturbing the Pairing of Bivalents with Colcemid

The first model deals with the matter of chromosome pairing during mammalian oocyte development, and the apparently essential structure of this pairing—the synaptonemal complex. The organization of events for the accurate pairing of homologous chromosomes and the subsequent molecular events of recombination, particularly in mammals, are not well understood (Stern & Hotta, 1977). Major treatises dealing with theoretical aspects have been written by Catchside (1977), Holliday (1974), Maguire (1979), Meselson and Radding (1975), Moses, (1968), and Whitehouse (1973), and some experimental evidence has been produced that supports portions of each concept. Approaches toward understanding the pairing aspect have included ultrastructural dissection of synaptonemal complex formation (Westergaard & Wettstein, 1972), structure (LaCour & Wells, 1977), and behavior (Maguire, 1982), or induced or spontaneous mutants (Carpenter, 1979; Jones, 1973) wherein pairing was perturbed.

One novel approach to studying the events of the pairing process and the formation of the synaptonemal complex was initially presented by Derman (1938), in *Rheo*, and Levan (1939), in *Allium*, who reported that the mitotic inhibitor colchicine disrupted prophase and affected subsequent crossing-over. This surprising effect appeared to be quite distinct from its well-known microtubule inhibitory effects. Levan felt that this agent acted specifically by interfering with the progress of synapsis.

Little was done with this finding until the experiments of Driscoll, Darvey, and Barben (1967) and Driscoll and Darvey (1970), who extended the work of Feldman (1966) with the 5B chromosome of wheat (*T. aestivum*). The separation of the proposed effect of the microtubule inhibitor on either the earliest spatial relationships of chromosome pairing or on synapsis and chiasma formation was attempted with hexaploid wheat containing an iso-chromosome. With this species, the effect was thought to be on the attainment of the spatial proximity.

Thereafter, again studying colchicine effects on wheat, Dover and Riley (1973) demonstrated the importance of the timing of inhibitor application in the meiotic cycle. They, and later, Bennett, Rao, Smith, and Baylise (1973), showed clearly that in wheat the effect on synapsis was induced between the last premeiotic anaphase and early premeiotic GI.

However, studies with synchronous *Lillium* cells (Shepard, Boothroyd, & Stern, 1974) demonstrated alignment and meiotic commitment effects not only during premeiosis, but also during leptotene and early zygotene. A reduced chiasma frequency, univalents, and pachytene pairing gaps were observed in this system. These were ascribed to prealignment effects and the authors noted synaptonemal complexes with lateral elements in place, but absent central elements. The authors also indicated variations from cell to cell in treated *Lillium*, apparent complete repair with a single treatment, inhibition of nucleolar fusion, and absence of a Vinblastin (another microtubule inhibitor) effect.

An important sequelae of the observed pairing gaps at pachytene that resulted from treatment with colchicine at leptotene/zygotene were effects on diplotene. An additional "meiotic arrest" was noted with treatment of anthers at late interphase/early leptotene. Cells that were in the S-phase when treated became arrested later at meiotic prophase. These data were felt to obviate a spindle inactivation as a primary effect, and an effect on a nuclear membrane component that bound colchicine was believed to underly these observations. Biochemical analysis of the effects of colchicine on meiosis in *Lillium* by this same group (Hotta & Shepard, 1973) revealed nil effects on DNA, RNA, or protein synthesis during early prophase, but a marked reduction in DNA synthesis at pachytene in affected cells. Predictably, labeled colchicine was found in cytoplasm, but 20% was unexpectedly found in the nucleus. Separation of a DNA-binding protein and the colchicine heavy membrane binding component was demonstrated. It was thus concluded that colchicine affects pairing via an action(s) on this nuclear membrane protein in this species.

These experiments were re-examined by Bennett, Toledo, and Stern (1979) with an improved system for sustaining the treated *Lillium* through meiotic division. A putative effect on intercellular transport of nucleosides between tapetum microsporocytes was suggested and larger chromosomes were noted to be more resistant to pairing effects than smaller ones. Also very important was the finding that the treated bivalents behaved as though chiasmata were redistributed among the total genome.

Salonen, Paranko, and Parvinen (1982), studying the effects of Colcemid on rat spermatocytes with time-lapse photography, noted inhibition of the rotary pairing movements of the chromosomes of zygotene spermatocytes. They concluded that such movement restriction interfered with homologue pairing and synaptonemal complex formation by altering nuclear attachment plaques.

Also germane to interpreting these reports on colchicine effects are the papers of Ierardi, Moss, and Bellvé (1981) and Li, Meistrich, Brock, Hsu, and Kuo (1983). Ierardi et al. (1981) used sequential extraction of CD-1 mouse pachytene spermatocytes to obtain synaptonemal complex matrices with protein constituents different from somatic nuclear matrices, as well as to demonstrate similar matrix proteins in pachytene spermatocytes and spermatids. They also demonstrated the absence of the three characteristic laminin proteins of somatic cells. Li et al. (1983) reported isolation of rat pachytene spermatocyte synaptonemal complexes and called attention to the integral role of the SNC as a support for chromatin domains and to its common characteristics with the nuclear matrix. Since some DNA synthesis occurs during pachytene apparently at the SNC, the need for correct SNC alignment and composition becomes more definite. Stick and Schwarz (1982) also reported the absence of nuclear laminae in chicken pachytene oocytes.

It seemed reasonable to the authors of this chapter to try to use the Colcemid probe as a tool in examining pairing characteristics in the fetal mammalian oocyte since successful perterbation of this essential function has been demonstrated in lower forms and male germ cells. The strategy required acceptance of the idea that disruption of the formation of the synaptonemal complex would result in alterations in genetic exchange, and that the alteration of genetic exchange seen as chiasmata would be predicted to alter disjunction ultimately, if Mather's original hypotheses were correct (1938).The *in vivo* experiments tested female Swiss mice at gestational ages of 12–15 days. Injections of 0.2 μg of Colcemid per gram of body weight were given intraperitoneally. Mice were sacrificed subsequently at day 17 of gestation and preparations of fetal pachytene and diplotene oocytes were made. The model assessed end points of oocyte pachytene chromomere maps and light microscopic analysis of whole mount spreads of synaptonemal complexes to evaluate pairing integrity. Analysis of diplotene oocytes for chiasma number served as a monitor for possible effects on recombination.

The findings in the preliminary experiments with this model were encouraging. The well-known appearance of the normal whole mount spread synaptonemal complex was markedly disturbed. Single locations of pairing failure in a bivalent, multiple pairing failures in register in several bivalents, or total disruption of pairing were seen in the treated oocytes (see Figures 1, 2, and 3). Disruption of the central element and the nuclear interface of the synaptonemal complex was seen as well. Analysis of chiasmata in diplotene cells indicated that disruption and presumed repair of pairing fidelity interfered with recombination as defined by chiasma frequencies (21.85/genome in treated oocytes and 27.80/genome in controls). These were significant at

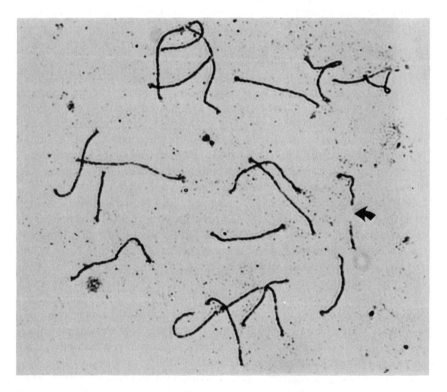

Figure 1. Photomicrograph of a whole mount spread synaptonemal complex of treated mouse oocytes with single pairing failure in a bivalent (2500×).

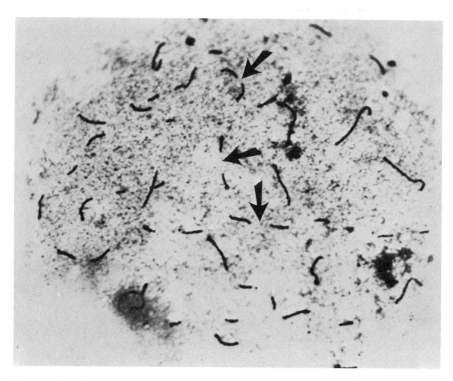

Figure 2. Photomicrograph of a whole mount spread synaptonemal complex of treated mouse oocytes with multiple pairing failures in register in several bivalents (arrows) (2500×).

the $p < 0.001$ level [t-test]. It is the authors' belief that the nature of the disturbance in the formation of the synaptonemal complex seen as a structural representation of the effects of Colcemid remains unknown. It would, however, appear to be coincidental with or preceded by a disruption of the exchange of genetic units. The data acquired in this preliminary study, when considered with similar fundamental studies by Moses (1985), who has used cyclophosphamid and mitomycin C to attempt evaluation of premeiotic "S" damage and subsequent aneuploidy, present new tools for understanding the delayed effects of influences acting during fetal mammalian oogenesis on subsequent chiasma behavior and disjunction.

Using Cold to Disrupt Pairing

A second research model that the authors developed dealt in some detail with this same meiotic sequence. In these experiments, a physiological condition, hibernation, was used to alter the timing of the meiotic cycle, and particularly the DNA synthesis ["S"] time period. The proposed cascade of effects on chiasmata and disjunction could then be examined.

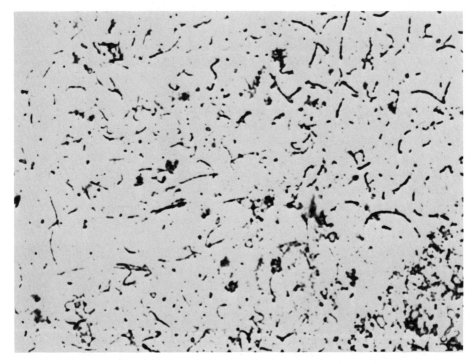

Figure 3. Photomicrograph of a whole mount spread synaptonemal complex of treated mouse oocytes with total disruption of pairing (2500×).

This model offered the distinct advantage of avoiding complex injury to the individual cell populations such as is caused by irradiation or chemical damage, two modalities that were previously studied *in extenso* for their effects on disjunction. This model proposed that with a core body temperature decrease the total meiotic cycle in the hamster gonad becomes longer than at normal body temperature, a phenomenon that has been well described in lower animal forms and plants (Henderson, 1966; Peacock, 1970) and that can result in significantly decreased chiasmata (Henderson, 1970).

The experiments involved placing adult male Golden hamsters, which are permissive hibernators, in an 8°C controlled environment with 2 hours of light and 22 hours of darkness in November. The animals were caged individually and allowed access to minimal food and water. Hibernation, with its accompanying decrease in body temperature, as monitored by Tele-thermometer, began in the cold-exposed animals in late December. Testicular histology of sacrificed males revealed a decline of spermatogenesis to stem cell stages in both the control and treated animals (Smit-Vis & Akkerman-Belaart, 1967).

In the subsequent months, the first wave of spermatogenesis to the stage of sperm returned in both populations. Samples of testicular epithelium were obtained in late February and early March for assessment of the DNA synthesis ["S"] period, diplotene chiasmata scores, and metaphase II ploidy. The "S" phase was measured by a modification of the method of Ghosal and Mukherjee (1971), by the injection of [^{3}H]thymidine, with samples of testicular tissue removed 4 hours, 48 hours, and 5 days later. Histological and cytogenetic preparations were made and leptotene nuclei were photographed before preparing autoradiographs. These were developed 7 days later and leptotene nuclei were scored for the presence of 20 or more grains as an indication of the incorporation of [^{3}H]thymidine into DNA. Plots of the percentage of activity in letptotene nuclei versus time were used to calculate the duration of DNA "S." Cytogenetic examination of diplotene spermatocyte chiasmata and second metaphase chromosome complements was carried out at 125X in Giemsa-stained preparations by three observers using coded slides.

The results of the studies of DNA synthesis revealed that at a body temperature of 33.2°C the "S" phase was 56 hours long, while in the hibernators at a core temperature of 13.5°C, the "S" phase had increased to 86 hours. A significantly reduced chiasmata frequency of 21.84 was found in the cold-exposed animals versus a control of 24. Startling nondisjunction was detected in second metaphase spermatocytes. Sixty per cent of the cells from the hibernating hamsters had chromosomal aneuploidy of 21 or 23 chromosomes compared to the control number of 22.

These preliminary data suggest that this model is a potentially useful one. It allows examination of the separate features of mechanisms between preleptotene "S" and disjunction at meiosis I in a physiological, synchronized state, a paradigm heretofore not available to the study of the etiology of mammalian nondisjunction.

An Epidemiological Theory

The third model relates to the general problem of trisomy as perceived by epidemiologists, and is the work of Stein, Stein and Susser (1986). The fundamental notion is that there is an association of trisomy 21 with advanced maternal age in all *recognized* pregnancies. This association arises from the attrition of unrecognized anomalies in the period between fertilization and implantation; this attrition declines in intensity as the age of the mother increases.

The essential phenomenon for this model is the evaluation of the marker studies reported thus far and shown in Table 3. It is clear that the ratio of marker-identified maternal to paternal origins in 266 cases of trisomy 21 reported thus far does not increase notably with increasing maternal age (del Mazo, Castillo, & Abrisqueta, 1982; Hansson & Mikkelsen, 1978; Magenis

Table 3.   Ratio in Down syndrome of maternal to paternal origin (M/P), and number of informative cases (n), by maternal age at birth.

Maternal age group	<20	20–24	25–29	30–34	35–39	40–44	45–
M/P rounded (no)	7(8)	3(48)	3(65)	3(58)	6(35)	3(39)	∞(5)

Sources: del Mazo, Castillo, and Abrisqueta (1982), Spain, = 37; M/P = 1.3. Hansson and Mikkelsen (1978), Copenhagen, n = 26. M/P = 2.7. Magenis and Chamberlin (1981), Portland, n = 39, M/P = 4.0. Mattei, Ayme, Mattei, and Giraud (1980), Marseilles, n = 51, M/P = 4.1. Mikkelsen, Poulson, Grinsted, and Lange (1980), Funen, n = 45, M/P = 8.0; Zealand, n = 34, M/P = 3.25. Wagenbichler, Killan, Rett, and Schnedl (1976), Vienna, n = 34, M/P = 1.8. (Adapted from Stein, Stein, and Susser, 1986.)

& Chamberlin, 1981; Mattei, Ayme, Mattei, & Girand, 1980; Mikkelsen, Poulsen, Grinsted, & Lange, 1980; Wagenbichler, Killan, Rett, & Schnedl, 1976). The calculated incidence of trisomy at fertilization is also constant, thus excluding an association of maternal age with disomies before fertilization. The maternal age effect seen with aborted trisomies must arise, therefore, after fertilization. Verification of this hypothesis must await cytogenetic findings in chorionic villus samples and *in vitro* fertilization work.

FUTURE BIOLOGICAL EXPLORATIONS

Much of the previous discussion can be considered history. The possibilities for new explorations of potential causes for human nondisjunction are set out in Table 4 and return to the concept of a primary developmental defect. Clearly, in the main, they are focused on the question of etiologies not related to chiasma formation, number, position, and terminalization, but rather on the structures or mechanisms of the chromosome distribution process as it occurs during the preovulatory completion of meiosis I in the human oocyte.

First on this list is the possibility of studying the marmoset as a model for human nondisjunction. This species more nearly approaches the conundrum of trisomy seen in the human being; thus, better understanding of the reproductive biology and mechanisms of haploid genome formation in this species would be very valuable for translation to the human abnormality.

Table 4.   New horizons

1. Marmoset as a model for human nondisjunction
2. Cloned chromosome DNA—Unique sequences
3. Centromere proteins; centriole: Tubulin
4. Intraspindle membranes and Ca^{2+}
5. Mutations of distribution apparatus
6. Mitochondria
7. Nuclear, cytoplasmic matrices

Cloned chromosomal DNA can aid immeasurably with identifying parental origins unavailable by other markers. The use of these cloned markers for testing the aforementioned epidemiological model is obvious.

Examination of the characteristics of centromere proteins may lead us to unique and vulnerable properties of this structure; considerable effort is being expended by investigators in this area (Earnshaw & Rothfield, 1985). The apparent absence of the centriole in mammalian oocytes is a unique circumstance that must be explored along the lines of an alternate disjunctional mechanism, perhaps involving the mid-zone.

Studies of the mid-body or intraspindle apparatus, so important to correct progession of anaphase I, or detection of mutations of any of the apparatus of distribution, so well described in lower forms, must be sought in the human (where they no doubt exist). Outside of the complete spindle area lie important organelles such as the "mitochondrial cage," which surrounds the first metaphase plate in oocytes and theoretically produces the energy of chromosome movement, or the nuclear and cytoplasmic matrices whose complex structures provide transport and direction for molecular movement. The opportunity to begin to search in these unexplored areas with the new tools of molecular science seems promising—one may find the answer or answers to the ancient and vexing problem of human aneuploidy, and especially trisomy 21.

REFERENCES

Alberman, E. (1972). Parental exposure to X-irradiation and Down's syndrome. *Annals of Human Genetics, 36,* 195–208.

Ayme, S., & Lippman-Hand, A. (1982). Maternal age effects in aneuploidy: Does altered embryo selection play a role? *American Journal of Human Genetics, 34,* 558–565.

Bennett, M. D., Rao, K., Smith, J. B., & Baylise, M. W. (1973). Cell development in the anther, the ovule, and the young seed of *Triticum aestivum L.* var-Chinese Spring. *Philosophical Transactions of the Royal Society of London, Series B, 266,* 39–81.

Bennett, M. D., Toledo, L. A., & Stern, H. (1979). The effect of colchicine on meiosis in *Lillium speciosum* cv. "Rosemede." *Chromosoma (Berl.), 72,* 175–189.

Bodmer, W. F. (1961). Effects of maternal age in the incidence of congenital abnormalities in mouse and man. *Nature (Lond.), 190,* 1134–1135.

Bond, D. J., & Chandley, A. C. (1983). The origin and causes of aneuploidy in man. *Aneuploidy: Oxford monographs on medical genetics.* Oxford: Oxford University Press.

Carpenter, A. T. C. (1979). Recombination nodules and synaptonemal complex in recombination-defective female of *Drosophila melanogaster. Chromosoma (Berl.), 75,* 259–292.

Catchside, D. G. (1977). *The genetics of recombination.* Baltimore: University Park Press.

Chandley, A. C. (1968). The effect of X-rays on female germ cells of *D. melanogaster*. A comparison with heat treatment on crossing over in the X chromosome. *Mutation Research, 5*, 93–107.

Crowley, P. H., Gulati, D. K., Hayden, T. L., Lopez, P., & Dyer, R. (1979). A chiasma-hormonal hypothesis relating Down's syndrome and maternal age. *Nature (Lond.), 280*, 417–418.

del Mazo, J., Castillo, A. M., & Abrisqueta, J. A (1982). Origin of nondisjunction. *Human Genetics, 62*, 316–320.

Derman, H. (1938). A cytological analysis of polyploidy. *Journal of Heredity, 29*, 211–229.

Dover, G. A., & Riley, R. (1973). The effect of spindle inhibitors applied before meiosis on meiotic chromosome pairing. *Journal of Cell Science, 12*, 143–161.

Driscoll, C. J., & Darvey, N. L. (1970). Chromosome pairing: Effect of colchicine on an isochromosome. *Science, 169*, 290–291.

Driscoll, C. J., Darvey, N. L., & Barben, H. N (1967). Effects of colchicine on meiosis of hexaploid wheat. *Nature (Lond.), 216*, 687–688.

Earnshaw, W. C., & Rothfield, N. (1985). Identification of a family of human centromere proteins using autoimmune sera from patients with scleroderma. *Chromosoma (Berl.), 91*, 313–321.

Evans, H. J. (1967). The nucleolus, virus infection, and trisomy in man. *Nature (Lond.), 214*, 361–363.

Feldman, M. (1966). The effect of chromosomes 5D and 5A on chromosomal pairing in *Triticum aestivum. Proceedings of the National Academy of Science (USA), 55*, 1447–1453.

German, J. (1968). Mongolism, delayed fertilization, and human sexual behavior. *Nature (Lond.), 217*, 516–518.

Ghosal, S. K., & Mukherjee, B. B. (1971). Chronology of DNA synthesis, meiosis, and spermiogenesis in the male mouse and golden hamster. *Canadian Journal of Genetics and Cytology, 13*, 672–682.

Hansson, A., & Mikkelsen, M. (1978). The origin of the extra chromosome 21 in Down syndrome. *Cytogenetics and Cell Genetics, 20*, 194–203.

Harlap, S., Shiono, P. H., Pellegrin, F., Golbus, M., Bachman, R., Mann, J., Schmidt, L., & Lewis, J. P. (1979). Chromosome abnormalities in oral contraceptive breakthrough pregnancies. *Lancet, i*, 1342–43.

Hassold, T., & Jacobs, P. (1984). Trisomy in man. *Annual Review of Genetics, 18*, 69–97.

Henderson, S. A. (1966). The time of chiasma formation in relation to the time of DNA synthesis. *Nature (Lond.), 211*, 1043.

Henderson, S. A. (1970). The time and place of meiotic crossing-over. *Annual Review of Genetics, 4*, 295–324.

Henderson, S. A., & Edwards, R. G. (1968). Chiasma frequency and maternal aging in mammals. *Nature (Lond.), 218*, 22–28.

Holliday, R. (1974). Molecular aspects of genetic exchange and gene conversion. *Genetics, 78*, 273–287.

Hook, E. B. (1983). Down syndrome, its frequency in human populations and some factors pertinent to variation in rates. In F. F. de la Cruz & P. S. Gerald (Eds.), *Down syndrome perspectives* (pp. 4–23). Baltimore: University Park Press.

Hook, E. B. (1985, March 25–29). Parental age and chromosome abnormalities in human [Abstract No. 15]. *Proceedings of the Symposium on Aneuploidy: Etiology and Mechanisms*. Washington, DC: U.S. Environmental Protection Agency, National Institute of Environmental Health Sciences, Council for Research Planning in Biological Sciences.

Hotta, Y., & Shepard, J. (1973). Biochemical aspects of colchicine action on meiotic cells. *Molecular and General Genetics, 122,* 243–260.

Ierardi, L., Moss, S. B., & Bellvé, A. R. (1981). The nuclear matrices of pachytene spermatocytes and spermatids: Their isolation and biochemical characterization. *Journal of Cell Biology, 91,* 65a.

Jagiello, G. M., & Fang, J. S. (1979). Analysis of diplotene chiasma frequencies in mouse oocytes and spermatocytes in relation to aging and sexual dimorphisms. *Cytogenetics and Cell Genetics, 23,* 53–60.

Jones, G. H. (1973). Modified synaptonemal complex in spermatocytes of *Stethophyma grossum. Cold Spring Harbor Symposium on Quantitative Biology, 38,* 109–115.

LaCour, L. F., & Wells, B. (1977). Some morphological aspects of the synaptonemal complex in higher plants. *Philosophical Transactions of the Royal Society of London, Series B, 277,* 259–266.

Levan, A. (1939). The effect of colchicine on meiosis in *Allium. Hereditas, 25,* 9–26.

Li, S., Meistrich, M. L., Brock, W. A., Hsu, T. C., & Kuo, M. T. (1983). Isolation and preliminary characterization of the synaptonemal complex from rat pachytene spermatocytes. *Experimental Cell Research, 144,* 63–72.

Magenis, R. E., & Chamberlin, J. (1981). Parental origin of nondisjunction. In F. F. de la Cruz & P. S. Gerald (Eds.), *Trisomy 21 (Down syndrome): Research perspectives* (pp. 77–93). Baltimore: University Park Press.

Maguire, M. P. (1979). An indirect test for a role of the synaptonemal complex in the establishment of sister chromatid cohesiveness. *Chromosoma (Berl.), 70,* 313–321.

Maguire, M. P. (1982). Evidence for a role of the synaptonemal complex in provision for normal chromosome disjunction at meiosis II in *Maize. Chromosoma, (Berl.), 84,* 675–686.

Mailhes, J. B., Preston, R. J., & Lavappa, K. S. (1985, March 25–29). Whole mammals—female germ cells (Abstract No. 105). *Proceedings of the Symposium on Aneuploidy: Etiology and Mechanisms.* Washington, DC: U.S. Environmental Protection Agency, National Institute of Environmental Health Sciences, Council for Research Planning in Biological Sciences.

Martin, R. H., Dill, F. J., & Miller, J. R. (1976). Nondisjunction in aging female mice. *Cytogenetics and Cell Genetics, 17,* 150.

Mather, K. (1938). Crossing-over. *Biological Review, 13,* 252–292.

Mattei, J. F., Ayme, S., Mattei, M. G., & Giraud, F. (1980). Maternal age and origin of nondisjunction in trisomy 21. *Journal of Medical Genetics, 17,* 368–372.

Meselson, M., & Radding, C. M. (1975). A general model for genetic recombination. *Proceedings of the National Academy of Science (USA), 72,* 358–361.

Mikkelsen, M., Poulsen, H., Grinsted, J., & Lange, A. (1980). Nondisjunction in trisomy 21. Study of chromosomal heteromorphisms in 110 families. *Annals of Human Genetics, 44,* 17–28.

Moses, M. J. (1968). Synaptonemal complex. *Annual Review of Genetics, 2,* 363–412.

Moses, M. (1985, March 25–29). Synaptonemal complex in meiosis: Significance of induced perturbations (Abstract No. 29). *Proceedings of the Symposium on Aneuploidy: Etiology and Mechanisms.* Washington, DC: U.S. Environmental Protection Agency, National Institute of Environmental Health Sciences, Council for Research Planning in Biological Sciences.

Peacock, W. J. (1970). Replication, recombination, and chiasmata in *G. Australasiae*. *Genetics, 65*, 593–617.

Polani, P. E., Biggers, J. H., Ford, C. E., Clark, C. M., & Berg, D. J. (1960). A mongol girl with 46 chromosomes. *Lancet, i*, 721–724.

Polani, P. E., & Jagiello, G. M. (1976). Chiasmata, meiotic univalents, and age in relation to aneuploid imbalance in mice. *Cytogenetics and Cell Genetics, 16*, 505–529.

Rundle, A., Coppen, A., & Cowie, V. (1961). Steroid excretion in mothers of mongols. *Lancet, ii*, 846–848.

Salonen, K., Paranko, J., & Parvinen, M. (1982). A Colcemid-sensitive mechanism involved in regulation of chromosome movements during meiotic pairing. *Chromosoma (Berl.), 85*, 611–618.

Shepard, J., Boothroyd, R., & Stern, H. (1974). The effect of colchicine on synapsis and chiasmata formation in microsporocytes of *Lillium*. *Chromosoma, (Berl.), 44*, 423–437.

Smit-Vis, J. H., & Akkerman-Belaart, M. A. (1967). Spermiogenesis in hibernating golden hamsters. *Experientia, 23*, 844–846.

Speed, R. M. (1985). The prophase stages in human foetal oocytes studied by light and electron microscopy. *Human Genetics, 69*, 69–75.

Speed, R. M., & Chandley, A. C. (1983). Meiosis in the foetal mouse ovary. II. Oocyte development and age-related aneuploidy. Does a production line exist? *Chromosoma (Berl.), 88*, 184–89.

Stein, Z., Stein, W., & Susser, M. (1986). Attrition of trisomies as a screening device. An explanation of the association of trisomies with maternal age. *Lancet, i*, 944–946.

Stern, H., & Hotta, Y. (1977). Biochemistry of meiosis. *Philosophical Transactions of the Royal Society of London, Series B, 277*, 277–294.

Stick, R., & Schwarz, H. (1982). The disappearance of the nuclear lamina during spermatogenesis: An electron microscopic and immunofluorescence study. *Cell Differentiation, 11*, 235–243.

Uchida, I. (1979). Radiation induced nondisjunction. *Environmental Health Perspectives, 31*, 13–18.

Wagenbichler, P., Killan, W., Rett, A., & Schnedl, W. (1976). Origin of the extra chromosome No. 21 in Down syndrome. *Human Genetics, 32*, 13–16.

Wallace, M. E., MacSwiney, F. J., & Edwards, R. G. (1976). Parental age and recombination frequency in the house mouse. *Genetical Research, 28*, 241–251.

Westergaard, M., & Wettstein, D. von (1972). The synaptonemal complex. *Annual Review of Genetics, 6*, 71–110.

Whitehouse, H. L. K. (1973). *Towards an understanding of the mechanism of heredity* (3rd ed.). New York: St. Martin's Press.

Response

Further Notes
on the Etiology
of Down Syndrome

Horace C. Thuline

✛✛✛

Chapter 1 provides a remarkable review of the etiology of human trisomy 21, and there is no need to retrace each point. Three areas, however, may bear additional comment: 1) the "third model" for restudying nondisjunction, based on Stein and collaborators' epidemiological theory cited in Chapter 1; 2) nondisjunction; and 3) the plurality of mechanisms resulting in Down syndrome.

THE THIRD MODEL

The epidemiological theory as understood from Chapter 1 has two components. These are: 1) the rate for trisomy among conceptuses is not related to maternal age, 2) the observed maternal age effect for trisomy in spontaneously aborted embryos and fetuses is not a function of the embryo or fetus but of uterine factors.

The first proposition is based on the observation that for liveborn infants with trisomy 21 the ratio of maternal to paternal origin (M:P) for the trisomy does not appear to change with maternal age. This is derived from a review of several reports in the literature for a total of 266 individuals with Down syndrome. A recent study by Bricarelli et al. (1985) (reported in an abstract) of 177 families informative as to parent of origin for the trisomy 21 in an offspring found that 75% were maternal and 25% were paternal in origin. Meiosis I accounted for 92% of the maternal trisomies and 89% of the paternal. It would be of great interest to see the data from their series as to M:P ratio in relation to maternal age, since the series has the advantage of being done over a 2-year span, 1981–1983, by the same investigators.[1]

---

[1]Jagiello said that at a meeting where that study (Bricarelli et al., 1985) was reported, the authors gave data showing that the M:P ratio was not maternal age related. This is consistent with

From the hypothesis that the frequency of trisomy in conceptuses is not related to maternal age arises the implication that the observed increase for prevalence of trisomy 21 in relation to increasing maternal age is a function of decreasing loss in the preimplantation period. As yet, there are no mechanisms proposed for such a phenomenon.

Although data on the preimplantation frequency of human trisomy 21 and the M:P ratio related to maternal age for such conceptuses would seem to be excluded from being obtained by prospective experimental study, the postimplantation ratio for M:P origin has been determined for 17 fetuses with trisomy 21. Hassold, Chiu, and Yamane (1984) reviewed prior reports and added their own series to obtain the total of 17. Thirteen of these were maternal and 4 were paternal in origin. This is consistent with the M:P ratio found for live births in which trisomy 21 is present; however, the maternal age relationship of the M:P ratio for the period from implantation to delivery is still undescribed.

This question is relevant to the second hypothesis, which implies that after implantation of a trisomic embryo there are uterine factors that are maternal age related and lead to increasing frequency of spontaneous abortion with increasing maternal age. This is an observed phenomenon in the human that is supported by experimental data from the laboratory mouse. In their review, Schneider and Kram (1981) cited the evidence for a maternal age effect on the frequency of aneuploidy in 10.5-day-old mouse embryos.

However, data for 3.5 day preimplantation mouse embryos, from the experiments by Brook, Gosden, and Chandley (1984) show a preimplantation maternal age effect with increased frequency of aneuploidy (including trisomy) for biologically aged mice. This does not provide support for the first hypothesis cited in the beginning of this section since, in the mouse, the rate for aneuploidy at fertilization was not found constant with no age effect. Perhaps the mouse is suitable as an animal model to study postimplantation factors relating to pregnancy with trisomic fetuses, but it may not be equally suitable for preimplantation factors in humans.

As to maternal age effect, there may be another way to look at it. Traditionally, maternal age effect is described for the prevalence of Down syndrome in a general population or for the age of mothers at the time the child with Down syndrome is born. There is at present no proven technique for identifying prospectively the population of women who will bear a child with Down syndrome. However, there is a population of women who have borne a child with Down syndrome which the author studied. The unpublished data for nearly 600 families is represented in Figures 1 and 2.

Figure 1 shows the percentage of live births at given maternal age quinquenniums for a 25-year period (1940–1965) in the state of Washington. The

---

the review data cited in Chapter 1. Jagiello said the authors plan to publish the M:P/maternal age relationship data.

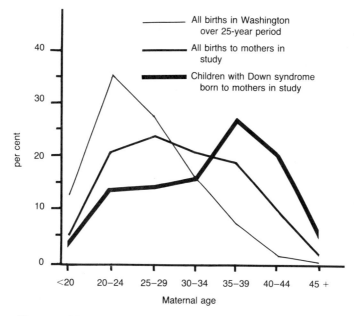

Figure 1.   Maternal age at birth of children in the state of Washington.

two other curves are for the study population. It is apparent that the highest percent in a 5-year maternal age period for all children being born to these mothers was in the 25–29 year age period. The figure also shows the typical rise in prevalence for children with Down syndrome, which peaks at age 35–39. Both of these are familiar curves.

Figure 2 uses the same data but shows the percentage of children with Down syndrome among all children born in a given maternal age period. For children with Down syndrome, the curve is J-shaped; this implies that more than a single etiological factor is operating. More significant is that for this population of mothers, known to be able to carry a child with Down syndrome to term, 20% of the children born at the maternal age of under 20 had Down syndrome. This was the age period when only 5% of all their children were born. Further, in the 25–29 year age period, when 24% of all children were born to these mothers, the prevalence for Down syndrome was the lowest (15%). Also, for these mothers, as they aged, the proportion of their offspring with Down syndrome increased from 20% at age 30–34 to 53% at 40–44, and, in a much smaller number of births, at age 45 or older, to 61%.

The implication from these data is that women who give birth to a child with Down syndrome are a specific population and carry factors that either predispose to nondisjunctions in their conceptions, allow them to carry trisomic fetuses to term, or both. In the population being cited, 25% of 2,424 children had Down syndrome.

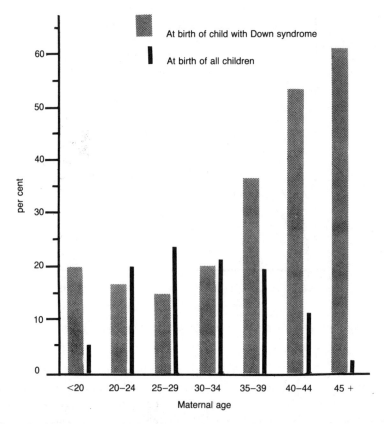

Figure 2. Maternal age at birth of children for study population of 600 families in the state of Washington.

This raises the matter of urgency in identifying the factors that might identify these women as at risk. A hypothesis proposed by Emanuel, Sever, Milham, and Thuline (1972) may warrant further consideration through the use of current technology. The hypothesis suggests that the maternal age effect is related to biological aging and its effect on the reproductive process. Mothers giving birth to a child with Down syndrome at younger ages may be manifesting the same mechanisms as operate in older women, but represent one end of a frequency distribution curve for aging. The primary age factor would be biological rather than chronological.

Some support for this concept has been obtained by the studies in the laboratory mouse by Brook et al. (1984). They found the increase in aneuploidy for preimplantation embryos to be significantly related to factors of biological aging rather than chronological aging of the dams. It would be of interest to see the concept developed.

NONDISJUNCTION

As to the mechanisms of nondisjunction, there seems to be a focus on the centromere as the chromosome structure of interest. However, Sybenga (1972), in describing the process of mitosis, describes the separation of the chromatids as relating to a release between small chromosomal segments on both sides of the centromeres rather than at the centromeres. It seems worthwhile to note the work of Kurnit et al. (1984) on the characteristics of the DNA in pericentromeric regions of human acrocentric chromosomes as being of possible future significance to the mechanisms of chromosome 21 disjunction or nondisjunction.

A PLURALITY OF MECHANISMS

The last item for comment is the plurality of mechanisms resulting in Down syndrome. Most of the research emphasis is on mechanisms hypothesized for the major portion of the population with Down syndrome. However, there are significant segments of that population in which the mechanisms leading to trisomy of the long arm of 21 (called 21q) can be described from cytogenetic findings.

In contrast to the aforementioned comments about the possibility that centromeres are not etiologically involved in nondisjunction, there is good evidence for involvement of the centromere in the trisomy of 21q from isochromosome formation. This is of significance to the data for the occurrence of "21/21 translocations." In a review of 4,760 patients with Down syndrome, Giraud and Mattei (1975) found 4.8% with translocations (about 230) and of these, 40.9% (about 94) were 21qDq with 96% arising *de novo*. Of the 21qGq, 83.3% were 21q21q (about 78). It is these *de novo* 21q21q findings that are of interest in terms of the cytogenetic mechanics that may be deduced from karyotype findings.

The first mechanism is an apparent instability of the centromere, resulting in misdivision in mitosis and mosaicism for 21p- and normal 21s. The next step is formation of an isochromosome 21q from the 21p- with a consequent cell line trisomic for 21q. Case reports describing 46,21p-/46,i21q mosaicism have appeared in the literature. The author had an opportunity to do cytogenetics for a child with clinical Down syndrome and her parents. The following karyotypes were found:

Proband	47,XXX,21p-/47,XXX,-21p-,+i21q
Father	46,XY (normal 21p)
Mother	46,XX (normal 21p)

A second patient referred for possible Down syndrome was found to have:

Proband	45,XX,-13,-21,+t(13;21)(p11;q11)/47,XXX,13p-,21p-/
	47,XXX,13p-,-21p-,+i21q
Father	46,XY (normal 21p, no translocation)
Mother	46,XX (normal 21p, no translocation)

These two patients both show abnormal X numbers as well as evidence for an unstable centromere. In the first patient, the XXX finding is in all cells, in the second there is XX/XXX mosaicism. In the first patient, a *de novo* 21p- has apparently formed an i21q early enough in development to give her unquestioned Down syndrome. For the second girl, the primary line appears to be the *de novo* 13q:21q translocation which broke down into the 13p-, 21p- containing line with a third cell line showing 13p-;i21q. This last is a minor cell line and is consistent with Down syndrome remaining as a clinical question.

The third child to illustrate the point being made had a firm clinical diagnosis of Down syndrome. Her karyotype was found to be:

$$46,XX/46,XX,-21,+i21q$$
(Parents' karyotypes not obtained)

In her 46,XX cell line, each cell examined showed normal 21s although, in theory, a 21p- cell line could be present and give rise to the 46,XX,-21,+i21q line that was found. However, since the ratio of normal to i21q lines is essentially 1:1, it is more probable that the i21q arose from a centromere division error in first cleavage division with loss of the i21p derivative.

The finding of these karyotypes in a single service cytogenetic laboratory experience suggests that centromere instability may be more common than thought. The counseling implication is that 21p- in a parent may be as important in assessing recurrence risk as a minor mosaicism of i21q. Prudence dictates that parents of a child with an apparent 21q21q translocation should be checked for 21p- even though they have normal children and a 21q21q carrier state seems to have been ruled out.

REFERENCES

Bricarelli, F. D., Arslanian, A., Coviello, D. A., Ferro, M. A., Frateschi, M., Gessaga, M., Pierluigi, M., & Strigini, P. (1985). Origin of non-disjunction and "de novo" translocation in trisomy 21 syndrome: A study of 267 families. *Clinical Genetics, 27,* 298–299.

Brook, J. D., Gosden, R. G., & Chandley, A. C. (1984). Maternal aging and aneuploid embryos—Evidence from the mouse that biological and not chronological age is the important influence. *Human Genetics, 66,* 41–45.

Emanuel, I., Sever, L. E., Milham, S., Jr., & Thuline, H. C. (1972). Accelerated aging in young mothers of children with Down's syndrome. *Lancet, 2,* 361–363.

Giraud, F., & Mattei, J. F. (1975). Aspects epidemiologics de la trisomy 21 [Epidemiological aspects of trisomy 21]. *Journal de Genetique Humaine, 23,* (supplement 1), 1–30.

Hassold, T., Chiu, D., & Yamane, J. A. (1984). Parental origin of autosomal trisomies. *Annals of Human Genetics, 48,* 129–144.

Kurnit, D. M., Neve, R. L., Morton, C. C., Bruns, G. A. P., Ma, N. S. F., Cox, D. R., & Klinger, H. P. (1984). Recent evolution of DNA sequence homology in the pericentromeric regions of human acrocentric chromosomes. *Cytogenetics and Cell Genetics, 38,* 99–105.

Schneider, E. L., & Kram, D. (1981). Animal models for studying parental age effects. In F. F. de la Cruz & P. S. Gerald (Eds.), *Trisomy 21 (Down syndrome): Research perspectives* (pp. 275–280). Baltimore: University Park Press.

Sybenga, J. (1972). *General cytogenetics* (pp. 26–27). New York: American Elsevier Publishing Co.

Chapter 2

Somatic Cell Molecular Genetics of Chromosome 21

David Patterson, Sharon Graw, James Gusella, and Paul Watkins

Down syndrome, first identified in 1866 (Down), is the most common specifically identified genetic cause of mental retardation and congenital heart disease in the United States, afflicting 1 in 800 to 1 in 1,100 live births (Adams, Erickson, Layde, & Oakley, 1981). Over 70% of conceptuses with Down syndrome end as spontaneous abortions (Boue, Deluchat, Nicolas, & Boue, 1981).

It was first suggested that the disorder might involve a chromosomal defect due to nondisjunction in 1932 (Waardenberg), and that a trisomy might be involved in 1934 (Bleyer). It was not until 1959, after the correct chromosome number in humans had been determined, that Lejeune was able to show that trisomy of a G-group chromosome was in fact associated with Down syndrome (Lejeune, Gauthier, & Turpin, 1959; Tjio & Levan, 1956). In 1960 (Polani, Briggs, Ford, Clarke, & Berg), the first translocation patient with Down syndrome was described and in 1961 (Clarke, Edwards, & Smallpiece), the first child with trisomy 21 mosaicism was identified.

THE PATHOLOGY OF DOWN SYNDROME

Types of Pathogenic Conditions

A number of pathogenic conditions are seen with greater frequency among

This is contribution #578 of the Eleanor Roosevelt Institute for Cancer Research. This work was supported by National Institutes of Health Grants HD07197, HD13423, HD17449, HD06470; National Institute of Aging Grant AG00029; and the Reynolds Foundation. The authors are grateful to Dr. Margaret Van Keuren for valuable discussions, advice and assistance, and to Dr. Jeffrey Davidson, Dr. Yoram Groner, and Dr. Bernard Forget for providing DNA probes for use in this work.

persons with Down syndrome than in the normal population. Certain examples are discussed in the following section.

Development of banding techniques and study of individuals with translocations have allowed a narrowing of the pathogenetic region of chromosome 21 to band 21q22 (Neibuhr, 1974; Rethore, Dutrillaux, & Lejeune, 1973) and possibly even to subbands of this region (Habedank and Rodewald, 1982; Mattei, Mattei, Baeteman, & Giraud, 1981; Sinet et al., 1976; Taysi, Sparkes, O'Brien, & Dengler, 1982). In some cases in which band q22.1 or band q22.3 was found not to be trisomic, patients were described as having moderate or partial Down syndrome (Habedank & Rodewald, 1982; Mattei et al., 1981; Taysi et al., 1982). These studies depend upon difficult cytogenetic analysis without molecular or biochemical markers so that, at least at present, it may still be possible that trisomy of the entire q22 band of chromosome 21 is essential for classic Down syndrome.

Infection and Leukemia   Some individuals with Down syndrome have a compromised immune system (Tolksdorf & Wiedemann, 1981), a finding possibly related to their increased susceptibility to various types of infection and for development of leukemia (Balarajan, Donnan, & Adelstein, 1982; Carter, Mikkelson, & Nelson, 1964; Evans, 1970; Oster, Mikkelson, & Nielsen, 1975; Rosner & Lee, 1972; Scoggin & Patterson, 1982; Sturm, Staneck, & Myers, 1980; Tolksdorf & Weideman, 1981; Weinberger & Olenik, 1970). For a child with Down syndrome, the risk of leukemia is estimated at 1 in 95, compared to 1 in 2,900 for normal children (Rowley, 1981). Children with Down syndrome also have a tendency to develop a transient leukemoid reaction that is seen in virtually no other syndrome (Barak, Mogilner, Karov, Schlesinger, & Levin, 1982; Lazarus, Heerema, Palmer & Baehner, 1981; Miller & Cosgriff, 1983). Children with Down syndrome who experience a transient leukemoid reaction do not seem to have an elevated risk of later developing leukemia. The types of leukemia seen in Down syndrome are similar to those seen in the general population (Miller & Cosgriff, 1983; Scholl, Stein, & Hansen, 1982), although there may be a tendency toward specific types of acute myeloid leukemia in children with Down syndrome with acute nonlymphocytic leukemia (Kaneko et al., 1981).

Alzheimer Disease   Down syndrome is considered to be a progeroid syndrome (Balarajan et al., 1982; Barak et al., 1982; Carter et al., 1964; Evans, 1970; Kaneko et al., 1981; Lazarus et al., 1981; Miller & Cosgriff, 1983; Oster et al., 1975; Rosner & Lee, 1972; Rowley, 1981; Scholl et al., 1982; Sturm et al., 1980; Weinberger & Olenik, 1970). Of particular interest is the association of Alzheimer disease with Down syndrome (Dalton, Crapper, & Schlotter, 1974; Ellis, McCulloch, & Corley, 1974; Glenner, 1983; Glenner & Wong, 1984; Heston, 1976; Heston & Mastri, 1977; Olson & Shaw, 1969; Tolksdorf & Wiedemann, 1981). Alzheimer disease is one of the most commonly identified causes of premature senility in the United States. Commonly, Alzheimer disease does not occur in the normal population until after age 50 (Tolksdorf & Wiedemann, 1981). Neuropathological evidence of Alzheimer-type changes can be found in virtually all brains examined of persons with Down syndrome who die after the age of 35 years (Glenner, 1983; Glenner & Wong, 1984; Tolksdorf & Wiedemann, 1981). Amyloid protein from Alzheimer disease patients and patients with Down syndrome showing the signs of Alzheimer disease has been compared and found to be identical, thus strengthening the connection between the two diseases (Glenner & Wong, 1984).

Hyperuricemia Individuals with Down syndrome often show hyperuricemia (Fuller, Luce, & Mertz, 1962). In a particularly complete and well-controlled study, Pant, Moser, and Krane (1968) examined 280 patients with Down syndrome and 298 control patients. Serum uric acid levels were elevated in all age groups and both sexes in the Down syndrome population. Hyperuricemia was not observed in 27 patients with Klinefelter syndrome or in parents of patients with Down syndrome. Patients with Down syndrome with trisomy 21 or translocations showed similar serum uric acid elevations. Urinary excretion of uric acid was elevated in 80% of subjects. These results are highly suggestive that the hyperuricemia in patients with Down syndrome is related to overproduction of purines. The ratio of urate in serum of persons with Down syndrome to normal persons is remarkably close to that predicted if a gene or genes on chromosome 21 was rate-limiting for purine synthesis and expressed according to gene dosage, 1.45 times normal in females and 1.55 times normal in males over the age of 20.

The hyperuricemia of persons with Down syndrome is not known to be pathogenic. However, defects in purine metabolism, especially increases in the concentration of certain purine nucleotides, are harmful to normal fetal development in a wide variety of animal species from *Drosophila* to humans (Bazelon, Stevens, Davis, Seegmiller, & Greene, 1968; Becker, 1976; Becker, Kostel, Meyer, & Seegmiller, 1973; Dagg, Karnofsky, Lacon, & Roddy, 1957; Giblett, Ammann, Sandman, Wara, & Diamond, 1975; Giblett, Anderson, Cohen, Pollara, & Meuwissen, 1972; Green & Kochhar, 1975; Henderson, Rosenbloom, Kelley, & Seegmiller, 1968; Ho et al., 1984; Hooft, Van Nevel, & De Schaepdryver, 1968; Kelley, Rosenbloom, Henderson, & Seegmiller, 1967; Konrad & Harris, 1971; Lesch and Nyhan, 1964; Nyhan, James, Seberg, Sweetman, & Nelson, 1969; Parkman, Gelfand, Rosen, Sanderson, & Hirschhorn, 1975; Seegmiller, Rosenbloom, & Kelley, 1967; Theirsch, 1957; Valentine, Palgia, Tartaglia, & Gilsanz, 1977). Aberrant purine metabolism is associated with immune deficiency and with mental retardation (Bazelon et al., 1968; Becker, 1976; Becker et al., 1973; Giblett et al., 1975; Giblett et al., 1972; Kelley et al., 1967; Lesch & Nyhan, 1964;

Parkman et al., 1975; Seegmiller et al., 1967), two of the pathologies seen in Down syndrome. Therefore, it may well be that defects in purine metabolism are significant in the aberrant development noted in individuals with Down syndrome.

Biochemical Basis of the Pathology

Although there is no conclusive information on the biochemical basis of any of the pathology seen in Down syndrome, the idea that an excess of specific genes on chromosome 21 is responsible for the pathology in the syndrome is an attractive one and offers a place to start a molecular analysis. For example, the virtual 100% association between Alzheimer disease and persons with Down syndrome who die as young adults, recently confirmed on a bio-chemical level, suggests that specific genes on chromosome 21 may lead to this aspect of the pathology (Glenner & Wong, 1984).

It has been proposed that genes on chromosome 21 may be involved in the development of leukemia in normal individuals (Rowley, 1981), a pro-posal consistent with the involvement of specific genes on chromosome 21 in specific aspects of the pathology of Down syndrome. Collaborative work between the authors' and Rowley's laboratories is consistent with this hypoth-esis (Drabkin et al., 1985). They have isolated in a somatic cell hybrid one of the rearranged chromosomes from a patient with AML subtype M2 with an 8;21 chromosomal translocation. It is clear from these studies that the c-*mos* oncogene, cytogenetically located at the breakpoint band on chromosome 8 (Neel, Jhanwar, Chaganti, & Hayward, 1982; Prakash et al., 1982), does not have to be translocated to chromosome 21 for the development of AML. This leaves open the possibility that there are genes on chromosome 21, perhaps in the q22.3 region, claimed to be the breakpoint in this type of leukemia (Yunis, 1984), that are important in the development of leukemia in otherwise normal individuals. In recent studies, Dayton et al. (1984) have reported similar findings in a patient with poorly differentiated leukemia containing a (17;21) chromosomal translocation and have also mentioned the possibility of a role for chromosome 21 specific sequences in leukemia.

That individuals with Down syndrome are at a markedly increased risk for development of leukemia, but not necessarily for other types of malignan-cy (Rowley, 1981; Scholl et al., 1982) is reminiscent of other chromosomal disorders. For example, deletions on chromosome 13 or on chromosome 11 increase the risk of retinoblastoma and Wilms tumor, respectively. It can thus be argued that at least some of the pathology seen in Down syndrome is related to specific genes on chromosome 21.

The transient leukemoid response sometimes seen in infants with Down syndrome also suggests that genes on chromosome 21 may be significant for hematopoietic development and maintenance (Barak et al., 1982; Lazarus et al., 1981; Miller & Cosgriff, 1983). Also, patients with mosaic trisomy or tetrasomy 21 show a much lower frequency of trisomic cells in blood than in other tissues (Hunter, Clifford, Speevak, & MacMurray, 1982; Kwee, Barth, Arwert, & Madan, 1984; Wilson, Towner, & Forsman, 1980). This observation of selective mosaicism has recently been extended to chimeric mice that are trisomic for the parts of mouse chromosome 16 analogous in part to human chromosome 21 (Cox, Smith, Epstein, & Epstein, 1984).

For any gene to be pathogenetic for all or part of the phenotype of Down syndrome, it would have to be regionally mapped to the q22 band of chromosome 21. So far, there are five genes whose assignment to chromosome 21 has been confirmed and five whose assignment is provisional (de Grouchy & Turleau, 1984; Skovby, Krassikoff, & Francke, 1984; Vora & Francke, 1981). One, the ribosomal RNA gene, located on the short arm of the chromosome, is thought not to be relevant to the pathology of Down syndrome. Of the other four, three—superoxide dismutase-1 (SOD-1), phosphoribosylamine-glycine ligase (GARS), and phosphofructokinase liver form (PFKL)—may be in the q22 region (Bradley, Patterson, & Robinson, 1986; Chadefaux, et al., 1984; Cox, Kawashima, Vora, & Epstein, 1984; Sinet et al., 1976; Yosimitsu et al., 1983) although recent evidence suggests that PFKL may not map to the pathogenetic segment (Chadefaux, Rethore, & Allard, 1984). The fourth, the interferon receptor, located from q21→qter, may also be in the q22 band (de Grouchy & Turleau, 1984). Two of the five genes provisionally assigned to chromosome 21, phosphoribosylformylglycinamidine cyclo-ligase (AIRS) and primary thrombocytosis (TAC) may also be on the long arm of chromosome 21.

PURINE BIOSYNTHESIS AND CHROMOSOME 21

Any of the genes currently known to be assigned to chromosome 21 might well be involved in one or another of the symptoms seen in persons with Down syndrome. For example, perturbation of oxygen radical metabolism levels because of elevated SOD-1 activity and altered response to viruses because of increased interferon receptors both might play a role in the pathology of Down syndrome (Sinet et al., 1976; Weil, Tucker, Epstein, L. B., & Epstein, C. J., 1983). The possibility that elevated levels of two or more of the enzymes of *de novo* biosynthesis of purines may be related to the observed hyperuricemia in individuals with Down syndrome and perhaps to developmental abnormalities is of major interest in the authors' laboratory. From the work of the authors' laboratory and at least two others, the enzyme activity for

GARS is in fact elevated by a factor of 1.5 in patients with trisomy for the q22 band and probably for the q22.1 band of chromosome 21 (Barkley & Epstein, 1980; Bradley et al., 1985; Chadefaux, Allard et al., 1984).Measurement of AIRS levels has not yet been carried out due to the lack until recently of a sufficiently reliable and sensitive assay.

It has been argued that dosage of these enzymes will not lead to increased levels of purine synthesis since neither is hypothesized to be the rate-limiting step. However, the rate of purine synthesis may be regulated by many different mechanisms (Henderson, 1972). In fact, evidence has been presented implicating AIRS as the rate-limiting step of IMP synthesis (Rowe, McCairns, Madsen, Sauer, & Elliott, 1978). The authors have preliminary evidence that the specific activity of GARS may be the lowest of the 10 purine biosynthetic enzymes that they have assayed in Chinese hamster ovary (CHO) cells (Patterson, unpublished data).

In recent collaborative studies with Henikoff, the authors have obtained evidence that in *Drosophila,* and probably in other animals, GARS, AIRS, and a third gene for purine biosynthesis (see Figure 1 for a simplified representation of this biochemical pathway), phosphoribosylglycineamide formyltransferase (GARFT), are coded for by a single genetic locus and within a 12 kb stretch of DNA. This means that these three enzymes of purine synthesis are all encoded by DNA within the 21q22 band (Henikoff et al., 1986).

It may well be that elevated purine biosynthetic levels are related to the developmental anomalies seen in Down syndrome in addition to the hyperuricemia. This is a conclusion that a number of investigators reached independently. For example, Chadefaux, Allard et al. (1984) stated: ". . . trisomy for band q22 is known to determine the phenotype of trisomy 21. It is reasonable to conclude that the excess of GARS may contribute to the manifestations of the syndrome."

A valuable series of experiments relevant to gene dosage effects employed 2-dimensional protein gel electrophoresis. These studies suggested that there is not a gross alteration in type or amount of proteins found in individuals with Down syndrome (Van Keuren, Merril, & Goldman, 1983; Weil & Epstein, 1979). It appears that transcription of chromosome 21 genes is altered according to gene dosage in Down syndrome (Kurnit, 1979).

A complicating factor in understanding the role of gene dosage and expression in Down syndrome is that it may not be necessary for a gene to be located within the pathogenetic segment of chromosome 21 for its expression to be altered by the presence of an extra chromosome. That is, there may be genes on other chromosomes whose expression is altered by the presence of extra copies of genes on chromosome 21. Moreover, altered gene expression may not be strictly according to gene dosage. These points have been the subject of experimentation by Epstein and co-workers (Weil, Epstein, & Epstein, 1980; Weil et al., 1983). Finally, it may be that there is temporal and

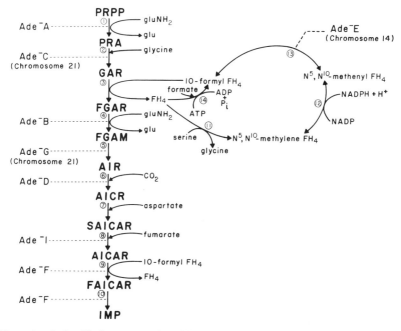

Figure 1. A simplified representation of the enzyme steps of purine biosynthesis, including synthesis of required tetrahydrofolate cofactor. Ade⁻A, Ade⁻B, etc. represent the designations of Chinese hamster cell mutants defective in the indicated enzymatic steps. Human chromosomal localizations for genes coding for certain enzymes are indicated in parentheses. (Abbreviations: glu NH_2, glutamine; glu, glutamate; PRA, β-phosphoribosylamine; GAR, phosphoribosylglycineamide; FGAR, phosphoribosylformylglycineamide; FGAM, phosphoribosylformylglycineamidine; AIR, phosphoribosylaminoimidazole; AICR, phosphoribosylaminoimidazole carboxylic acid; SAICAR, phosphoribosylaminoimidazolesuccinocarboxamide; AIC, aminoimidazolecarboxamide; FAICAR, phosphoribosylformamidoimidazolecarboxamide; IMP, inosine monophosphate; FH_4, tetrahydrofolate.)

tissue specificity of alterations in gene expression in Down syndrome that might be missed by most experimental procedures.

Experimental efforts in the authors' laboratory have focused on attempting to gain a better understanding of the physical organization of DNA in chromosome 21 and in generating a molecular map of the chromosome, with particular emphasis on defining at the molecular level the pathogenetic segment of the chromosome. The approaches they used took advantage of the location of genes coding for enzymes of purine synthesis in or near the 21q22 band. Specifically, this fact allowed us to isolate the intact chromosome 21 translocation chromosomes containing the 21q22 band and hybrids containing small fractions of the 21q22 band in CHO/human hybrids as the only detectable human genetic information. The authors then used recombinant DNA approaches and, in particular for these studies, human low repeat DNA sequences to begin to derive a molecular map of the 21q22 chromosomal region.

MATERIALS AND METHODS

Details of the procedures examining the production of somatic cell hybrids between CHO and human cells containing chromosome 21 as their only human genetic material have been published in Moore, Jones, Kao, and Oates (1977).

Production of Irradiation Reduction Hybrids

The procedure used closely follows that of Cirullo, Dana, and Wasmuth (1983), as depicted in Figure 2. In this approach, human/hamster hybrid cells containing chromosome 21 as their only recognizable human genetic information (with an Ade^-C mutant hamster background) were subjected to 3, 8, or 10 kiloroentgens of gamma irradiation. This kills virtually all of the cells and introduces breaks into the chromosomes of the hybrid cells. After this irradiation treatment, these nonviable hybrid cells were again fused with the hamster Ade^-C mutant cells and Ade^+ hybrids were selected. Viable hybrids should contain the chromosome fragment required for synthesis of human GARS but need not contain any other genetic information from the parental hybrid cell. Surviving colonies, called irradiation reduction hybrids, were picked and grown for analysis in a purine-free medium after such a treatment. All of the clones were analyzed by G-11 cytogenetic procedures in which human chromosomal material stained blue while hamster material stained magenta (Alhadeff, Velivasakis, & Siniscalco, 1977; Patterson & Schandle, 1983).

Analysis of DNA from Hybrids

It is possible to assess the human DNA content of irradiation reduction hybrids by Southern blot analysis, using as probes unique or repeated sequences isolated from the human genome which recognize human DNA in a

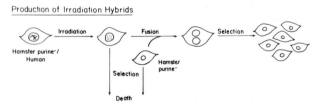

Figure 2. Production of irradiation hybrids. (Hamster purine-/human hybrid cells are killed by high doses of radiation, fused again with the same hamster mutant cell used to create the original hybrid cells, and selected for ability to grow without purines.)

Table 1. DNA probes used

	From	Size EcoR1 fragmented detected
pPW233F	J. Gusella and P. Watkins[a]	1.5 Kb
pPW231C	J. Gusella and P. Watkins[a]	2.1 Kb
pPW236B	J. Gusella and P. Watkins[a]	1.85 K[h]
pPW245D	J. Gusella and P. Watkins[a]	2.0 Kb
520-10R	J. Gusella and P. Watkins[a]	4.1 Kb
CP2	J. Davidson[b]	6.5 Kb
CP21G1	J. Davidson[b]	5.1 Kb
SOD-1	Y. Groner[c]	17.7 (chromosome 21 specific)
A36Fc	B. Forget[d]	multiple

[a]Gusella et al. (1985).
[b]Davidson, Rumsby, & Niswander (1985).
[c]Levanon et al. (1985).
[d]Duncan et al. (1979).

species-specific fashion (Gusella, Jones, Kao, Housman, and Puck, 1982; Gusella et al., 1980; Law, Davidson, & Kao, 1982). The low repeat probe used in the studies reported in this chapter was a sequence isolated from the globin gene region of chromosome 11, A36Fc (Gusella et al., 1982).

The sources of the DNA sequence probes are listed in Table 1. DNA isolated by the method of Gusella et al. (1982) was digested by various restriction endonucleases as recommended by the manufacturer. Electrophoresis of DNA on agarose gels was carried out according to Patterson and Schandle (1983). Southern blot hybridization analysis was carried out according to previously published procedures (Southern, 1975) with nick translated probes prepared as described by Rigby, Diekmann, Rhodes, & Berg (1977). Autoradiographs of Southern blots were analyzed and compared visually or, in some cases, were scanned using a densitometer.

EXPERIMENTAL RESULTS

The collection of CHO hybrids available for the studies mentioned in this section is described in Table 2.

To understand a genetic disease such as Down syndrome, it is vital to be able to map genes and DNA sequences to specific chromosomes and chromosome regions. The mapping of genes to regions of chromosomes is facilitated by using cells in which a translocation has occurred. For example, even

Table 2. Hybrids containing chromosome 21 specific material and parental and segregant cells

Cells: Parents	
CHO-K1	Chinese hamster ovary (fibroblasts).
A9	Mouse (fibroblasts).
Hybrids with chromosome 21 (as only human chromosome)	
153-E9a	Ade⁻C CHO × human.
153-E7b	Sister clone of 153-E9a; contains 21q.
72532X-6	Ade⁻G CHO × human.
2Fu^{r}1	CHO × human; contains 21q.
WAVR4dF9-4a	A9 × human from F. Ruddle; also subclones WA3 and WA17 (from R. Dutkowski) contain two and three 21s per cell, respectively.
SCC16-5	A9 × human from D. Cox.
ThyB1-33-6-1	Mouse × human suspension cells from C. Bostock.
ACEM	Ade⁻C × human, contains 21;21 translocation described in the first part of this chapter.
Segregants	
153-E9a-R4	Segregants of 153-E9a.
Q290-7a Q290-8c	Segregants of 1Fu^{4}1.
Hybrid with 8;21 (21q+) translocation chromosome	
21-8	Gly⁻B CHO × human AML cells; contains translocation 21pter→21q22;8q22→8qter.

though most persons with Down syndrome have a whole extra chromosome 21, some have only a translocation involving chromosome 21 and consequently only part of chromosome 21 is trisomic. The chromosomes of these individuals are useful not only in identifying which regions of chromosome 21 are responsible for Down syndrome but also in regional mapping. The rearranged chromosome can be isolated and studied in rodent/human hybrids.

The disadvantage of this method is that it relies on an informative rearrangement occurring in a patient and on this rearrangement being detected, usually through a morbid phenotype. There is no way to induce the formation of potentially valuable rearrangements if these do not occur in nature, or if they cannot be identified. The authors circumvented these obstacles by artifically inducing breaks in the genome and then selecting for the phenotype of interest, as described in the section discussing materials and methods.

The following hybrids have been produced using this protocol:

	No. in series	Hybrid parent	Hamster parent	Dose
1 × series	18	153-E9a	Ade⁻C(J162)	3,000 Roent.
3 × series	5	153-E7b	Ade⁻C(J162)	8,000 and 10,000 Roent.

These 23 hybrids were examined to determine the amount and nature of human chromosome 21 DNA they contained. This examination included cytogenetic analysis; biochemical analyses, such as SOD-1 isozyme analysis and thermal lability of the GARS enzyme; and DNA analyses, such as probing for the presence of unique sequences, low repeat sequence pattern, and middle repetitive (Alu) sequence pattern.

Cytogenetic Analysis

The 23 irradiation hybrids were examined with the G-11 staining technique. Of the 18 in the 1 × series, 8 had human chromosomal material resembling that of the parent cell and were thus excluded from further study. The remaining 10 of the 1 × series and all of the 3 × series had only fragments of human material. The remainder of this section includes only these hybrids. All cells examined had an approximately tetraploid chromosome constitution.

Biochemical Analyses

SOD-1 Isozyme Analysis   The 1 × series of hybrids was analyzed for human soluble SOD-1. When analyzed shortly after production, all 1 × hybrids had human SOD-1. Upon further cultivation, one of these (1 × 18c9) had lost human SOD-1. This indicated that some sort of stabilization process might have occurred after the initial formation of the irradiation hybrids. SOD-1 has been mapped to 21q22.1 (Sinet et al., 1976). In several patients with partial trisomy 21, however, SOD-1 has been dissociated from the complete Down syndrome phenotype. GARS has also been mapped to the 21q22.1 region (Chadefaux, Allard et al., 1984).

Thermal Lability of GARS   The authors' laboratory previously showed that human GARS is more heat labile than hamster GARS (Patterson & Schandle, 1983). Thus, preincubation of a cell extract at an increased temperature followed by measuring the GARS activity can indicate whether the enzyme is from a human or hamster source. Although only human GARS should be present in this system, there exists the potential for hamster GARS activity to be produced through reversion. The most highly reduced irradiation hybrid (1 × 18c9) has been tested in this fashion and shown to have a human-type heat lability. The results with 1 × 18c9 have been especially reassuring to the authors in light of the paucity of other markers found in this hybrid.

DNA Analyses

Single Copy Sequences   A number of cloned single-copy sequences have been mapped to chromosome 21. Clones used in this study are explained in Table 1. The results of Southern blot hybridization analysis of DNA from 15 irradiation hybrids using 5 of these unique sequence probes is shown in Table 3. Since the order of the cloned sequences on chromosome 21 is known, these data allowed the authors to define which regions of chromo-

Table 3. Southern blot hybridization analysis of irradiation reduction hybrids

Hybrid or parental cell line	DNA sequence or isozyme marker designation				
	236	245	SOD-1	21G1	231
1×3	+	+	+	+	+
1×4	−	−	+	+	+
1×5	+	+	+	+	+
1×8c1	+	+	+	+	+
1×9	+	+	+	+	+
1×12c2	−	+	+	−	−
1×15	+	+	+	+	+
1×16	+	+	+	+	+
1×17	+	+	+	+	+
1×18c9	−	−	−	−	−
3×1	+	+	+	−	−
3×5	+	+	+	+	+
3×11	+	+	+	+	+
3×12	+	+	+	+	+
3×19	+	+	+	+	+
Q511	−	−	−	+	+
153-E9a	+	+	+	+	+
Human	+	+	+	+	+
Hamster	−	−	−	−	−

A plus (+) indicates the presence of a particular marker in a particular cell line, a minus (−), its absence.

some 21 are found in each of these irradiation hybrids. Most (7 of 10 of the 1 × series and 4 of 5 of the 3 × series) have all the markers and were excluded from further study. Five clones of interest are summarized in Table 4. Also included is Q511, a derivative of 725-32X6 in which some chromosome 21 material was selected against by complement-mediated cytotoxicity

Table 4. Molecular hybridization map of chromosome 21 using irradiation reduction hybrids

Hybrid cell line	DNA sequence or isozyme marker designation						
	233	236	245	SOD-1	21G1	231	520
1×4	−	−	−	+	+	+	+
1×12c2	−	−	+	+	−	−	−
1×18c9	−	−	−	−	−	−	−
3×1	+	+	+	+	−	−	−
Q511	−	−	−	−	+	+	+

A plus (+) indicates the presence of a particular human marker in a particular hybrid cell line, a minus (−), its absence. Markers are listed from centromere to telomere on the long arm of chromosome 21.

in the presence of an antibody directed against a human chromosome 21 encoded fetal antigen (Miller, Jones, Scoggin, & Patterson, in press). Q511 retained some chromosome 21 markers, including the ability to confer purine prototrophy on AIRS deficient cells (Ade⁻G). Since the authors had previously shown the close association between the GARS and AIRS activities (Patterson, Graw, & Jones, 1981), it was included in the study described in this section. These five hybrids are divided into one encompassing the proximal half, two the distal half, one the central region, and one with no identified single copy chromosome 21 sequence. (The authors' analysis of the four informative irradiation hybrids and Q511 with additional chromosome 21 markers is currently underway.)

Low Repeat Sequences Certain DNA sequences are repeated fairly infrequently in the human genome. One of the sequences is A36Fc. The authors have previously reported studies on the use of this probe to study chromosome 21, and others have used it to study chromosome 11 (Gusella et al., 1982; Patterson & Schandle, 1983). Figure 3 shows a comparison of the bands detected with this probe in parental cell lines and irradiation hybrids. In 153-E9a, this sequence is found about 22 times. Probing the irradiation hybrids with the A36Fc sequence probe is the equivalent of probing with 22 sequences at one time and allows the correlation of specific bands with the specific regions of chromosome 21. All irradiation hybrids display a much simpler pattern than that of the parent, 153-E9a. Indeed, 1 × 18c9 has lost all A36Fc sequences. 1 × 4 has some of the bands but is missing others. Those missing bands probably are found proximally to SOD-1. Analyses of the complete set of irradiation hybrids and their parents will allow the authors to regionally map a large number of specific bands in a fashion similar to that of single copy sequences.

Middle Repetitive Sequences Alu sequences are repeated approximately 500,000 times in the human genome. Probing 153-E9a with nick translated human genomic DNA produces an intense hybridization signal along the entire length of the blot. The pattern seen was greatly simplified when hybrid 1 × 18xc9 was analyzed. Most of the high molecular weight bands were gone and only a few low molecular weight bands could be seen distinctly. The rest of the informative irradiation hybrids await analysis.

CONCLUSIONS AND DISCUSSION

It seems clear that altered expression of genes in the pathogenetic section of chromosome 21 is of critical importance for the symptoms observed in persons with Down syndrome. Such expression may be temporally regulated during development, may be tissue specific, or may be temporally and spatially constitutive. Moreover, expression may be altered according to gene dosage or may be altered in a more complex way and may affect genes on chromosomes other than 21. At present, there is no conclusive evidence that

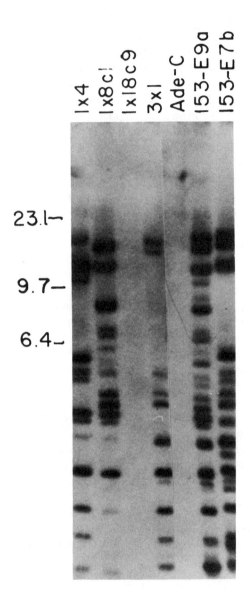

Probe: A36Fc

Figure 3. Southern blot hybridization analysis of DNA from human/hamster hybrid cells containing fragments of chromosome 21.

altered dosage of any gene found on chromosome 21 is significant for the pathology seen in Down syndrome.

Of particular interest in the authors' laboratory has been the possibility that elevation in the dosage of genes coding for enzymes of *de novo* purine synthesis may be relevant for the pathology of Down syndrome. One of these genes, GARS, has been shown to map to the q22 region of chromosome 21 (Chadefaux, Allard, et al., 1984). In at least some studies, purine levels appear to be elevated in what would appear to be a gene dosage dependent manner (Pant et al., 1968). This chapter has presented evidence that in animals, and perhaps in humans, two additional purine biosynthetic enzymes are coded for by a locus on chromosome 21, and that the same genetic locus encodes all three enzyme activities (Henikoff et al., 1986). It could be argued that an increase in gene dosage would not be significant unless the genes involved were rate limiting for purine synthesis. The authors and others have obtained evidence that this may indeed be the case, at least in certain conditions.

It seems reasonable that an increase to 150% of the levels of the normal rate of purine synthesis might be important in animal development. In this regard, the purine *de novo* biosynthetic pathway appears to be present at a level that is not sufficient for normal growth and development of at least some animals, notably *Drosophila melanogaster*. Thus, growth and development of this animal is markedly delayed if purines are not supplied in the food (Hinton, Ellis, & Noyes, 1951). Apparent deficiencies in synthesis of purines depress growth and development further (Falk & Nash, 1974). Additionally, a relatively small increase in dietary purines (less than 3-fold) results in embryonic death of *Drosophila* (Ho et al., 1984). These observations suggest that relatively small alterations in purine synthesis, such as those that might arise from an alteration in the dose of one or more genes coding for rate-limiting steps of the pathway, might indeed cause developmental problems in other organisms, such as humans. Clearly, similar arguments could be made regarding other metabolic enzymes whose genes might be in the region of chromosome 21 pathogenetic for Down syndrome.

Of critical importance in understanding this complex situation is a rigorous definition of the region of chromosome 21 that is important for Down syndrome and information on the genes in this region, including a linkage map of DNA sequences and genes in this chromosomal band. This chapter has presented the beginning of the authors' attempts to devise approaches to obtain this information.

The authors have shown the techniques described in this chapter to be an effective way of producing hybrids containing only selected fragments of specific chromosomes. This technique is applicable to any region of any chromosome for which a selection exists.

With the informative irradiation hybrids discussed in this chapter, it should be a relatively simple matter to regionally map any chromosome marker from chromosome 21. Thus, in addition to the obvious utility of this technique to mapping, the reduction of human material to a small selected region might facilitate cloning of the selected region. This should prove especially useful for those selectable genetic markers that have been refractory to cloning using other methods.

REFERENCES

Adams, M. M., Erickson, J. D., Layde, P. M., & Oakley, G. P. (1981). Down syndrome: Recent trends in the United States. *Journal of the American Medical Association, 246,* 758–760.

Alhadeff, B., Velivasakis, M., & Siniscalco, M. (1977). Simultaneous identification of chromatid replication and of human chromosomes in metaphases of man/mouse somatic cell hybrids. *Cytogenetics and Cell Genetics, 19,* 236–239.

Balarajan, R., Donnan, S. P. B., & Adelstein, A. M. (1982). Mortality and cause of death in Down's syndrome. *Journal of Epidemiology and Community Health, 36,* 127–129.

Barak, Y., Mogilner, B. M., Karov, Y., Schlesinger, E. N. M., & Levin, S. (1982). Transient acute leukaemia in a newborn with Down's Syndrome. *Acta Paediatrica Scandinavica, 71,* 699–701.

Barkley, J. A., & Epstein, C. J. (1980). Gene dosage effect for glycinamide ribonucleotide synthetase in human fibroblasts trisomic for chromosome 21. *Biochemical and Biophysical Research Communications, 93,* 1286–1289.

Bazelon, M., Stevens, H., Davis, M., Seegmiller, J. E., & Greene, M. (1968). Mental retardation, self-mutilation, and hyperuricemia in females. *Neurology Association, 93,* 187.

Becker, M. A. (1976). Patterns of phosphoribosylpyrophosphate and ribose 5-phosphate concentration and generation in fibroblasts from patients with gout and purine overproduction. *Journal of Clinical Investigation, 57,* 308.

Becker, M. A., Kostel, P. J., Meyer, L. J., & Seegmiller, J. E. (1973). Human phosphoribosylpyrophosphate synthetase: Increased enzyme specific activity in a family with gout and excessive purine synthesis. *Proceedings of the National Academy of Science (USA), 70,* 2749.

Blattner, F. R., Blechl, A. E., Denniston-Thompson, K., Faber, H. E., Richards, J. E., Slightom, J. L., Tucker, P. W., & Smithies, O. (1978). Cloning human fetal globin and mouse-type globin DNA: Preparation and screening of shotgun collections. *Science, 202,* 1279–1284.

Bleyer, A. (1934). Indication that mongoloid imbecility is a gametro mutation of degressive type. *American Journal of Diseases of Childhood, 47,* 342–348.

Boue, J., Deluchat, C., Nicolas, H., & Boue, A. (1981). Prenatal losses of Trisomy 21. In G. R. Burgio, M. Fraccaro, L. Tiepolo, & U. Wolf (Eds.), *Trisomy 21: An international symposium* (pp. 183–193). (Convento delle Clarisse, Rapallo, Italy, Nov. 8–10, 1979.) Berlin: Springer-Verlag.

Bradley, C. M., Patterson, D., & Robinson, A. (1986). Somatic cell genetic studies on a family with Down syndrome due to an unusual translocation (21q22→21qter). *Trisomy 21, 1,* 41–52.

Carter, J., Mikkelson, M. & Nelson, A. (1964). The mortality and causes of death in a patient with Down syndrome. *International Copenhagen Conference for the Scientific Study of Mental Retardation, 1,* 231.

Chadefaux, B., Allard, D., Rethore, M. O., Raoul, O., Poissonnier, M., Gilgenkrantz, S., Cheruy, C., & Jerome, H. (1984). Assignment of human phosphoribosylglycinamide synthetase locus to region 21q22.1. *Human Genetics, 66,* 190–192.

Chadefaux, B., Rethore, M. O., & Allard, D. (1984). Regional mapping of liver type 6-phosphofructokinase isoenzyme on chromosome 21. *Human Genetics, 68,* 136–137.

Cirullo, R. E., Dana, S., & Wasmuth, J. (1983). Efficient procedure for transferring specific human genes into Chinese hamster cell mutants: Interspecific transfer of the human genes encoding leucyl- and asparginyl-tRNA synthetases. *Molecular Cell Biology, 3,* 892–902.

Clarke, C. M., Edwards, J. H., & Smallpiece, V. (1961). 21 trisomy/normal mosaicism in an intelligent child with Mongoloid characteristics. *Lancet, 1,* 1028–1030.

Coburn, S. P., Seidenberg, M., & Mertz, E. T. (1967). Clearance of uric acid, urea, and creatinine in Down syndrome. *Journal of Applied Physiology, 23,* 579–580.

Coburn, S. P., Sirlin, E. M., & Mertz, E. T. (1968). Metabolism of N^{15} labeled uric acid in Down syndrome. *Metabolism, 17,* 560–562.

Cox, D. R., Kawashima, H., Vora, S., & Epstein, C. J. (1984). Regional mapping of SOD-1, PRGS and PFK-L on human chromosome 21. *Cytogenetics and Cell Genetics, 37,* 441–442.

Cox, D. R., Smith, S. A., Epstein, L. B., & Epstein, C. J. (1984). Mouse trisomy 16 as an animal model of human trisomy 21 (Down syndrome): Production of viable trisomy 16 ↔ diploid mouse chimeras. *Developmental Biology, 101,* 416–424.

Dagg, C. O., Karnofsky, D. A., Lacon, C., & Roddy, J. (1957). Comparative effects of 6-diaza-5-oxo-L-norleucine and O-diasoacetyl-L-serine in the chick embryo. *Proceedings of the American Association of Cancer Research, 2,* 101.

Dalton, A. J., Crapper, D. R., & Schlotter, C. R. (1974). Alzheimer's disease in Down syndrome: Visual retention defects. *Cortex, 10,* 366–377.

Davidson, J. N., Rumsby, G., & Niswander, L. A. (1985). Expression of genes on human chromosome 21. *Annals of the New York Academy of Sciences, 450,* 43–54.

Dayton, A. I., Selden, J. R., Laws, G., Dorney, D. J., Finan, J., Tripputi, P., Emanuel, B. S., Rovera, G., Nowell, P. C., & Croce, C. M. (1984). A human c-*erb*A oncogene homologue is closely proximal to the chromosome 17 breakpoint in acute promyelocytic leukemia *Proceedings of the National Academy of Science (USA), 81,* 4495–4499.

de Grouchy, J., and Turleau, C. (Eds.). (1984). *Clinical atlas of human chromosomes* (2nd ed., p. 337). New York: John Wiley & Sons.

Down, J. L. H. (1866). Observations on an ethnic classification of idiots. *Clinical Lecture Reports, London Hospital, 3,* 259–262.

Drabkin, H. A., Diaz, M., Bradley, C. M., Le Beau, M. M., Rowley, J. D., & Patterson D. (1985). Isolation and analysis of the 21q+ chromosome in the AML 8;21 translocation: Evidence that c-*mos* is not translocated. *Proceedings of the National Academy of Science (USA), 82,* 464–468.

Duncan, C., Biro, P. A., Choudary, P. V., Elder, J. T., Wang, R. R. C., Forget, B. G., de Riel, J. K., & Weissman, S. M. (1979). RNA polymerase III transcriptional units are interspersed among human non-α-globin genes. *Proceedings of the National Academy of Science (USA), 76,* 5095–5098.

Ellis, W. G., McCulloch, J. R., & Corley, C. L. (1974). Presenile dementia in Down's syndrome: Ultrastructural identity with Alzheimer's disease. *Neurology, 24,* 101–106.

Evans, D. I. K. (1970). Acute myelofibrosis in children with Down syndrome. *Archives of the Disabled Child, 50,* 458.

Falk, D. R., & Nash, D. (1974) Sex-linked auxotrophic and putative auxotrophic mutants of *Drosophila melanogaster. Genetics, 76,* 755–766.

Fuller, R. W., Luce, M. M., & Mertz, E. T. (1962). Serum uric acid and Mongolism. *Science, 137,* 868–869.

Giblett, E. R., Ammann, A. J., Sandman, R. S., Wara, D. W., & Diamond, L. K. (1975). Nucleotide-phosphorylase deficiency in a child with severely defective T-cell immunity and normal B-cell immunity. *Lancet, I,* 1010–1013.

Giblett, E. K., Anderson, J., Cohen, T., Pollara, B., & Meuwissen, J. H. (1972). Adenosine deaminase deficiency in two patients with severely impaired cellular immunity. *Lancet, 2,* 1067–1069.

Glenner, G. G. (1983). Biological aspects of Alzheimer's disease. *Banbury Report, 15,* 137–144.

Glenner, G. G., & Wong, C. W. (1984). Alzheimer's disease and Down's syndrome: Sharing of a unique cerebrovascular amyloid fibril protein. *Biochemistry and Biophysics Research Communications, 122* (3), 1131–1135.

Goodman, H. O., Lafland, H. B., & Thomas, J. J. (1966). Serum uric acid levels in Mongolism. *American Journal of Mental Deficiency, 71,* 437–446.

Green, R. M., & Kochhar, D. M. (1975). Limb development in mouse embryo: Protection against teratogenic effects of 6-diazo-5-oxo-L-norleucine (DON) *in vivo* and *in vitro. Journal of Embryology and Experimental Morphology, 33,* 355–370.

Gusella, J. F., Jones, C., Kao, F. T., Housman, D., & Puck, T. T. (1982). Genetic fine structure mapping in human chromosome 11 by use of repetitive DNA sequences. *Proceedings of the National Academy of Science (USA), 79,* 7804–7808.

Gusella, J. F., Keyes, C., Varsanyi-Breiner, A., Kao, F. T., Jones, C., Puck, T. T., & Housman, D. (1980). Isolation and localization of DNA segments from specific human chromosomes. *Proceedings of the National Academy of Science (USA), 77,* 2829–2833.

Gusella, J. F., Tanzi, R. E., Watkins, P. C., Gibbons, K. T., Hobbs, W. J., Faryniarz, A. G., Healy, S. T., & Anderson, M. A. (1985). Genetic linkage map for chromosome 21. *Annals of the New York Academy of Sciences, 450,* 25–31.

Habedank, M., & Rodewald, A. (1982). Moderate Down's syndrome in three siblings having partial trisomy 21q22.2→qter and therefore no SOD-1 excess. *Human Genetics, 60,* 74–77.

Henderson, J. F. (1972). Regulation of purine biosynthesis. *American Chemical Society Monograph, 170.*

Henderson, J. F., Rosenbloom, F. M., Kelley, W. N., & Seegmiller, J. E. (1968). Variations in purine metabolism of cultured skin fibroblasts from patients with gout. *Journal of Clinical Investigation, 47,* 1511–1516.

Henikoff, S., Patterson, D., Sloan, J. S., Bleskan, J., Hards, R., & Keene, M. A. (1986). Multiple purine pathway activities are encoded on a single genetic locus in *Drosophila. Proceedings of the National Academy of Science (USA). 83,* 720–724.

Heston, L. L. (1976). Alzheimer's disease, trisomy 21, and myeloproliferative disorders: Associations suggesting a genetic diathesis. *Science, 196,* 322–323.

Heston, L. L., & Mastri, A. R. (1977). The genetics of Alzheimer's disease. *Archives of General Physiology, 34,* 976–981.

Hinton, T., Ellis, J., & Noyes, D. T. (1951). An adenine requirement in a strain of *Drosophila. Proceedings of the National Academy of Science (USA), 37,* 293–303.

Ho, Y. K., Clifford, C. K., Sobieski, R. J., Cummings, K., Odokara, G., & Clifford, A. J. (1984). Effect of dietary purines and pyrimidines on growth and development of *Drosophila. Comparative Biochemical Physiology, 77A*(2), 389–395.

Hooft, C., Van Nevel, C., & De Schaepdryver, A. F. (1968). Hyperuricosuric encephalopathy without hyperuricemia. *Archives of Disease in Childhood, 43,* 734–736.

Hunter, A. G. W., Clifford, B., Speevak, M., & MacMurray, S. B. (1982). Mosaic tetrasomy 21 in a liveborn male infant. *Clinical Genetics, 21,* 228–232.

Irwin, M., Oates, D. C., & Patterson, D. (1979). Biochemical genetics of Chinese hamster cell mutants with deviant purine metabolism. Isolation and characterization of a mutant deficient in the activity of phosphoribosylaminoimidazole synthetase. *Somatic Cell Genetics, 5* (2), 203–216.

Jones, C., Kao, F. T., & Taylor, R. L. (1980). Chromosomal assignment of the gene for folylpolyglutamate synthetase to human chromosome 9. *Cytogenetics and Cell Genetics, 28,* 181–194.

Kaneko, Y., Rowley, J. D., Variakojis, D., Chilcote, R. R., Moohr, J. W., & Patel, D. (1981). Chromosome abnormalities in Down's syndrome patients with acute leukemia. *Blood, 58,* 459–466.

Kelley, W. N., Rosenbloom, F. M., Henderson, J. F., & Seegmiller, J. E. (1967). A specific enzyme defect in gout associated with overproduction of uric acid. *Proceedings of the National Academy of Science (USA), 57,* 1735–1739.

Konrad, P. N., & Harris, S. P. (1971). Nonspherocytic hemolytic anemia, high red cell ATP and ribosephosphate pyrophosphokinase (RPK, E.C. 2.7.6.1) deficiency. *Clinical Research, 19,* 567.

Kurnit, D. (1979). Down syndrome: Gene dosage at the transcriptional level in skin fibroblasts. *Proceedings of the National Academy of Science (USA), 76,* 2372–2375.

Kwee, M. L., Barth, P. G., Arwert, F., & Madan, K. (1984). Mosaic tetrasomy 21 in a male child. *Clinical Genetics, 26,* 150–155.

Law, M. L., Davidson, J. N., & Kao, F. T. (1982). Isolation of a human repetitive sequence and its application to regional chromosomal mapping. *Proceedings of the National Academy of Science (USA), 79,* 7390–7394.

Law, M. L., Kao, F. T., Patterson, D., & Davidson, J. N. (1980). Isolation of recombinant clones containing DNA segments from human chromosomes 12 and 21. *Cell Biology, 87,* 109A.

Lazarus, K. H., Heerema, N. A., Palmer, G. P., & Baehner, R. L. (1981). The myeloproliferative reaction in a child with Down syndrome: Cytological and chromosomal evidence for a transient leukemia. *American Journal of Hematology, 11,* 417–423.

Lejeune, J., Gauthier, M., & Turpin, R. (1959). Genetique—Les chromosomes humains en culture de tissues [Genetics—The human chromosomes in tissue culture]. *Comptes Rendus de Seances de L'Academie des Sciences, 248,* 602–603.

Lesch, M., & Nyhan, W. L. (1964). A familial disorder of uric acid metabolism and central nervous system function. *American Journal of Medicine, 36,* 561–570.

Levanon, D., Leiman-Hurwitz, J., Dafni, N., Wigderson, M., Sherman, L., Bernstein, Y., Laver-Rudich, Z., Danciger, E., Stein, O., & Groner, Y. (1985). Architecture and anatomy of the chromosomal lows in human chromosomal encoding the Cu/Zn superoxide dismutase. *The EMBO Journal, 4,* 77–84.

Martin, G. (1978). Genetic syndromes in man with potential relevance to the pathobiology of aging. In D. Bergsma & D. E. Harrison (Eds.), *Genetic effects on aging* (The National Foundation March of Dimes Birth Defects Original Article Series Vol. XIV[1]; pp. 5–39). New York: Alan R. Liss.

Mattei, J. F., Mattei, M. G., Baeteman, M. A., & Giraud, F. (1981). Trisomy 21 for the region 21q22.3: Identification by high-resolution R-banding patterns. *Human Genetics, 56* (3), 409–411.

Miller, M., & Cosgriff, J. M. (1983). Hematological abnormalities in newborn infants with Down syndrome. *American Journal of Medical Genetics, 16,* 173–177.

Miller, Y. E., Jones, C., Scoggin, C. H., & Patterson, D. (in press). A chromosome 21 associated cell surface antigen present on fetal brain. *Trisomy 21.*

Moore, E. E., Jones, C., Kao, F. T., & Oates, D. C. (1977). Synteny between glycinamide ribonucleotide synthetase and superoxide dismutase (soluble). *American Journal of Human Genetics, 29,* 389–396.

Neel, B. G., Jhanwar, S. C., Chaganti, R. S., & Hayward, W. S. (1982). Two human c-onc genes are located on the long arm of chromosome 8. *Proceedings of the National Academy of Science (USA), 79,* 7842–7846.

Neibuhr, E. (1974). Down syndrome, the possibility of a pathogenetic segment on chromosome #21. *Human Genetics, 21,* 99–101.

Nyhan, W. F., James, J. A., Seberg, A. J., Sweetman, L., & Nelson, L. G. (1969). A new disorder of purine metabolism with behavioral manifestations. *Journal of Pediatrics, 74,* 20–27.

Oates, D. C., Vannais, D., & Patterson, D. (1980). A mutant of CHO-K1 cells deficient in two nonsequential steps of *de novo* purine biosynthesis. *Cell, 20,* 797–805.

Olson, M. I., and Shaw, C. W. (1969). Pre-senile dementia and Alzheimer's disease in Down syndrome. *Brain, 92,* 147–156.

Oster, J., Mikkelsen, M., & Nielsen, A. (1975). Mortality and life-table in Down's syndrome. *Acta Paediatrica Scandinavica, 64,* 322–326.

Pant, S. S., Moser, H. W., & Krane, S. M. (1968). Hyperuricemia in Down's syndrome. *Journal of Clinical Endocrinology, 28,* 472–478.

Parkman, R., Gelfand, E. W., Rosen, F. S., Sanderson, A., & Hirschhorn, R. (1975). Severe combined immunodeficiency and adenosine deaminase deficiency. *New England Journal of Medicine, 292,* 714–719.

Patterson, D., Graw, S., & Jones, C. (1981). Demonstration, by somatic cell genetics, of coordinate regulation of genes for two enzymes of purine synthesis assigned to human chromosome 21. *Proceedings of the National Academy of Science (USA), 78,* 405–409.

Patterson, D., & Schandle, V. B. (1983). A comparison of Chinese hamster/human hybrid cells containing different fragments of chromosome 21 using cytogenetic, biochemical, and molecular approaches. *Banbury Report, 14,* 215–223.

Polani, P. E., Briggs, J. H., Ford, C. E., Clarke, C. M., & Berg, J. M. (1960). A Mongol girl with 46 chromosomes. *Lancet, 1,* 721–724.

Prakash, K., McBride, D. W., Swan, D. C., Devare, S. G., Tronick, S. R., & Aaronson, S. A. (1982). *Proceedings of the National Academy of Science (USA), 79,* 5210–5214.

Rethore, M. O., Dutrillaux, B., & Lejeune, J. (1973). Translocation 46, XX, t(15;21) (q13;q22,I) chez la mere de deux enfants atteints de trisomie 15 et de monosomie 21 partielles [Translocation 46, XX, t(15;21)(q13;q22.1) in a mother of two children with trisomy 15 and partial monosomy 21]. *Annales de Genetiques, 16* (4), 271–275.

Rigby, P. W. J., Diekmann, M., Rhodes, C., & Berg, P. (1977). Labeling deoxynucleic acid to high specific activity *in vitro* by nick-translation with DNA polymerase I. *Journal of Molecular Biology, 113,* 237–251.

Rosner, F., & Lee, S. L. (1972). Down syndrome and acute leukemia: Myeloblastic or lymphoblastic? *American Journal of Medicine, 53,* 203–218.

Rowe, P. B., McCairns, E., Madsen, G., Sauer, D., & Elliott, H. (1978). *De novo* purine synthesis in avian liver: Co-purification of the enzymes and properties of the pathway. *Journal of Biological Chemistry, 253,* 7711–7721.

Rowley, J. D. (1981). Down syndrome and acute leukaemia: Increased risk may be due to trisomy 21. *Lancet, 2,* 1020–1022.

Scholl, T., Stein, A., & Hansen, H. (1982). Leukemia and other cancers, anomalies and infections as causes of death in Down's syndrome in the United States during 1976. *Developmental Medicine and Child Neurology, 24,* 817–829.

Scoggin, C. H., Gabrielson, E., Davidson, J. N., Jones, C., Patterson, D., & Puck, T. T. (1981). Two-dimensional electrophoresis of human CHO cell hybrids containing human chromosome 11. *Somatic Cell Genetics, 7,* 389–398.

Scoggin, C., & Patterson, D. (1982). Down syndrome as a model disease: A review. *Archives of Internal Medicine, 142,* 462–464.

Seegmiller, J. E., Rosenbloom, F. M., & Kelley, W. N. (1967). An enzyme defect associated with a sex-linked human neurological disorder and excessive purine synthesis. *Science, 155,* 1682–1684.

Sinensky, M., Torget, R., & Edwards, P. (1981). Radioimmune precipitation of 3-hydroxy-3-methyl glutaryl coenzyme A reductase from Chinese hamster fibroblasts effect of 25-hydroxycholesterol. *Journal of Biological Chemistry, 256,* 11774–11779.

Sinet, P. M., Couturier, J., Dutrillaux, B., Poissonier, M., Raoul, O., Rethore, M. O., Allard, D., Lejeune, J., & Jerome, H. (1976). Trisomic 21 et superoxide dismutase, tentative de localisation sur la sous bande 22q22.1 [Trisomy 21 and superoxide dismutase: Attempt to map to the subband 22q22.1]. *Experimental Cell Research, 97,* 47–55.

Skovby, F., Krassikoff, N., & Francke, U. (1984). Assignment of the gene for cystathionine β-synthase to human chromosome 21 in somatic cell hybrids. *Human Genetics, 65,* 291–294.

Southern, E. M. (1975). Detection of specific sequences among DNA fragments transferred to nitrocellulose. *Journal of Molecular Biology, 98,* 503–517.

Sturm, R., Staneck, J. L., & Myers, J. P. (1980). Legionellosis in a child. *Kentucky Morbidity and Mortality Weekly Report,* p. 203.

Taysi, K., Sparkes, R. S., O'Brien, T. J., & Dengler, D. R. (1982). Down's syndrome phenotype and autosomal gene inactivation in a child with presumed (X-21) *de novo* translocation. *Journal of Medical Genetics, 19,* 144–148.

Thiersch, J. B. (1957). Effect of 6-diazo-5-oxo-L-norleucine (DON) on the rat litter *in utero. Proceedings of the Society of Experimental Biological Medicine, 94,* 33–35.

Tjio, J. H., & Levan, A. (1956). The chromosome number of man. *Hereditas, 42,* 1–6.

Tolksdorf, M., & Wiedemann, H. (1981). Clinical aspects of Down's syndrome from infancy to adult life. In G. R. Burgio, M. Fraccaro, L. Tiepolo, & U. Wolf (Eds.) *Trisomy 21:* An international symposium (pp. 1–31). (Convento delle Clarisse, Rapallo, Italy, Nov. 8–10, 1979.) Berlin: Springer-Verlag.

Valentine, W. N., Palgia, D. E., Tartaglia, A. P., & Gilsanz, F. (1977). Hereditary hemolytic anemia with increased red cell adenosine deaminase (45- to 70-fold) and decreased adenosine triphosphate. *Science, 195,* 783–785.

Van Keuren, M., Merril, C. R., & Goldman, D. (1983). Proteins affected by chromosome 21 and aging *in vitro.* In J. E. Celis & R. Bravo (Eds.), *Gene expression in normal and transformed cells* (pp. 349–378). New York: Plenum.

Vora, S., & Francke, U. (1981). Assignment of the human gene for liver-type 6-phosphofructokinase isozyme (PFKL) to chromosome 21 by using somatic cell hybrids and monoclonal anti-L antibody. *Proceedings of the National Academy of Science (USA), 78,* 3738–3742.

Waardenberg, P. J. (1932). *Das menschliche Auge und seine Erbanlagen* [The human eye and its genetic structure]. Haag: Martinus Nijhoff.

Weil, J., & Epstein, C. J. (1979). The effect of trisomy 21 on the patterns of polypeptide synthesis in human fibroblasts. *American Journal of Human Genetics, 31,* 478–488.

Weil, J., Epstein, L. B., & Epstein, C. J. (1980). Synthesis of interferon induced polypeptides in normal and chromosome 21 fibroblasts: Relationship to relative sensitivities in antiviral assays. *Journal of Interferon Research, 1,* 111–124.

Weil, J., Tucker, G., Epstein, L. B., & Epstein, C. J. (1983). Interferon induction of (2′–5′) oligoisoadenylate synthetase in diploid and trisomy 21 human fibroblasts: Relation to dosage of the interferon receptor gene (IFRC). *Human Genetics, 65,* 108–111.

Weinberger, M. M., & Olenik, A. (1970). Congenital marrow dysfunction in Down syndrome. *Journal of Pediatrics, 77,* 273–279.

Wilson, M. G., Towner, J. W., & Forsman, I. (1980). Decreasing mosaicism in Down's syndrome. *Clinical Genetics, 17,* 335–340.

Yosimitsu, K., Hatano, S., Kobayashi, Y., Takeoka, Y., Hayashidani, M., Ueda, K., Nomura, K., Ohama, K., & Usui, T. (1983). A case of 21 q− syndrome with half normal SOD-1 activity. *Human Genetics, 64,* 200–202.

Yunis, J. J. (1984). In A. Fazal et al. (Eds.), Advances in gene technology: Human genetic disorders. Proceedings of the 16th Miami Winter Symposium. *KSU Short Reports, 1,* 27–29.

Response

The Consequences of Altered Gene Dosage in Trisomy 21

Charles J. Epstein

The ability to identify which basic processes are involved in the pathogenesis of the manifestations of trisomy 21 depends on several factors. First, it is necessary to know exactly what is abnormal in Down syndrome. In particular, the lesions, both anatomical and functional, present in the central nervous system need to be more fully defined. In addition, the psychological deficits—the actual abnormalities of cognition that result in mental retardation—must be characterized in such a manner that they can ultimately be related to the neurobiological alterations. Second, knowledge of the identities and functions of the specific genes on chromosome 21 will make it possible to focus on particular developmental and functional processes that are likely to be perturbed by the presence of an extra copy of chromosome 21. (How this approach can be used is discussed in the following section.) Third, there needs to be an expansion of information in the general fields of neurobiology and psychology, as well as an increased understanding of the interrelationships between the two. It is this information and understanding that will ultimately make it possible to explain exactly what has gone wrong in Down syndrome (Epstein, 1986b).

At present, it is not really possible to identify the developmental and functional processes that are perturbed in Down syndrome, but it is possible to venture a guess about which ones might be particularly affected by a trisomic state. Based on a consideration of mechanisms by which extra doses of genes might alter structure and function, it has been inferred that certain processes might be particularly vulnerable to perturbation (Epstein, 1986a). Chief among these are processes involving cellular interaction (recognition, adhe-

This work was supported by grants from the National Institutes of Health (HD-17001), the American Cancer Society (CD-119), and the March of Dimes Birth Defects Foundation (1-760).

sion, communication), growth factors and morphogens, and receptors (particularly those concerned with growth factors and morphogens). Precedent for the potential involvement of cellular interaction factors already exists for Down syndrome. Wright, Orkin, Destrempes, and Kurnit (1984) have demonstrated that the adhesivity of fibroblasts from the hearts and lungs of fetuses with trisomy 21 is increased (see Table 1). Kurnit, Aldridge, Matsuoka, and Matthyse (1985) have provided theoretical arguments showing how such a change could lead to the occurrence of congenital heart disease. Likewise, both experimental studies (Hoffman & Edelman, 1983) and theoretical considerations (Epstein, 1986a; Rutishauser, 1986) have shown how small changes in the concentration of a cell surface recognition or adhesion molecule can have a profound impact on cellular interactions.

None of the considerations just discussed necessarily eliminates macromolecules, metabolic pathways (enzymes), transport systems, or regulatory systems from consideration as sites of abnormalities resulting from trisomy. In fact, particular attention has been devoted to such systems, particularly enzymes, in the study of trisomy 21. However, the experimental and theoretical information available suggests that these systems are, in general, less likely than those listed earlier to be of great importance in a condition such as trisomy 21 (Epstein, 1986a).

Table 1. The genes on human chromosome 21

Gene symbol	Gene name	Regional assignment
	Confirmed[a]	
CBS	Cystathionine β-synthase	q21-q22.1
IFNRA	Interferon-α receptor	q21-qter
PRGS	Phosphoribosylglycinamide synthetase	q22.1
SOD-1	Superoxide dismutase-1	q22.1
PFKL	Phosphofructokinase, liver type	q22
BCE-1	Breast cancer, estrogen inducible gene	q22.3
	Provisional	
PAIS	Phosphoribosylaminoimidazole synthetase	
CRYA1	Crystallin, alpha-A2 polypeptide	
MF13	Antigen (glycoprotein, MW 86K)	
MF14	Antigen (glycoprotein, MW 145K)	
MF17	Leukocyte-cell adhesion molecule (phorbol ester induced, MW 90K)	
S14	Surface antigen	

Source: Data from Human Gene Mapping 8 (1985).
[a]Assignment to chromosome 21 made by two independent methods or investigators.

IMBALANCE OF SPECIFIC LOCI ON HUMAN CHROMOSOME 21

The approach to the investigation of the abnormalities present in Down syndrome in which the author has been most interested is the analysis of the effects of unbalancing genes or loci known to be present on human chromosome 21. Of particular interest are those genes present on the distal half of the long arm of chromosome 21, in the region (21q22.1→q22.2) that is specifically implicated in the genesis of the phenotype of Down syndrome (Rethoré, 1981; Summitt, 1981). The relatively small list of genes definitely or provisionally mapped to human chromosome 21 is given in Table 1, and several of these genes appear to be in the Down syndrome region.

For the most part, studies of the genes on chromosome 21 have taken the form of determinations of the quantities of gene products and have demonstrated, for five known chromosome 21 genes, that the presence of an extra gene copy in trisomic cells is reflected in a proportional increase in the quantity of gene product, whether enzyme or receptor (see Table 2). These "gene dosage effects" for chromosome 21 genes, with an overall mean increase of 1.55 fold, are consonant with the gene dosage effects observed for many other trisomies (Epstein, 1986a). An increase of 50%, to 1.5 times the value present in nontrisomic (diploid) cells, is, of course, what would be expected in a trisomic state if, as appears to be the case, no system for dosage compensation exists.

Further explorations of the consequences of the increased dosage of chromosome 21 genes have been concerned with whether the extra amounts of gene products are reflected in detectable metabolic alterations. For the IFN-α receptor, trisomy 21 fibroblasts have the expected ~1.5 times the normal amount of receptor, as demonstrated by a 1.57-fold increase in the binding of IFN-α, and show proportional increases in the induction by IFN-α of the enzyme (2'-5') oligoisoadenylate synthetase and of eight intracellular peptides of unknown function (see Table 3). However, when the physiologi-

Table 2. Gene dosage effects in trisomy 21

Locus	Function	Ts/2n[a]
CBS	Cystathione β-synthase activity in stimulated lymphocytes	1.61
IFNRA	Interferon-α binding to fibroblasts	1.57
PFKL	Phosphofructokinase activity in red cells	1.47
PRGS	Phosphoribosylglycinamide synthetase activity in fibroblasts	1.56
SOD-1	Superoxide dismutase-1 activity in red cells, fibroblasts, platelets, lymphocytes, brain, granulocytes	1.52

Source: Data from Epstein (1986a) and Arias, Paradisi, and Rolo (1985).
[a]Ratio of activities in trisomic (Ts) and diploid (2n) cells.

Table 3. Primary and secondary effects of increased dosage of the interferon-α receptor in trisomy 21 cells

Effect	Mean responsiveness of trisomic cells
Primary effect	
Binding of interferon-α	1.57[a]
Secondary effects	
Induction of eight intracellular peptides	1.57[a]
Induction of (2'-5') oligoisoadenylate synthetase	1.69[b]
Protection of cells against viral challenge	6.3[b]
Inhibition of proliferation of fibroblasts	6.7[b]
Inhibition of maturation of monocytes to macrophages	3.7[b]
Inhibition of lectin-induced lymphocyte mitogenesis	4.0[b]

Source: Data summarized in Epstein and Epstein (1983).
[a] Ratio of binding, synthesis, or activity in trisomic and diploid cells.
[b] Ratio of amounts of interferon required to produce same biological effect in diploid and trisomic cells.

cal effects of interferon treatment are examined, the responsiveness or sensitivity of trisomic cells to the antiviral effect of IFN-α is increased anywhere from 3- to 15-fold (mean = 6.3) and to all effects by ~5 fold. This functional amplification has been attributed to the extra dose of the IFN-α receptor (Epstein, 1986a; Weil, Tucker, Epstein, & Epstein, 1983), although it still remains to be proven that this is in fact the case.

Much has been written about the increased concentration of superoxide dismutase-1 (SOD-1) in trisomic cells and tissues and its potential role in the pathogenesis of certain of the neurological abnormalities of Down syndrome (Sinet, 1982; Sinet, Lejeune, & Jerome, 1979). SOD-1 catalyzes the conversion (dismutation) of O_2^- radicals to H_2O_2 and O_2. However, the evidence for functional alterations in the metabolism of oxygen compounds as a result of increased SOD-1 activity is quite sketchy. The most persuasive results are those of Groner and his collaborators (1985). They found that cells overexpressing SOD-1 by 2- to 6-fold (after transfection with cloned SOD-1 genes) are more resistant to paraquat, an agent that leads to the generation of superoxide radicals. By contrast, it has been claimed by others that trisomic fibroblasts, with only 1.5 times more SOD-1 than normal, are more sensitive to the toxic effects of 95% oxygen, which are also attributed to superoxide generation, in terms of both decreased survival and increased lipid peroxidation (Mayes, Muneer, & Sifers, 1984). These contradictory results remain to be reconciled, but they lead to the possibility that an increase in SOD-1 activity could indeed have functional consequences, at least under conditions of oxidative stress that lead to the generation of superoxide.

The results obtained from studies of the interferon receptor and superoxide dismutase-1 systems in trisomy 21, as well as from the other genes studied both in trisomy 21 (Table 2) and in other trisomies and monosomies (Epstein, 1986a), indicate that the primary effects of all aneuploid states, which are themselves conditions in which there are abnormalities of gene dosage, are proportional alterations in the rates of synthesis of messenger RNAs (mRNAs) coded for by the unbalanced chromosome or chromosome region. Although one might expect that systems for regulating the rates of synthesis of mRNAs would exist, so that constant synthetic rates are maintained, no evidence for such regulatory systems has been obtained (Epstein, 1986a). Similarly, the 50% increases in synthetic rates found in trisomies, in all cases examined so far, appear to result in 50% increases in the concentrations of gene products. Post-translational regulation of gene product concentration does not appear to occur. Since virtually all of the products examined were enzymes, it is conceivable that the synthesis of other types of gene products might be more tightly regulated. However, no data in support of such a notion have been obtained as yet.

How are such proportional gene dosage effects translated into abnormalities of development and function? At the present time, any discussion of how gene dosage effects result in developmental or functional abnormalities must be considered as being highly speculative in nature. However, the major inference that can be drawn is not. Any mechanism proposed to explain how trisomy 21 causes mental retardation, or hypotonia, or Alzheimer disease, must ultimately be able to begin with one or more specific chromosome 21 genes present in an extra dose, proceed through the demonstration of the existence of 50% more of the gene product or products coded for by these genes, and then relate the increased amount(s) of product to the genesis of a specific functional or morphogenetic abnormality (see Figure 1). The last relationship, of increased gene product to specific abnormality, may be either a direct one or, more likely, an indirect one involving a series of intermediate events. Stated the other way around, any proposed pathogenetic mechanisms for neurological or other abnormalities in trisomy 21 must ultimately lead

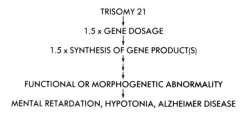

Figure 1. The chain of events relating the presence of an extra chromosome 21 to the neurological manifestations of Down syndrome.

back to the quantitative imbalance of a specific gene or set of genes. Down syndrome, like the other aneuploid conditions, is a genetic disease resulting from abnormal gene dosage, not abnormal gene structure, and must ultimately be explicable as such.

Calculations based on the sizes of chromosome 21 and of individual genes suggest that the number of genes potentially involved in the neurological and other abnormalities of Down syndrome is anywhere from 100 to 1000 (Epstein, 1986a). Such estimates might lead one to be pessimistic about being able to identify a set of genes responsible for the neurological abnormalities associated with trisomy 21, but this need not be the case. There is nothing implicit in the existence of such a large number of genes that excludes the possibility that a relatively small number of genes may play a disproportionately great role in determining the fate of the nervous system and other affected tissues and organs, at least under conditions of genetic imbalance.

A MOUSE MODEL OF HUMAN TRISOMY 21

The notion of developing mouse models for human autosomal aneuploidy became tenable when Gropp, Giers, and Kolbus (1974), Gropp, Kolbus, and Giers (1975), and White, Tjio, Van de Water, and Crandall (1974) first described methods for generating trisomic mice. With this ability to generate aneuploid mice with predictable types of chromosomal imbalance at a high frequency, it became possible to consider the production of trisomic mice that could constitute a model for human trisomy 21 (Epstein, 1981).

The reasons for wanting to develop such a model were several. In general terms, one of the principal difficulties in studying human disorders of development, particularly if the nervous system is involved, is the inability, for both technical and ethical reasons, to study more than a very restricted number of tissues and developmental processes. The developing human fetus is inaccessible to any type of systematic study, and the brain can only be approached postmortem or, during life, by a limited number of noninvasive techniques. Therefore, to be able to study the mechanisms discussed above that underlie the development of abnormalities associated with trisomy 21, abnormalities both of prenatal somatic and neurological development and probably of postnatal neurological development and function as well, it is necessary to have experimental systems that lend themselves to convenient analysis. While initially directed toward issues of mechanism, such analysis could, if specific metabolic lesions are identified, ultimately turn also to considerations of therapy; again, a model system would be most useful.

The decision to attempt the development of a mouse model for human trisomy 21 was based on the premise that it should be possible to study the effects of increased doses of particular human chromosome 21 genes, or sets of such genes, by using mice that are trisomic for the particular mouse chromosome or chromosomes that carry the human chromosome 21 homologous loci. Therefore, the basic approach was to map genes known to be on human chromosome 21 onto the mouse genome, using conventional somatic cell genetic techniques. Of the quite limited number of identified loci now known to be present on human chromosome 21, three (SOD-1, PRGS, and IFRC [IFNRA]) have so far been mapped in the mouse, and all three are on mouse chromosome 16 (Cox, Epstein, & Epstein, 1980; Cox, Goldblatt, & Epstein, 1981; Francke & Taggart, 1979; Lin, Slate, Lawyer, & Ruddle, 1980) (see Figure 2). That all three of these human chromosome 21 genes are present on the same mouse chromosome, and that two of them (SOD-1 and PRGS) are present on defined small regions of each chromosome (Cox & Epstein, 1985) strongly suggest that a human chromosome 21 region of significant size has, as hoped, been evolutionarily conserved between man and

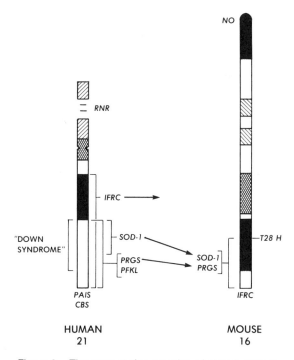

Figure 2. The comparative mapping of mouse chromosome 16 and human chromosome 21. The regional localization of SOD-1 and PRGS to the distal segment of mouse chromosome 16, beyond the breakpoint of the T28H translocation, is shown. (From Epstein, C. J. [1986a]. *The consequences of chromosome imbalance. Principles, mechanisms, and models.* New York: Cambridge University Press; reprinted by permission.)

mouse. This region is the same one to which the phenotype of Down syndrome has been localized (Figure 2). It also seems reasonable to infer that other homologous loci are also present on the two chromosomes in question and that there are many more than just the three genes mapped to date.

The salient aspects of the phenotype of mouse fetuses with trisomy 16 are summarized in Table 4, as is a comparison of the features of mouse trisomy 16 with those of human chromosome 21. Many interesting parallels between the mouse and human phenotypes can be drawn, including the congenital heart disease (endocardial cushion defect) (Miyabara, Gropp, & Winking, 1982; Rehder, 1981), the retarded development of the brain and craniofacies with deficiencies in numbers of neurons, and the thymus and T-lymphocyte abnormalities. Nevertheless, the author certainly does not mean to imply that Down syndrome has actually been fully reproduced in the mouse.

While the trisomic embryos and fetuses are appropriate for studies on prenatal morphogenesis and development, they are not, of course, suitable for investigations of behavior and other aspects of postnatal central nervous system function. Therefore, to make the latter possible, trisomic cells have been combined with diploid ones in the form of postnatally viable trisomy 16 ↔ 2n chimeras or mosaics (Cox, Smith, Epstein, & Epstein, 1984). These chimeras, which constitute the second form of the model, are the equivalent of human trisomy 21/2n mosaics which, when the proportion of trisomy 21 cells is high enough, display the functional and morphological phenotype of Down syndrome (Kohn, Taysi, Atkins, & Mellman, 1970). The trisomy 16 ↔ 2n chimeras that were prepared were normal in appearance and grossly normal in behavior, although systematic tests of behavior were not performed. In many organs, including the brain, kidney, liver, and heart, significant proportions (30%–60%) of trisomy 16 cells were present. However, not surprisingly, in view of the immunological and hematopoietic cell deficits found in the trisomy 16 fetuses, the thymus, spleen, blood, bone marrow, and coat (pigment cells) of the chimeras were characterized by a marked deficiency of trisomy 16 cells. These findings suggested that the trisomic cells in the hematopoietic, lymphoid, and pigment cell lineages were unable to compete in a normal manner with diploid cells of the same type.

Coyle, Gearhart, Oster-Granite, Singer, and Moran (1986) recently reported preliminary data on the behavior of two trisomy 16 ↔ 2n chimeras that they prepared. In comparison to both chimeric and wild-type controls, these animals displayed increased spontaneous motor activity. This increased activity was particularly evident during the hours of darkness. These results indicated that behavior differences may actually exist in the trisomy 16 ↔ 2n chimeras, thereby fulfilling one of the major objectives for developing the model system in the first place.

Table 4. The phenotype of mouse trisomy 16 compared with that of human trisomy 21

	Mouse trisomy 16 (fetal)	Human trisomy 21 (postnatal)
Survival beyond term	None	≤30% of conceptions
Growth *in utero* (weight)	Decreased 10%–25%	Reduced ~10% at birth
Edema *in utero*	Transient massive generalized edema	Transient edema of neck
Facies	Flat snout, short neck, open eyelids; retarded craniofacial development	Flat face, short neck, epicanthal folds
Congenital heart disease	Present in 96%, with aortic arch anomalies in >80% and endocardial cushion defect in ~50%	Present in ~45% with endocardial cushion defect in ~32% and aortic lesions in ~15%
Brain development	Weight reduced ~65%	Head circumference decreased ~2% at birth
	Decreased cell proliferation and migration in cortex	Deficiencies of cells in cortical layers
	Retarded development of cerebellar foliation and hippocampal fissure formation	Disproportionately small cerebellum; decreased neuron density in hippocampus
	Reductions in several neuronal neurotransmitter markers	Reduction in cholinergic markers in later life (associated with Alzheimer disease)
	Structural alterations of cochlear and vestibular portions of the inner ear	Anomalies of the inner ear
Immunological and hematological	Severe thymic hypoplasia	Thymic hypoplasia at birth
	Delayed maturation of thymic lymphocytes *in vitro*	Reduced T lymphocyte responses
	Reduction in pre-B and B lymphocytes	Decreased antibody responses
	Reduced stem cell populations in liver (erythroid, granulocyte-macrophage, multipotential)	? Decreased circulating granulocyte-macrophage stem cells
	Poor lymphoid and erythroid cell survival in radiation and aggregation chimeras	Reduced proportion of trisomic lymphocytes in blood of trisomy 21/2n mosaics

Source: Modified from Epstein, Cox, and Epstein (1985). See also Epstein, Hofmeister et al. (1985).

The mouse trisomy 16 model for human trisomy 21 now permits the study of several problems related to the presence of extra copies of known human chromosome 21 genes, as well as analysis of phenotypic similarities, such as congenital heart disease (endocardial cushion defect), for which mechanisms have been suggested even though the responsible locus or loci have not yet been identified (Wright et al., 1984). Nevertheless, since trisomy for all of mouse chromosome 16, as is produced in the current models, results in a degree of genetic imbalance more extensive than occurs in human trisomy 21, an improved model would be an animal with a duplication of just the distal part of chromosome 16, the region in which SOD-1 and PRGS are located, or an animal with an extra dose of a single human chromosome 21 gene. The latter would permit an examination of the phenotypic consequences of the imbalance of individual loci and, in theory, a dissection of the aneuploid phenotype and assignment of features to specific loci or sets of loci (see Epstein, 1986a for a discussion of the theoretical basis of this assertion). If the degree of genetic imbalance were not too great, such animals would probably be viable beyond birth. However, the approaches now being used for the creation of transgenic mice (Brinster et al., 1983) provide a basis for work in this direction, and the successes obtained so far give hope that it will eventually be possible to achieve the integration into the mouse genome and expression of sets of individual mouse genes homologous to genes on human chromosome 21. This would permit the realization of the prediction made by Lederberg (1966) that:

> Human nuclei, or individual chromosomes and genes, will also be combined with those of other animal species . . . . Before long we are bound to hear of tests of the effect of dosage of the human twenty-first chromosome on the development of the brain of the mouse or the gorilla . . . . They need . . . just a small step in cell biology. (p. 10)

REFERENCES

Arias, S., Paradisi, I., & Rolo, M. (1985). Cystathionine beta-synthase (CBS) location excluded from 21pter→q11, but confirmed to 21q, by gene dosage in trisomy 21. *Cytogenetics and Cell Genetics, 40*, 570.

Brinster, R. L., Ritchie, K. A., Hammer, R. E., O'Brien, R. L., Arp, B., & Storb, U. (1983). Expression of a microinjected immunoglobulin gene in the spleen of transgenic mice. *Nature, 306*, 332–336.

Cox, D. R., & Epstein, C. J. (1985). Comparative gene mapping of human chromosome 21 and mouse chromosome 16. *Annals of the New York Academy of Science, 450*, 169–177.

Cox, D. R., Epstein, L. B., & Epstein, C. J. (1980). Genes coding for sensitivity to interferon (IfRec) and soluble superoxide dismutase (SOD-1) are linked in mouse and man and map to mouse chromosome 16. *Proceedings of the National Academy of Science (USA), 77*, 2168–2172.

Cox, D. R., Goldblatt, D., & Epstein, C. J. (1981). Chromosomal assignment of mouse PRGS: Further evidence for homology between mouse chromosome 16 and human chromosome 21. *American Journal of Human Genetics, 33,* 145A.

Cox, D. R., Smith, S. A., Epstein, L. B., & Epstein, C. J. (1984). Mouse trisomy 16 as an animal model of human trisomy 21 (Down syndrome): Formation of viable trisomy 16 ↔ diploid mouse chimeras. *Developmental Biology, 101,* 416–424.

Coyle, J. T., Gearhart, J. D., Oster-Granite, M. L., Singer, H. S., & Moran, T. H. (1986). Brain neurotransmitters: Implications for Down syndrome from studies of mouse trisomy 16. In C. J. Epstein (Ed.), *The neurobiology of Down syndrome* (pp. 153–169). New York: Raven Press.

Epstein, C. J. (1981). Animal models for human trisomy. In F. F. de la Cruz & P. S. Gerald (Eds.) *Trisomy 21 (Down syndrome): Research perspectives* (pp. 263–273). Baltimore: University Park Press.

Epstein, C. J. (1986a). *The consequences of chromosome imbalance. Principles, mechanisms, and models.* New York: Cambridge University Press.

Epstein, C. J. (Ed.) (1986b). *The neurobiology of Down syndrome.* New York: Raven Press.

Epstein, C. J. (1986c). Trisomy 21 and the nervous system: From cause to cure. In C. J. Epstein (Ed.), *The neurobiology of Down syndrome* (pp. 1–15). New York: Raven Press.

Epstein, C. J., Cox, D. R., & Epstein, L. B. (1985). Mouse trisomy 16: An animal model of human trisomy 21 (Down syndrome). *Annals of the New York Academy of Science, 450,* 157–168.

Epstein, C. J., & Epstein, L. B. (1983). Genetic control of the response to interferon in man and mouse. In E. Pick & M. Landy (Eds.), *Lymphokines,* (Vol. 8, pp. 277–301). New York: Academic Press.

Epstein, C. J., Hofmeister, B. G., Yee, D., Smith, S. A., Philip, R., Cox, D. R., & Epstein, L. B. (1985). Stem cell deficiencies and thymic abnormalities in fetal mouse trisomy 16. *Journal of Experimental Medicine, 162,* 695–712.

Francke, U., & Taggart, R. T. (1979). Assignment of the gene for cytoplasmic superoxide dismutase (SOD-1) to a region of the chromosome 16 and of Hprt to a region of the X chromosome in the mouse. *Proceedings of the National Academy of Science (USA), 76,* 5230–5233.

Groner, Y., Lieman-Hurwitz, J., Dafni, N., Sherman, L., Levanon, D., Bernstein, Y., Danciger, E., & Elroy-Stein, O. (1985). Molecular structure and expression of the gene locus on chromosome 21 encoding the Cu/Zn superoxide dismutase and its relevance to Down syndrome. *Annals of the New York Academy of Science, 450,* 133–156.

Gropp, A., Giers, D., & Kolbus, U. (1974). Trisomy in the fetal backcross progeny of male and female metacentric heterozygotes of the mouse. I. *Cytogenetics and Cell Genetics, 13,* 511–535.

Gropp, A., Kolbus, U., & Giers, D. (1975). Systematic approach to the study of trisomy in the mouse. II. *Cytogenetics and Cell Genetics, 14,* 42–62.

Hoffman, S., & Edelman, G. M. (1983). Kinetics of homophilic binding by embryonic and adult forms of the neural cell adhesion molecule. *Proceedings of the National Academy of Science (USA), 80,* 5762–5766.

Human Gene Mapping 8. (1985). Eighth International Workshop on Human Gene Mapping. *Cytogenetics and Cell Genetics, 40,* (1–4).

Kohn, G., Taysi, K., Atkins, T. E., & Mellman, W. J. (1970). Mosaic mongolism. I. Clinical correlations. *Journal of Pediatrics, 76,* 874–879.

Kurnit, D. M., Aldridge, J. F., Matsuoka, R., & Matthyse, S. (1985). Increased adhesiveness of trisomy 21 cells and atrioventricular malformations in Down syndrome: A stochastic model. *American Journal of Medical Genetics, 20,* 385–399.

Lederberg, J. (1966). Experimental genetics and human evolution. *Bulletin of the Atomic Scientists, 22*(8), 4–11.

Lin, P.-F., Slate, D. L., Lawyer, F. C., & Ruddle, F. H. (1980). Assignment of the murine interferon sensitivity and cytoplasmic superoxide dismutase genes to chromosome 16. *Science, 209,* 285–287.

Mayes, J., Muneer, R., & Sifers, M. (1984). Superoxide dismutase activity and oxygen toxicity in Down syndrome fibroblasts. *American Journal of Human Genetics, 36,* 15S.

Miyabara, S., Gropp, A., & Winking, H. (1982). Trisomy 16 in the mouse fetus associated with generalized edema, cardiovascular, and urinary tract anomalies. *Teratology, 25,* 369–380.

Rehder, H. (1981). Pathology of trisomy 21—with particular reference to persistent common atrioventricular canal of the heart. In G. R. Burgio, M. Fraccaro, L. Tiepolo, & U. Wolf (Eds.), *Trisomy 21: An international symposium* (pp. 57–63). Berlin: Springer-Verlag.

Rethoré, M. O. (1981). Structural variation of chromosome 21 and symptoms of Down's syndrome. In G. R. Burgio, M. Fraccaro, L. Tiepolo, & U. Wolf (Eds.), *Trisomy 21: An international symposium* (pp. 173–182). Berlin: Springer-Verlag.

Rutishauser, U. (1986). The potential effects of gene dosage on cell-cell interactions during development. In C. J. Epstein (Ed.), *The neurobiology of Down syndrome* (pp. 171–178). New York: Raven Press.

Sinet, P. M. (1982). Metabolism of oxygen derivatives in Down's syndrome. *Annals of the New York Academy of Science, 396,* 83–94.

Sinet, P. M., Lejeune, J., & Jerome, H. (1979). Trisomy 21 (Down syndrome). Glutathione peroxidase, hexose monophosphate shunt, and IQ. *Life Sciences, 24,* 29–34.

Summitt, R. L. (1981). Chromosome specific segments that cause the phenotype of Down syndrome. In F. F. de la Cruz & P. S. Gerald (Eds.) *Trisomy 21 (Down syndrome): Research perspectives* (pp. 225–235). Baltimore: University Park Press.

Weil, J., Tucker, G., Epstein, L. B., & Epstein, C. J. (1983). Interferon induction of (2′-5′) oligoisoadenylate synthetase in diploid and trisomy 21 fibroblasts: Relation to dosage of the interferon receptor gene (*IFRC*). *Human Genetics, 65,* 108–111.

White, B. J., Tjio, J.-H., Van de Water, L. C., & Crandall, C. (1974). Trisomy 19 in the laboratory mouse. I. Frequency in different crosses at specific developmental stages and relationship of trisomy to cleft palate. *Cytogenetics and Cell Genetics, 13,* 217–231.

Wright, T. C., Orkin, R. W., Destrempes, M., & Kurnit, D. M. (1984). Increased adhesiveness of Down syndrome fetal fibroblasts *in vitro. Proceedings of the National Academy of Science (USA), 81,* 2426–2430.

Chapter 3

Inborn Errors
of Morphogenesis
in Down Syndrome
A Stochastic Model

David M. Kurnit and Rachael L. Neve

Characteristic features of the inborn errors of morphogenesis in Down syndrome include hypoplasia, specificity, variability among subjects, and early onset during gestation. Inborn errors of cardiogenesis and pulmonogenesis are also seen in persons with Down syndrome.

HYPOPLASIA

Hypoplasia is a striking feature in many of the malformations in Down syndrome. The most apparent outward sign is that linear growth is deficient (Cronk, 1978). Further, most internal organs in infants with Down syndrome show diminished weight at birth (Naeye, 1967). Total brain size and head circumference are deficient, with the anteroposterior diameter more severely affected than the biparietal diameter, giving rise to microbrachycephaly (Roche, 1966). The diminished anteroposterior growth results in midface hypoplasia, yielding a flat nasal bridge, epicanthal folds, upward slanting palpebral fissures, and tongue protrusion (Smith, 1982; Zellweger, 1977). In addition to being smaller, morphometric measurements among persons with Down syndrome show greater variation than for normal individuals; this increased variability is seen most frequently in traits that tend to show the greatest diversity among normal persons. Such increased variability has been termed ''amplified developmental instability'' (see Shapiro, 1983).

Preparation of this chapter was supported by NIH grants HD 20118, HD 18658, HD 06276, and the American Heart Association, Massachusetts Division. Kurnit is the recipient of a Research Career Development Award from NICHD and Neve is the recipient of a National Down Syndrome Society fellowship.

SPECIFICITY

The phenotype of trisomy 21 is distinct from other syndromes, both chromosomal and nonchromosomal, that are also associated with hypoplasia (Smith, 1982; Zellweger, 1977). Although some malformations seen frequently in Down syndrome are nonspecific in that they are seen in a number of other syndromes (e.g., four-finger line in the palm, reflecting hypoplastic metacarpals; clinodactyly of the fifth finger, reflecting hypoplasia of the second phalanx on this digit), the overall phenotype is specific enough to permit clinical diagnosis. Many malformations are highly over-represented in Down syndrome. These include: atrioventricular (AV) canal defects in 40% of persons with Down syndrome (Park et al., 1977; Perry, Meidgerly, Galioto, Shapiro, & Scott, 1980; Rowe & Uchida, 1961; Tandon & Edwards, 1973); pulmonary acinar hypoplasia in 7 out of 7 persons examined (Cooney & Thurlbeck, 1982); microbrachycephaly and midface hypoplasia, yielding the characteristic facies of Down syndrome (Smith, 1982; Zellweger, 1977); and duodenal obstruction in 1% of persons with Down syndrome, accounting for 30% of all neonates with duodenal atresia/stenosis (Fonkalsrud, De Lorimier, & Hays, 1969).

Neuropathology of the brains of persons with Down syndrome has not, as yet, yielded a simple hypothesis to explain the inborn errors of neurogenesis that presumably underly the mental deficiency associated with the syndrome. As summarized in a recent review (Ross, Galaburda, & Kemper, 1984, p. 909), gross examination shows the brains of persons with Down syndrome to be "underweight showing a rounded cerebrum, simplicity of convolutional pattern, small cerebellum and brainstem, shortened anteroposterior diameter with steep inclinations of the occipital lobes, and a cuboidal thalamus." On microscopic examination, they noted neuronal paucity, particularly of small neurons (? aspinous stellate cells). They postulate that a migration defect involving such small neurons may play a role in the neural pathogenesis of Down syndrome (Ross et al., 1984).

VARIABILITY AMONG SUBJECTS

Most infants with Down syndrome may be diagnosed by physical examination, as most such infants have a number of the characteristic constellation of defects. However, except for the microbrachycephaly and midface hypoplasia that are (almost) uniformly seen, as just stated, most of the other defects are seen in only a proportion of persons with Down syndrome. Further, as just noted, the increased variation among subjects with Down syndrome for metric analysis of morphometric traits is well documented. The salient points are that: 1) all subjects with Down syndrome share the same underlying genetic defect, that is, trisomy for chromosome 21 (Jacobs, Baikie, Court-Brown, &

Strong, 1959; Lejeune, Gautier, & Turpin, 1959); 2) virtually all subjects with Down syndrome share enough clinically appreciable stigmata to be identifiable at birth; and 3) although the phenotype is usually recognizable, there remains great variation among individuals with Down syndrome for the expression of many of the characteristically observed defects. Taken together, these points argue for a probabilistic or stochastic model, whereby persons with Down syndrome have a greater chance of showing certain defects, but that any given individual may or may not have these defects.

EARLY ONSET

As expected in a disorder such as Down syndrome in which the error (trisomy 21) is present constitutively from the time of zygote formation, the errors of morphogenesis in Down syndrome begin early in development. Most of these errors can readily be dated to times in development well before prenatal diagnosis is feasible, even with chorionic biopsy techniques. Since neural development both precedes and continues after the time frame during which prenatal diagnosis is possible, it remains an open question whether genetic manipulations to ameliorate the neurological deficits of affected individuals will be feasible.

INCREASED ADHESIVENESS OF TRISOMY 21 CELLS

The increased adhesiveness of trisomy 21 cells may explain cardiac and pulmonary malformations in Down syndrome.

Gene Dosage

As outlined in Chapter 2 and its Response in Section I of this book, the primary biochemical error in trisomy 21 appears to be gene dosage: the increase in dosage (three copies rather than the normal two copies) for genes on chromosome 21 is reflected in a generalized increase of approximately 50% more messenger RNA from genes on chromosome 21 (Kurnit, 1979). Transcriptional dosage has been verified for the one structural gene on chromosome 21, superoxide dismutase-1, that has been cloned (Sherman, Dafni, Lieman-Hurwitz, & Groner, 1983). As reviewed earlier in this book, by Epstein and Patterson et al., gene dosage for a number of enzymes encoded by chromosome 21 indeed results in 50% higher specific activities of such enzymes. It is not clear that dosage for such enzymes would result in the phenotypic defects of trisomy 21, especially in view of the dampening effect of kinetic networks on dosage for genes in those networks and in light of the fact that most enzymes are present normally "in excess" (Kacser & Burns, 1981).

Although dosage for both transcription and specific activity is the norm for chromosome 21–encoded genes examined to date, two exceptions have been noted. One protein putatively encoded by chromosome 21, a 68,000 molecular weight microtubule-associated protein with homology to the *Drosophila* heat shock protein (Lim, Hall, Leung, & Whatley, 1984), appears to show dosage at the transcriptional but not the protein level (Whatley, Hall, Davison, & Lim, 1984). Such dosage compensation has been described in a number of other eucaryotic systems (Aragoncillo, Rodriguez-Loperena, Salcedo, Carbonero, & Garcia-Olmedo, 1978; Devlin, Holm, & Grigliatti, 1982; Pearson, Fried, & Warner, 1982).

The second exception is that while the interferon receptor is encoded by chromosome 21, presumably resulting in a 50% increase of receptor molecules on the surface of trisomy 21 cells, responsiveness of trisomy 21 cells to interferon (as measured by antiviral response) is elevated in a nonlinear fashion (increased up to an order of magnitude over normal controls) (Tan, Schneider, Tischfield, Epstein, & Ruddle, 1974; Weil, Epstein, & Epstein, 1980). Given the many roles that interferon may play in regulating homeostasis and growth control (e.g., the effect of interferon on regulation of the c-myc gene; Jonak & Knight, 1984), the interferon receptor may turn out to have key roles in modulating dysharmonic growth, immune abnormalities, and the increased frequency of neoplasia in Down syndrome (see Zellweger, 1977).

Hypothesis

Based on the aforestated evidence, Kurnit, Aldridge, Matsuoka, and Matthysse (1985) proposed a model to explain some of the inborn errors of morphogenesis of Down syndrome. Their rationale was based on the following points:

1. Dosage for genes on chromosome 21 is the primary abnormality in Down syndrome.
2. Cell surface molecules are known to mediate morphogenesis in a variety of systems (Edelman, 1983; Frazier & Glaser, 1979).
3. Cell surface adhesion correlates negatively with cellular migration in some systems (Thiery, Duband, Rutishauser, & Edelman, 1982).

Kurnit, Aldrich, Matsuoka, and Matthysse (1985) proposed that increased dosage for cell surface molecules encoded by chromosome 21 involved in intercellular adhesion might inhibit migration of specific cells at specific times during development; in turn, this could explain the findings of hypoplasia and specificity, and the appearance of morphological defects during early gestation that characterize the malformations of Down syndrome.

Experimental Evidence

The primary prediction of the above model is that trisomy 21 cells in developing tissues should be more adhesive than normal controls. Wright, Orkin, Destrempes, and Kurnit (1984) set out to determine the validity of this prediction experimentally. Tissues from 20-week-old abortuses were explanted into tissue culture to obtain fibroblasts from lung, skin, and structures derived from the endocardial cushions that form the AV canal structures deficient in Down syndrome. Divalent cation-independent rates of aggregation of fibroblasts were compared for fibroblasts from trisomy 21 and age-matched normal controls. Fibroblasts from lung and from some cardiac cushion cultures aggregated more rapidly for the trisomy 21 samples than for the normal controls (Wright et al., 1984). No differences were observed between trisomy 21 and normal skin fibroblasts. The differences between trisomy 21 and normal fibroblasts were not due to differences in several factors known to affect intercellular adhesiveness; no differences were observed between normal and trisomy 21 lung fibroblasts for hyaluronic acid metabolism, membrane polarization (Wright et al., 1984), or glycosyl transferase activities (Figlewicz, Johnson, & Kurnit, unpublished observations). Kurnit, Aldridge, Matsuoka, and Matthysse (1985) concluded that, as predicted by their original hypothesis, there is evidence for tissue-specific increased adhesiveness among trisomy 21 fibroblasts from fetal lung and endocardial cushion–derived structures. The authors speculated that such adhesiveness defects might exist earlier in development as well, and might underly the pulmonary acinar hypoplasia and endocardial cushion AV canal defects seen frequently in persons with Down syndrome.

Stochastic Model

As noted earlier in this chapter, most of the "characteristic" defects of Down syndrome are not seen in all patients. This variation cannot simply be due to genetic differences, as all subjects with Down syndrome have the same underlying genetic defect, namely, trisomy 21; and monozygotic twins with Down syndrome have been described who are discordant for AV canal defects (Rehder, 1981). The discordance between monozygotic twins with trisomy 21 effectively rules out genetic differences as the basis for this phenomenon, and environmental factors are also difficult to implicate as both twins shared a common uterine environment. (Differences in monozygotic twin development secondary to environmental uterine differences are usually seen much later in gestation than the timing for AV canal development at roughly 5 weeks gestation. Differences in monozygotic twin development secondary to a late monozygotic twinning event that may affect the primitive streak [ca. 16 days] give rise to a number of mesodermal defects that constitute the VACTERL

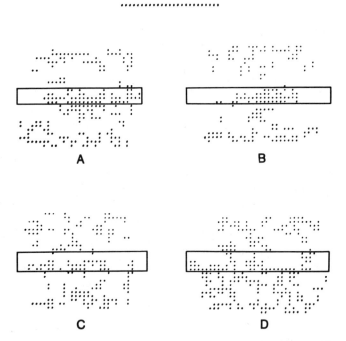

Figure 1.   Simulation of normal endocardial cushion-to-cushion fusion. The simulation begins with two lines of 25 cells located 25 spaces apart on a grid. In the panel labeled "Origin," the upper line of cells represents the superior endocardial cushion of the atrioventricular canal and the lower line of cells represents the inferior cushion of cells. The computer simulations and parameters, including intercellular adhesiveness, were run as defined in Kurnit, Aldridge, Matsuoka, and Matthysse (1985). Each panel is independent in that a different input seed number was given to a random number generator in the program. The spaces enclosed by the rectangular boxes indicate the region where superior and inferior cushion-to-cushion fusion should normally occur. At a low value of adhesiveness (0.2), cushion-to-cushion fusion consistently occurred normally as indicated by good filling of the rectangle with endocardial cells. (From Kurnit, D. M., Aldridge, J. F., Matsuoka, R., & Matthysse, S. [1985]. Increased adhesiveness of trisomy 21 cells and atrioventricular canal malformations in Down syndrome: A stochastic model. *American Journal of Medical Genetics, 20,* 393. Copyright © 1985 by Alan R. Liss, Inc.; reprinted by permission.)

association, but isolated AV canal defects are not typically involved in the VACTERL association [Schinzel, Smith, & Miller, 1979].) Taken together, these data suggest that random, probabilistic (stochastic) factors play an important role in the causation of AV canal defects in Down syndrome.

Kurnit, Aldridge, Neve, and Matthysse (1985) have elaborated a stochastic model to explain how increased adhesiveness among lung and endocardial cushion fibroblasts could explain pulmonary acinar hypoplasia and AV canal defects in Down syndrome. In their computer simulations of AV canal development, randomly walking endocardial cells were allowed to migrate, divide, and adhere with programmable probabilities. Low values of intercellular adhesiveness yielded simulations for normal AV canal development (see Figure 1); higher values of adhesiveness uniformly yielded abnormal AV canal development (see Figure 2); and moderately high levels of

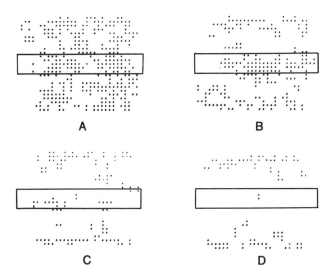

Figure 2. Effect of altering adhesiveness. In each of the panels, all parameters except adhesiveness were identical to those used in Figure 1. The values of adhesiveness used in this figure were: Panel A: 0.1; Panel B: 0.2; Panel C: 0.3; Panel D: 0.4. When adhesiveness is less (Fig. 2, Panel A) than the normal control (Fig. 1, Panel B; Fig. 2, Panel B), cushion-to-cushion fusion occurs, but cells are packed uniformly throughout the cardiac jelly of the endocardial cushions, in contrast with light microscopic data (Hay & Low, 1972). When adhesiveness is greater than the normal state, cushion-to-cushion fusion is either incomplete (Fig. 2, Panel C) or absent (Fig. 2, Panel D). (From Kurnit, D. M., Aldridge, J. F., Matsuoka, R., & Matthysse, S. [1985]. Increased adhesiveness of trisomy 21 cells and atrioventricular canal malformations in Down syndrome: A stochastic model. *American Journal of Medical Genetics, 20,* 394. Copyright © 1985 by Alan R. Liss, Inc.; reprinted by permission.)

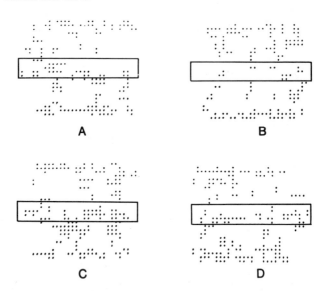

Figure 3. Stochastic effects. As in Fig. 1, independent simulations were performed by using different input seed numbers without changing the major parameters. In each of the panels from this figure, the same parameters have been used; a moderately elevated value of adhesiveness was used (0.25), and all other parameters were as used in Figs. 1 and 2. In this figure, whereas Panels A, C and D demonstrate examples of relatively complete cushion-to-cushion fusion, Panel B demonstrates a marked deficiency of cushion-to-cushion fusion. This difference represents the effects of stochastic (random) variations resulting from multiple independent runs of this probabilistic program. (From Kurnit, D. M., Aldridge, J. F., Matsuoka, R., & Matthysse, S. [1985]. Increased adhesiveness of trisomy 21 cells and atrioventricular canal malformations in Down syndrome: A stochastic model. *American Journal of Medical Genetics, 20,* 395. Copyright © 1985 by Alan R. Liss, Inc.; reprinted by permission.)

adhesiveness yielded abnormalities in only a proportion of multiple, independently performed simulations, as is the case in Down syndrome (see Figure 3). The model successfully predicted the anatomy of the AV canal lesions seen in Down syndrome, variability due solely to stochastic factors among individuals with the same genotype (viz., the monozygotic twins discussed earlier), and amplified developmental instability.

Future Research

Proof of the model will require isolation of genes encoding cell surface markers determined by chromosome 21. Toward that end, antibodies have been prepared that recognize cell surface markers encoded by human chromosome 21 (Kurnit, Aldridge, Neve, & Matthysse, 1985). These antibodies, as well as antibodies from other groups (Miller, Jones, Scoggin, & Patterson,

1981), will be used to screen genic libraries that the authors have constructed in specialized cloning vectors (Young & Davis, 1983); in this manner, it should be feasible to clone chromosome 21–specific genes that encode relevant cell surface markers. Antibodies prepared to gene products expressed by such cloned genes will be assayed to determine whether such antibodies can inhibit the abnormally high adhesiveness observed among trisomy 21 fibroblasts. Cloning such genes would present the opportunity to create a rodent model (Epstein, Epstein, & Cox, 1982; Miyabara, Gropp, & Winking, 1982) for inborn errors of morphogenesis due to increased adhesiveness among trisomy 21 cells. Dosage for such genes could be increased by expanding the gene copy number following transfection into early embryos, or decreased by injecting a cloned molecule dedicated to the production of "anti-sense" RNA (see Travers, 1984). The phenotype of animals with increased, normal, or decreased dosage for these genes could be compared to determine the effects of gene dosage for specific genes on morphogenesis.

REFERENCES

Aragoncillo, C., Rodriguez-Loperena, M. A., Salcedo, G., Carbonero, P., & Garcia-Olmedo, F. (1978). Influence of homoeologous chromosomes on gene-dosage effects in allohexaploid wheat (*Triticum aestivum L.*). *Proceedings of the National Academy of Science (USA), 75*, 1446–1450.

Cooney, T. P., & Thurlbeck, W. M. (1982). Pulmonary hypoplasia in Down's syndrome. *New England Journal of Medicine, 307*, 1170–1173.

Cronk, C. E. (1978). Growth of children with Down's syndrome: Birth to age 3 years. *Pediatrics, 61*, 564–568.

Devlin, R. H., Holm, D. G., & Grigliatti, T. A. (1982). Autosomal dosage compensation in *Drosophila melanogaster* strains trisomic for the left arm of chromosome 2. *Proceedings of the National Academy of Science (USA), 79*, 1200–1204.

Edelman, G. M. (1983). Cell adhesion molecules. *Science, 219*, 450–457.

Einat, M., Resnitzky, D., & Kimchi, A. (1985). Close link between reduction of c-myc expression by interferon and G_0/G_1 arrest. *Nature, 313*, 597–600.

Epstein, C. J., Epstein, L. B., & Cox, D. R. (1982). Mouse model for trisomy 21. *Down's Syndrome: Papers and Abstracts for Professionals, 5*, 1–4.

Fonkalsrud, E. W., De Lorimier, A. A., & Hays, D. M. (1969). Congenital atresia and stenosis of the duodenum. *Pediatrics, 43*, 79–83.

Frazier, W., & Glaser, L. (1979). Surface components and cell recognition. *Annual Reviews of Biochemistry, 48*, 491–523.

Hay, D. A., & Low, F. N. (1972). The fusion of dorsal and ventral endocardial cushions in the embryonic chick heart. *American Journal of Anatomy, 133*, 1–24.

Jacobs, P. A., Baikie, A. G., Court-Brown, W. M., & Strong, J. A. (1959). The somatic chromosomes in mongolism. *Lancet, I*, 710–711.

Jonak, G. J., & Knight, E., Jr. (1984). Selective reduction of c-myc mRNA in *Daudi* cells by human beta interferon. *Proceedings of the National Academy of Science (USA), 81*, 1747–1750.

Kacser, H., & Burns, J. A. (1981). The molecular basis of dominance. *Genetics, 97*, 639–666.

Kurnit, D. M. (1979). Down syndrome: Gene dosage at the transcriptional level in skin fibroblasts. *Proceedings of the National Academy of Science (USA), 76,* 2372–2376.

Kurnit, D. M., Aldridge, J. F., Matsuoka, R., & Matthysse, S. (1985). Increased adhesiveness of trisomy 21 cells and atrioventricular canal malformations in Down syndrome: A stochastic model. *American Journal of Medical Genetics, 20,* 385–399.

Kurnit, D. M., Aldridge, J. F., Neve, R. L., & Matthysse, S. (1985). Genetics of congenital heart malformations: A stochastic model. *Annals of the New York Academy of Science, 450,* 191–204.

Lejeune, J., Gautier, M., & Turpin, R. (1959). Etudes des chromosomes somatiques de neuf enfants mongoliens [Studies of somatic chromosomes in nine mongoloid children]. *Comptes Rendues Academies Sciences (Paris), 248,* 1721–1722.

Lim, L., Hall, C., Leung, T., & Whatley, S. (1984). The relationship of the rat 68 kDa microtubule-associated protein with synaptosomal plasma membranes and with the *Drosophila* 70 kDA heat-shock protein. *Biochemical Journal, 224,* 677–680.

Miller, Y. E., Jones, C., Scoggin, C. H., & Patterson, D. (1981). A chromosome 21 encoded fetal brain antigen. *Journal of Cell Biology, 91,* 35a.

Miyabara, S., Gropp, A., & Winking, H. (1982). Trisomy 16 in the mouse fetus associated with generalized edema and cardiovascular and urinary tract anomalies. *Teratology, 25,* 369–380.

Naeye, R. L. (1967). Prenatal organ and cellular growth with various chromosomal disorders. *Biological Neonatology, 11,* 248–260.

Osley, M. A., & Hereford, L. M. (1981). Yeast histone genes show dosage compensation. *Cell, 24,* 377–384.

Park, S. C., Mathews, R. A., Zuberbuhler, J. R., Rowe, R. D., Neches, W. H., & Lenox, C. C. (1977). Down syndrome with congenital heart malformations. *American Journal of Diseases in Childhood, 131,* 29–33.

Pearson, N. J., Fried, H. M., & Warner, J. R. (1982). Yeast use translational control to compensate for extra copies of a ribosomal protein gene. *Cell, 29,* 347–355.

Perry, L., Meidgerly, F., Galioto, F., Shapiro, S., & Scott, L. (1980). Down's syndrome and cardiovascular disease. *Down's Syndrome: Papers and Abstracts for Professionals, 3,* 1–4.

Rehder, H. (1981). Pathology of trisomy 21, with particular reference to persistent common atrioventricular canal of the heart. In G. M. Burgio, M. Fraccaro, L. Tiepolo, & U. Wolf (Eds.), *Trisomy 21: An international symposium* (pp. 57–73). Berlin: Springer-Verlag.

Roche, A. F. (1966). The cranium in mongolism. *Acta Neurologica, 42,* 62–78.

Ross, M. H., Galaburda, A. M., & Kemper, T. L. (1984). Down's syndrome: Is there a decreased population of neurons? *Neurology, 34,* 909–916.

Rowe, R., & Uchida, I. (1961). Cardiac malformations in mongolism: A prospective study of 184 mongoloid children. *American Journal of Medicine, 31,* 726–735.

Schinzel, A. A. G. L., Smith, D. W., & Miller, J. R. (1979). Monozygotic twinning and structural defects. *Journal of Pediatrics, 95,* 921–930.

Shapiro, B. L. (1983). Down syndrome—a disruption of homeostasis. *American Journal of Medical Genetics, 14,* 241–269.

Sherman, L., Dafni, N., Lieman-Hurwitz, J., & Groner, Y. (1983). Nucleotide sequence and expression of human chromosome 21–encoded superoxide dismutase mRNA. *Proceedings of the National Academy of Science (USA), 80,* 5465–5469.

Smith, D. W. (1982). *Recognizable patterns of human malformation* (3rd ed.). Philadelphia: W. B. Saunders.

Tan, Y. H., Schneider, E. L., Tischfield, J., Epstein, C. J., & Ruddle, F. H. (1974).

Human chromosome 21 dosage: Effect on the expression of the interferon induced antiviral state. *Science, 186,* 61–63.

Tandon, R., & Edwards, J. E. (1973). Cardiac malformations associated with Down's syndrome. *Circulation, 47,* 1349–1355.

Thiery, J.-P., Duband, J.-L., Rutishauser, U., & Edelman, G. M. (1982). Cell adhesion molecules in early chicken embryogenesis. *Proceedings of the National Academy of Science (USA), 79,* 6737–6741.

Travers, A. (1984). Gene expression: Regulation by anti-sense RNA. *Nature, 311,* 410.

Weil, J., Epstein, L. B., & Epstein, C. J. (1980). Synthesis of interferon-induced polypeptides in normal and chromosome 21–aneuploid human fibroblasts: Relationship to relative sensitivities in antiviral assays. *Journal of Interferon Research, 1,* 111–124.

Whatley, S. A., Hall, C., Davison, A. N., & Lim, L. (1984). Alterations in the relative amounts of specific mRNA species in the developing human brain in Down syndrome. *Biochemical Journal, 220,* 179–187.

Wright, T. C., Orkin, R. W., Destrempes, M., & Kurnit, D. M. (1984). Increased adhesiveness of Down syndrome fetal fibroblasts *in vitro. Proceedings of the National Academy of Science (USA), 81,* 2426–2430.

Young, R. A., & Davis, R. W. (1983). Efficient isolation of genes by using antibody probes. *Proceedings of the National Academy of Science (USA), 80,* 1194–1198.

Zellweger, H. (1977). Down syndrome. In P. J. Vinken & G. W. Bruyn (Eds.), *Handbook of Clinical Neurology* (Vol. 31, pp. 367–469). Amsterdam: North Holland.

RESPONSE

Development and Differentiation in the Embryo with Down Syndrome

Michael R. Cummings

Langdon Down first described the clinical entity that bears his name in 1866. It was not until 1959, however, that Jerome Lejeune discovered that Down syndrome was associated with the presence of an extra copy of chromosome 21. Since then, a great deal of work has focused on cytogenetic and biochemical aspects of Down syndrome in an attempt to explain how quantitative alterations in the genetic material can produce the characteristic pattern of physical and mental defects. Cytogenetic studies have provided evidence that a small segment of the long arm of chromosome 21 is responsible for the full array of clinical symptoms. At the biochemical level, a number of genes have been mapped to chromosome 21, and elevated levels of enzymes have been clearly demonstrated in several instances.

These latter observations, gathered over the past 25 years, have generated the current working hypothesis that states that increases in the copy number of certain genes, and, in turn, in the concentration of their gene products, in prenatal development lead to the deleterious effects seen in trisomy 21. What Kurnit and Neve have done with their work on the formation of the endocardial cushion is to redirect our attention from the metabolic to the developmental level.

An examination of the literature shows that one of the oldest observations about Down syndrome deals with developmental problems. In his book, *Down's Anomaly,* Smith cites an 1886 paper by Shuttleworth in which newborns with Down syndrome are regarded as "unfinished children" who, although brought to term, are developmentally incomplete. To further explore Down syndrome as a problem in development, consider the paradigm that is used in the study of development and differentiation. Developmental biology is a discipline that has borrowed the methods of many other fields including anatomy, histology, genetics, and molecular biology. This diverse array of techniques is used in the study of the processes involved in the assembly of a complex, multicellular organism from a fertilized egg.

Following fertilization, cell division produces an unorganized collection of cells. Subsequently, cell division is temporarily reduced, and these cells undergo a programmed set of cell migrations. After migration, cell-cell recognition and preferential adhesion lead to the formation of discrete fields within the embryo for differentiation. A complex series of molecular and biochemical events within and between cells then initiates the process of differentiation and the formation of recognizable structures. Each of these processes has been experimentally dissected in lower organisms, whereas understanding of these events in higher organisms, including humans, has been more limited.

RELEVANCE OF THE FINDINGS

The question now is whether Kurnit and Neve's findings of changes in cell adhesion are relevant to these developmental processes and to Down syndrome. The author believes that Kurnit and Neve's proposal is pertinent and important, first of all, because it supplies a link between gene product(s) and a developmental event. Cell adhesion is associated with a discrete set of gene products in the form of cell surface molecules. Changes in the type, number, or arrangement of these molecules can alter or abolish the ability of the cell to adhere to other cells or to a substrate. The computer model described in Chapter 3 suggests that alterations in adhesive properties can produce a range of defects in the formation of the endocardial cushion. The *in vitro* experiments demonstrate that there is, in fact, an alteration in the adhesiveness of cells from individuals with Down syndrome. With these observations in hand, it is possible to explore the surface of cells in Down syndrome using immunological and recombinant DNA techniques to recover and study cell surface proteins and the genes that encode them. Extension of these studies to the mouse trisomy 16 model system described by Epstein will allow a direct experimental approach to help elucidate the role of cell adhesion in specific developmental events such as the formation of the endocardial cushion. Regardless of whether these experiments are ultimately successful, they signal a new approach in basic research that is likely to be followed by others.

SUMMARY

Kurnit and Neve's proposal about cell adhesion is an important development in Down syndrome research for three reasons:

1. It provides a direct link between gene products and a specific developmental defect in Down syndrome.
2. It provides a means for the isolation and characterization of structural genes encoding an important class of proteins with developmental significance.
3. The idea can be transferred to the trisomy 16 mouse system that has been proposed as a model for Down syndrome. This will allow a direct experimental approach to study the role of cell-cell adhesion in the genesis of specific developmental defects.

A DIALOGUE BETWEEN AUTHORS: AFTERTHOUGHTS

Preparation of the response to Chapter 3 precipitated further discussion among authors about how the system works, and why the model is important. Their comments that follow provide additional insight.

Cummings: Dr. Kurnit, do you think that this cell-cell adhesiveness is specific to Down syndrome only in a quantitative way or is it possible that it is a qualitative system as well?

Kurnit: It is intended to start with quantity (gene dosage), and to illustrate how quantity can change into quality, reminiscent of the fundamental principle of dialectics.

Cummings: Is there any evidence that trisomy 21 cells adhere more strongly to each other than they do to, say, normal cells?

Kurnit: We did not do a mixing experiment, so that we examined solely the avidity with which trisomy 21 cells adhered to trisomy 21 cells, and normal cells to normal cells, respectively. I have no data concerning the adhesiveness between trisomy 21 and normal cells.

Cummings: Anatomic studies show an abnormal persistence of muscles and extra muscle groups in children with Down syndrome as a rather consistent finding. How does that tie in with your model?

Kurnit: It doesn't tie in overtly. We have kept "low to the ground" with this model, which was designed to explain specific visceral defects that are associated with Down syndrome. We deliberately set out to examine a relatively simple system, the developing endocardial cushions. Specifically, endocardial cushion outgrowth involves a defined cell type, migrating at a specified time during development, and does not appear to involve cell death. Thus, our model involves a simplification of a system that is moderately simple to start with. To extend this simplified model to ever more complex systems is intriguing, but hazardous.

Crocker: Dr. Kurnit is to be saluted for his statement about keeping low key with this until he gets a better platform for all of the potential pieces of it. I wonder whether he'd be willing to consider that it's possible that the adhesiveness concept is overly simplistic but that in this way of thinking and data gathering, some related phenomenon, perhaps more multiphasic or whatever, will tumble out which can lead to further exploration. I think of this as a first and critically valuable big cut at the larger question of how all of the aberration occurs in development. This one model may not be the payoff, but it may be the cousin to the one that is. Would you be willing to speculate on a stepwise strategy of how one might get there?

Kurnit: Our current goal is to see whether the model is indeed valid for the cases of deficient pulmonary and endocardial cushion outgrowth that define Down syndrome. We are laboring to isolate antibodies that recognize chromosome 21–encoded cell surface markers, and to use such antibodies to clone genes on chromosome 21 that might mediate the adhesive abnormalities we observed. If we do find such genes, their expression in a variety of organs, including the developing brain, could then be studied.

REFERENCES

Down, J. L. H. (1866). Observations on an ethnic classification of idiots. *Clinical Lectures and Reports, London Hospital, 3,* 259.

Lejeune, J., Gautier, M., & Turpin, R. (1959). Etude des chromosomes somatiques de neuf enfants mongoliens [Study of somatic chromosomes in nine mongoloid children]. *C. R. Acad. Sci. Paris, 248,* 1721–1722.

Smith, G. (1976). *Down's anomaly* (2nd ed.). New York: Churchill Livingstone.

Chapter 4

Epidemiology of Down Syndrome

Lewis Holmes

The term Down syndrome refers primarily to the occurrence of trisomy 21, as about 94% of the affected individuals have this chromosome abnormality. The translocation type occurs in 3%, mosaicism in 2%, and various rare abnormalities in the remaining 1%.

FREQUENCY

In discussing the epidemiology of Down syndrome, one must deal with the fact that this chromosome abnormality is more common among spontaneous abortuses and stillborn infants than liveborn children. Summarizing the findings from several studies, the frequencies in these three groups are: liveborn infants, 0.13%; stillborn infants, 1.3%; and spontaneous abortuses 2.3% (Hassold & Jacobs, 1984).

This means that epidemiological studies based on the findings in liveborn infants only consider the "tip of the iceberg." Of all spontaneous abortions, 50% have an associated chromosome abnormality, with about 25% of these being trisomies. This rate of chromosomal disorders among spontaneous abortuses is 80 times greater than the rate in newborn infants. Among abortuses, trisomy 16 is the most common trisomy, with trisomies 21 and 22 the next most common. The peak occurrence of trisomies is among spontaneous abortions at 11 to 12 weeks of gestation. Unfortunately, chromosome studies on spontaneous abortuses and stillborn infants are not available as a routine procedure at most major medical centers and are even more difficult to obtain at community hospitals.

Another complication of epidemiological studies of Down syndrome is the lack of reliable information on liveborn infants obtained from birth certifi-

The author thanks Dr. Ernest B. Hook, who provided him with a copy of his then unpublished manuscript and several previous publications, and Jody Bell, for typing this manuscript.

cates. For example, during the years 1965–1974, in Minnesota, only 48% of the infants confirmed by chromosome analysis as having Down syndrome had this diagnosis recorded on their birth certificate (Venters, Schacht, & ten Bensel, 1976). Huether and his associates (1981) found an average of 33.9% of the infants with Down syndrome born in Ohio between 1970 and 1979 were reported as having the disorder on their birth certificate. The author has found a similar degree of underreporting on birth certificates in Massachusetts. Unfortunately, while this problem is well known, no method for improving the accuracy of the reporting on birth certificates has been developed.

DEMOGRAPHIC CHANGES

The epidemiological studies done on the occurrence of Down syndrome have shown some dramatic demographic changes during the past 40 years. First, there has been a significant decrease in the number of pregnancies among women aged 35 years and older. In 1960, these women had 10.8% of all births; in 1978, they had 4.5% of all births (Adams, Erickson, Layde, & Oakley, 1981). Since the woman aged 35 and older has a greater likelihood of having a child with trisomy 21, the decreasing proportion of pregnancies among "older" women should lead to a shift in the percentage of infants with Down syndrome who are born to young women. This is the second major demographic change that has been observed. Studies in several parts of the world, including the United States (Adams et al., 1981), British Columbia (Lowry, Jones, Renwick, & Trimble, 1976), Copenhagen (Mikkelsen, 1977), and Japan (Kuroki, Yamamoto, Matsui, & Kurita, 1977), have shown a steady decline in the percentage of infants born to women aged 35 years or older. For example, in 1960, 43.8% of all infants with Down syndrome were estimated to have been born to "older" women, whereas by 1978, only 21.2% were born to women aged 35 years or older.

A third demographic change has been in the utilization of prenatal diagnosis by amniocentesis. This has occurred as a result of a greater awareness and availability of this type of prenatal diagnosis. It has been used primarily by women who are 35 years or older. A smaller group utilizing this technology is composed of couples who have had one child with trisomy 21 and are concerned about the recurrence in a subsequent pregnancy.

The author has seen the impact of the prenatal diagnosis of Down syndrome and the option of therapeutic abortion of affected fetuses in the frequency of Down syndrome among infants born at Brigham and Women's Hospital in Boston. Through a program of daily surveillance for malformed infants among liveborn and stillborn infants and among therapeutic abortuses, the author and his colleagues have identified all infants/fetuses with Down syndrome since 1979. There has been an increase in the frequency of Down syndrome among infants/fetuses at this hospital, reflecting the fact that many diagnosed elsewhere by amniocentesis have been transferred for an elective termination of pregnancy (Table 1).

From the increase in the utilization of prenatal diagnosis and the elective termination of pregnancies, a decrease in the frequency of the Down syndrome could occur. However, based on 1978 census figures, it has been estimated that 50% of women who are 35 years or older would have to use prenatal diagnosis for the incidence of Down syndrome in infants born to women of all ages to decrease from 0.99 per 1,000 births (rate at 0% utilization) to 0.88 (rate at 50% utilization) (Adams et al., 1981).

These predictions may be changed by new developments in routine serum alpha-fetoprotein (AFP) screening. Recent observations (Merkatz, Nitowsky, Macri, & Johnson, 1984) have suggested that there is an association between low maternal serum AFP levels and the presence of chromosome abnormalities in the fetus. The cause of this association is not known. More information is needed to determine the reliability of this observation. If true, as serum AFP screening at 16–18 weeks of gestation becomes a part of routine prenatal care, more fetuses with trisomy 21 will be identified in "young" pregnant women who would not otherwise have had prenatal testing by amniocentesis.

An increase in the incidence of infants born with Down syndrome is projected to occur in the 1980s and 1990s as women born in the "baby boom" that followed World War II reach age 35 (Huether, 1983). This increase will occur unless there is a significant increase in prenatal screening both by amniocentesis and serum AFP. At present, there are not enough facilities for carrying out these tests to meet the projected need. This may lead to an increase in the portion of prenatal testing done in commercial laboratories rather than academic institutions.

Table 1. Status of infants/fetuses at Brigham and Women's Hospital, 1979–1984

Classification	1979	1980	1981	1982	1983	1984
Infants/fetuses with Down syndrome (total)	13	17	10	10	24	23
Liveborn	12	13	6	4	7	10
Stillborn/neonatal death	1	0	1	1	0	1
Therapeutic abortion	0	4	2	5	17	11
Status unknown	0	0	1	0	0	1
All infants/fetuses	6,263	6,533	7,363	7,687	8,302	8,600
Frequency of Down syndrome per 1,000	2.1	2.6	1.4	1.3	2.9	2.7

SECULAR TRENDS

The possibility of a different frequency of Down syndrome in different ethnic and racial groups has been evaluated in only a few studies. Hook (1982) reported that there are no significant differences between blacks and whites in Atlanta. He noted two instances of variation: in New Zealand, a lower rate among Maoris than Europeans; and, in Israel, a lower rate among Jewish mothers of European origin in comparison to non-European mothers. In both of these examples, there are questions about the completeness of the information, and a need for further study.

Several studies have suggested that there is seasonality in the birth of infants with Down syndrome, while others have shown no such variation. The lack of consistency in the observations is the most impressive aspect (Hook, 1982).

Since the risk for Down syndrome increases with maternal age, a crude association with birth order is to be expected. However, after correcting for maternal age, there is no conclusive evidence of a birth order effect (Hook, 1982).

To date, socioeconomic factors have not been correlated with the occurrence of Down syndrome. Hook (1982) noted, as was cited earlier, that, in Israel, there was a higher rate of occurrence among non-European women than European women; the non-European women also had a lower socioeconomic status than did the European women. Unfortunately, it has been difficult to separate and identify ethnic, cultural, and economic factors in this population. In the United States, the National Collaborative Perinatal Project found no evidence of a significant socioeconomic association among 55,000 births between 1959 and 1965 (Sever, Gilkeson, Chen, Ley, & Edwards, 1970).

ETIOLOGICAL FACTORS

With the improvement in cytogenetic techniques, it has been possible in most families to determine whether the extra 21 chromosome came from the mother or the father. Among 369 cases of trisomy 21, maternal nondisjunction accounted for 79.1% and paternal nondisjunction for 20.9% (Juberg & Mowrey, 1983). Among those of maternal origin, the nondisjunction occurred at the first meiotic division in 77%; and among those of paternal origin, the nondisjunction occurred at the first meiotic division in 60% (Juberg & Mowrey, 1983). Among spontaneous abortuses with trisomy 21, the same pattern (i.e., a much higher frequency of maternal origin and errors in first meiotic division) is true (Hassold & Jacobs, 1984). This information about the origin of the extra chromosome should make it possible to identify the underlying etiological factors. Several have been proposed.

Maternal Age

Figure 1 shows an increase in the rate of births of infants with Down syndrome for each maternal age interval, a vivid reminder of the association with maternal age. To the author's knowledge, there is not enough data to draw a similar figure using information from families in which the maternal origin of the extra chromosome has been determined. The figure has been interpreted to

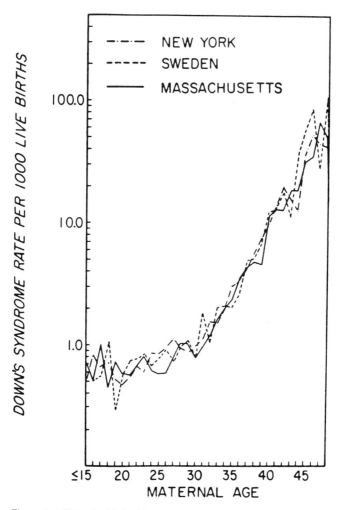

Figure 1.   Rates for birth of infants with Down syndrome by single-year maternal age intervals in three studies. (From: Hook, E. B. [1982]. Epidemiology of Down syndrome. In S. M. Pueschel & J. E. Rynders [Eds.], *Advances in biomedicine and the behavioral sciences*. Cambridge, MA: Ware Press; reprinted by permission.)

show three components of change: between ages 20 and 30 years, a slight increase; above 30, an exponential increase; and below 20, some fluctuation among data from different studies (Hook, 1982). The cause of the correlation with maternal age is not known.

The availability of information as to the parental source of the nondisjunction has not clarified the situation. As noted earlier, in the compilation of information on 369 cases of Down syndrome, the average age of all groups of parents was increased in comparison to controls (Juberg & Mowrey, 1983). When there was paternal origin of nondisjunction, there was no lower parental age (either maternal or paternal) as had been expected (Hook, 1985). Furthermore, one would have predicted that the maternal age would be higher for nondisjunctional errors that arose in the first meiotic division, as these errors have been attributed to the long interval between the time the eggs reached this stage *in utero* and the time after puberty when meiosis continued (Juberg & Mowrey, 1983). However, no increase in maternal age was observed for first meiotic division errors in comparison to second meiotic errors.

One possible explanation of the effect of maternal age is that with increasing age there is more fertilization of +21 gametes and/or a preferential survival *in utero* of trisomy 21 embryos and fetuses (Hook, 1985). More information is needed to determine whether this explanation is correct.

Paternal Age

It is difficult to separate the effect of the age of the father from the effect of the age of the mother. In families in which the paternal origin of the extra 21 chromosome was known, no advanced paternal age was demonstrated.

In two epidemiological studies (Matsunage & Maruyama, 1969; Stene et al., 1977), a strong paternal age effect was seen among men aged 55 years and older. However, several questions have been raised about the methods of analysis used (Hook, 1985), so the issue of paternal age effect remains unresolved.

Ionizing Radiation

Uchida (1981) and others have postulated that the cumulative effects of background radiation over time contribute to the observed increase in Down syndrome with increasing maternal age. However, Hook (1985) considers the evidence for an association with ionizing radiation to be variable and inconsistent.

Furthermore, there was no evidence that exposure to high levels of ionizing radiation at Hiroshima and Nagasaki, in August, 1945, had an effect on the occurrence of Down syndrome in these cities (Schull & Neel, 1962).

Genetic Predisposition

Parents who have had one child with trisomy 21 have an increased risk (about 1%) of having a second affected child. Penrose (1961) was the first to suggest that genes could predispose to nondisjunction. More recent studies have considered whether inbreeding, and presumably autosomal recessive genes, could cause a higher rate of occurrence of Down syndrome. Among the Amish population in the United States, two groups (Juberg & Davis, 1970; Kwitterovich, Cross, & McKusick, 1966) found no increase in the frequency of Down syndrome in comparison to outbred populations of similar European background.

Nucleolus Organizing Region

It has been suggested that the presence of double nucleolus organizing regions (NOR) variants in the chromosomes of parents can increase significantly their risk of having children with Down syndrome (Jackson-Cook, Flannery, Corey, Nance, & Brown, 1984). The evidence supporting this is the fact that there is a much higher frequency of double NOR variants among these parents in comparison to controls. Furthermore, the higher frequency is primarily in the parent from whom the extra 21 chromosome was derived.

The correlation with the size of the NOR is intriguing as this region is known to relate to nonrandom associations between chromosomes, especially chromosomes 13, 14, 15, 21, and 22. The five pairs of acrocentric chromosomes have these regions, which are sites of clusters of ribosomal RNA genes and are located primarily on the stalks of the satellites of these chromosomes. A persistence of nucleolar organizers in older women as a factor in the effect of aging was postulated by Evans in 1967.

If the role of the double NOR as a risk factor for nondisjunction is confirmed in future studies, one could propose screening of ''young'' couples to identify those with an increased risk. However, the technology needed to make this screening cost-effective is not yet available.

REFERENCES

Adams, M. M., Erickson, J. D., Layde, P. M., & Oakley, G. P. (1981). Down's syndrome: Recent trends in the United States. *Journal of the American Medical Association, 246,* 758–760.

Evans, H. J. (1967). The nucleolus virus infection and trisomy in man. *Nature, 214,* 361–363.

Hassold, T. J., & Jacobs, P. A. (1984). Trisomy in man. *Annual Review of Genetics, 18,* 69–97.

Hook, E. B. (1982). Epidemiology of Down syndrome. In S. M. Pueschel & J. E. Rynders (Eds.), *Advances in biomedicine and the behavioral sciences* (pp. 11–88). Cambridge, MA: Ware Press.

Hook, E. B. (1985). Maternal age, paternal age and human chromosome abnormality: Nature, magnitude, etiology, and mechanisms of effect. In V. L. Dellarco, P. E. Voytek, & A. Hollaender (Eds.), *Aneuploidy: Etiology and mechanisms* (pp. 117–132). New York: Plenum Press.

Huether, C. A. (1983). Projection of Down's syndrome births in the United States 1979–2000, and the potential effects of prenatal diagnosis. *American Journal of Public Health, 73,* 1186–1189.

Huether, C. A., Gummere, G. R., Hook, E. B., Dignan, P. St. J., Volodkevich, H., Barg, M., Ludwig, D. A., & Lamson, S. H. (1981). Down's syndrome: Percentage reporting on birth certificates and single year maternal age risk rates for Ohio 1970–79: Comparison with upstate New York data. *American Journal of Public Health, 71,* 1367–1372.

Jackson-Cook, C. K., Flannery, D. D., Corey, L. A., Nance, W. E., & Brown, J. A. (1984). The double NOR variant: A risk factor in trisomy 21. *American Journal of Human Genetics, 36* (Suppl.), 97S.

Juberg, R. C., & Davis, L. M. (1970). Etiology of nondisjunction: Lack of evidence for genetic control. *Cytogenetics, 9,* 284–293.

Juberg, R. C., & Mowrey, P. N. (1983). Origin of nondisjunction of trisomy 21 syndrome: All studies compiled, parental age analysis, and international comparisons. *American Journal of Medical Genetics, 16,* 111–116.

Kuroki, Y., Yamamoto, Y., Matsui, I., & Kurita, T. (1977). Down syndrome and maternal age in Japan, 1950–1973. *Clinical Genetics, 12,* 43–46.

Kwitterovich, P. O., Cross, H. E., & McKusick, V. A. (1966). Mongolism in an inbred population. *Bulletin of Johns Hopkins Hospital, 119,* 269–275.

Lowry, R. B., Jones, D. C., Renwick, D. H. G., & Trimble, B. K. (1976). Down syndrome in British Columbia, 1952–1973: Incidence and mean maternal age. *Teratology, 14,* 29–34.

Matsunage, E., & Maruyama, T. (1969). Human sexual behavior, delayed fertilization, and Down's syndrome. *Nature, 221,* 642–644.

Merkatz, I. R., Nitowsky, H. M., Macri, J. N., & Johnson, W. E. (1984). An association between low maternal serum α-fetoprotein and fetal chromosomal abnormalities. *American Journal of Obstetrics and Gynecology, 148,* 886–894.

Mikkelsen, M. (1977). Down syndrome: Cytogenetical epidemiology. *Hereditas, 86,* 45–50.

Penrose, L. S. (1961). Mongolism. *British Medical Bulletin, 17,* 184–189.

Schull, W. J., & Neel, J. V. (1962). Maternal radiation and mongolism. *Lancet, 1,* 537–538.

Sever, J. L., Gilkeson, M. R., Chen, T. C., Ley, A. C., & Edmonds, D. (1970). Epidemiology of mongolism in the collaborative project. *Annals of the New York Academy of Science, 171,* 328–340.

Stene, J., Fischer, G., Stene, E., Mikkelsen, M., & Petersen, E. (1977). Paternal age effect in Down syndrome. *Annals of Human Genetics, 40,* 299–306.

Uchida, I. A. (1981). Down syndrome and maternal radiation. In F. F. de la Cruz & P. S. Gerald (Eds.), *Trisomy 21 (Down syndrome): Research perspectives* (pp. 201–205). Baltimore: University Park Press.

Venters, M., Schact, L., & ten Bensel, R. (1976). Reporting of Down's syndrome from birth certificate data in the state of Minnesota. *American Journal of Public Health, 66,* 1099.

Demographic Projections for Down Syndrome

Carl Huether

In this response to the numerous items Holmes has covered in Chapter 4, three interrelated issues are considered, and then a brief statement is made on the further development of a new line of research that may be promising. The three issues are: 1) to reinforce Holmes's concern about the problem of obtaining accurate data; 2) to show a little more detail on the importance of demographic change in affecting the incidence and number of Down syndrome births over an 80-year period, 1920–2000; and 3) to show the current effect of prenatal diagnosis on preventing births of infants with Down syndrome, and to present a few models on what effect it may have during the next 15 years.

PROBLEMS IN OBTAINING ACCURATE DATA

To underline Holmes's statements concerning the problems of obtaining accurate data, a case in point is the percentages of both false negative and false positive diagnoses of Down syndrome found on Ohio birth certificates. (A false negative is not designating an individual as having Down syndrome when he or she, in fact, has that status; a false positive is when an individual stated to have the syndrome, in fact, does not.) False negatives were determined from the Ohio data for 1970–1984. Overall, 65.9% (1,070 out of 1,623) of chromosomally analyzed children with Down syndrome were not reported on their birth certificates as having Down syndrome. Statistically significant racial differences existed as well, in that 63% (890 out of 1,409) of whites were false negatives as opposed to 86% (150 out of 175) of blacks. Clearly, physicians are recording (and presumably recognizing) Down syndrome significantly less often in blacks than in whites. For the false negatives, 89.3% were reported as having no congenital malformation, 3.5% had vague diagnoses suggesting Down syndrome (e.g., "protrusion of tongue," "floppy baby," "chromosome abnormality"), and 7.2% had diagnoses that were not suggestive of Down syndrome (e.g., "breech," "cleft lip and palate," "hydrocephaly").

As for false positives, 7.8% (64 out of 824) of overall births were coded as having Down syndrome, but did not. Again, a significant difference existed between races, with 7% (53 out of 770) of whites being false positives, in contrast to 20% (11 out of 54) of blacks. Some individuals listed on their birth certificates as having a "Mongolian spot" or "Simian crease" were coded as having Down syndrome (most were black), while both normal individuals and those with other autosomal aneuploids (trisomies 13 and 18) were misdiagnosed as having Down syndrome. Besides race, maternal age also had a significant effect on whether a false positive occurred; a much higher false positive percentage was found for younger maternal ages than older ones. For mothers under age 30, the percentage was 8.8, while for those older than 30, it was 2.2%, a fourfold difference. (See Johnson et al., 1985 for more discussion of false positives.)

This has helped refine the estimates of single-year maternal age risk rates for Down syndrome in Ohio, some of which are compared in Table 1 to estimates from several different geographic and temporal periods. In all, the data show considerable consistency; the Ohio data are the most recent, and are generally in the middle ranges of the other estimates. The Ohio data base contains over 2,000 individuals with Down syndrome from a 15-year period (1970–1984), and seems to have produced firm maternal age risk rate estimates. One indication of this is that the addition of the last 4 years of data had little effect.

Table 1. Comparison of selected single-year maternal age regression derived risk rates for births of infants with Down syndrome (rates are per 1,000 live births)

Maternal age	Ohio[a] 1970–84	S. Australia[b] 1955–77	Massachusetts[c] 1958–65	Sweden[d] 1968–70	New York[e] 1970–74
20	0.65	0.49	0.57	0.64	0.73
25	0.76	0.67	0.74	0.83	0.87
30	1.22	0.91	0.90	1.08	1.43
35	3.08	2.21	2.53	2.51	3.62
40	10.66	7.64	8.52	9.57	12.20
45	41.44	26.43	28.71	36.55	45.45
≥49	126.00	71.34	75.89	106.76	142.86

[a]Data obtained from Goodwin and Huether (in press).
[b]Data obtained from Sutherland, Clisby, Bloor, and Carter (1979).
[c]Data obtained from Hook and Fabia (1978).
[d]Data obtained from Hook and Lindsjo (1978).
[e]Data obtained from Hook and Chambers (1977).

Table 2.   Comparison of changes in birth incidence of Down syndrome and percentage of such births to women 35 years of age and older among studies in different countries and time periods

Region	Period	Changes in incidence of Down syndrome (per 1,000 live births)	Percentage of births with Down syndrome to women age 35 years and older
United States[a]	1920–1979	2.42 → 1.14	64% → 25%
South Australia[b]	1955–1977	1.25 → 0.90	66% → 30%
England[c]	1961–1979	1.69 → 1.07	55% → 28%
Japan[d]	1962–1975	1.11 → 0.98	32% → 20%
South Belgium[e]	1971–1978	1.27 → 1.19	52% → 33%
British Columbia[f]	1952–1973	Constant	54% → 28%
Denmark[g]	1948–1972	Constant	50% → 33%

[a]Data obtained from Huether and Gummere (1981).
[b]Data obtained from Sutherland, Clisby, Bloor, and Carter (1979).
[c]Data obtained from Owens, Harris, Walker, McAllister, and West (1983).
[d]Data obtained from Tanaka (1969); Kuroki, Yamomoto, Matusi, and Kurita (1977).
[e]Data obtained from Koulischer and Gillerot (1980).
[f]Data obtained from Lowry, Jones, Renwick, and Trimble (1976).
[g]Data obtained from Mikkelson, Fischer, Stene, Stene, and Peterson (1976).

DEMOGRAPHIC CHANGES

To give an idea of just how important demographic changes in population age structure and maternal age birth rates can be, the predicted births of infants with Down syndrome from 1920 to 1979 were calculated on the basis of these two changes alone (Huether & Gummere, 1981). The results showed a dramatic decrease, from 64% to 25%, in births of infants with Down syndrome to women 35 years of age and older. They also showed an equally dramatic change in incidence rate, from over 2.4 per 1,000 live births in 1920 to 1.1 in the 1970s, and in the annual number of births of infants with Down syndrome, from 7,300 in 1957 to 3,800 in 1975. These data are consistent with results found in a number of other countries for various times within this period, as is shown in Table 2.

The latest Census Bureau live birth projection data, published in 1982, as well as the latest estimates of single-year maternal age risk rates from the Ohio data set, have been used to calculate projected births with Down syndrome for the United States to the year 2002 (Goodwin & Huether, in press). Women born in the post–World War II baby boom (i.e., those who were 23–38 years old in 1985) represent a bulge in the population age pyramid. This clearly suggests more births to older women in the future, in part because of their greater number, but also because of the recent trend by many women toward delaying childbearing. Taking these various changes into account, baseline projected births for infants with Down syndrome from 1970 to 2002 in the United States have been calculated, and are shown in Table 3 (these data assume no use of prenatal diagnosis). The projected number of annual births with Down syndrome rises to 5,100 in the 1990s, where it is close to equilibrium. The incidence rate per 1,000 live births also increases from 1.13 to 1.43 for this period; this closely parallels changes in the percentage of infants with Down syndrome born to women aged 35 years and older, which increases from a low of 26% in 1980 to a high of 39% in 2000.

In sum, the estimated number of births with Down syndrome in the United States for the decade of the 1970s was 39,000, with projected births rising to almost 46,000 for the 1980s, and 51,000 for the decade of the 1990s, increases of 17% and 30%, respectively, over the 1970s. Considered by maternal age quinquennia, the data show that the vast majority of the increase will occur in the age categories of 30–34 years and 35–39 years, in which the number of births with Down syndrome will more than double. However, it must be remembered that these are baseline projections that exclude the effect of prenatal diagnosis.

Table 3. Estimated and projected number, incidence, and percentage of births of infants with Down sydrome to women 35 years of age and older in the United States, 1970–2002

Year	Number	Incidence (per 1,000 live births)	Percentage of births with Down syndrome to women age 35 and older
1970	4,750	1.28	38.2
1972	3,950	1.22	34.9
1974	3,650	1.15	30.1
1976	3,600	1.13	27.8
1978	3,750	1.13	26.3
1980	4,100	1.14	25.8
1982	4,300	1.17	27.1
1984	4,550	1.20	28.2
1986	4,750	1.24	29.5
1988	4,950	1.28	30.8
1990	5,100	1.32	32.1
1992	5,150	1.37	33.8
1994	5,150	1.40	35.7
1996	5,100	1.43	37.4
1998	5,050	1.43	38.5
2000	4,950	1.42	38.7
2002	4,900	1.40	38.0

Adapted from Goodwin and Huether (in press).

PRENATAL DIAGNOSIS

What effect prenatal chromosome diagnosis may now be having has been calculated by using recent data on Ohio's amniocentesis utilization. While the literature (see Naber, Huether, & Goodwin, in press) shows Ohio utilization to be substantially less than the other states reported, it may be higher than those not reported; therefore, it may be more or less representative of the national average (Ohio is typically representative of the country for a number of demographic variables). Even though the numbers have increased dramatically since 21 amniocenteses were performed in 1972 to the 2,400 performed in 1983, the utilization by women 35 years of age and older has apparently begun to reach a plateau. The utilization ratio by these women changed from less than 2% in 1975 to 15.8% in 1980, with annual increases to 20.2% in 1981, 22.6% in 1982, and 23.4% in 1983.

In addition to calculating the effect of Ohio's 1983 utilization ratios on reducing projected births for infants with Down syndrome (designated model I), Goodwin and Huether (in press) also looked at the effect of two other amniocentesis utilization models. For women 30–34 years of age, they assumed utilization ratios of 25% and 50% for models II and III, respectively (whereas Ohio's 1983 utilization ratio for these women was 1.7%). For women aged 35 and older, Goodwin and Huether assumed utilization ratios of 50% and 70% relative to Ohio's 1983 utilization rate of 23%. The results given in Table 4 show a maximum reduction in projected births with Down syndrome, using Ohio's 1983 rates, of 9%; but that model II could have as much as a 25% reduction by the year 2000; and model III, up to a 38% reduction. These models may appear overly optimistic, but for at least some reported regions outside the United States, they are currently approaching these values, as suggested by several recent studies (Bell et al., 1985; Bo & Pedersen, 1982; Diernaes & Filtenborg, 1982).

Table 4. Reduction in estimated and projected births of infants with Down syndrome for the United States, assuming different levels of amniocentesis utilization among women age 30–34 and 35 and older, for selected years during 1983–2000

Year	Baseline projections	Model I reduction in:		Model II reduction in:		Model III reduction in:	
		#	(%)	#	(%)	#	(%)
1983	4,411	302	(6.8)	855	(19.4)	1,343	(30.4)
1985	4,653	332	(7.1)	942	(20.2)	1,479	(31.8)
1990	5,095	406	(8.0)	1,152	(22.6)	1,812	(35.6)
1995	5,137	463	(9.0)	1,273	(24.8)	1,982	(38.6)
2000	4,973	470	(9.5)	1,253	(25.2)	1,929	(38.8)

Adapted from Goodwin and Huether (in press).

Amniocentesis utilization may further increase because of the recent and exciting finding that maternal serum alpha-fetoprotein (MSAFP) assay enhances prenatal screening for Down syndrome. Since the initial observation reported by Merkatz, Nitowsky, Macri, and Johnson (1984), at least 10 additional reports have appeared in less than 2 years that have retrospectively compared MSAFP levels between cases of aneuploidy and controls (see Spencer & Carpenter, 1985, for references). The weighted median of these data as reported by Spencer and Carpenter is that the MSAFP for cases of Down syndrome is 0.79 multiple of the control median. As a result, several laboratories are beginning to use low MSAFP to prospectively screen women under 35 years of age, with one state (Connecticut) using a risk of at least 1 in 250 as the criterion for counseling about amniocentesis, based on maternal age, gestational age, MSAFP concentration, and the mother's weight (Baumgarten, Schoenfeld, Mahoney, Greenstein, & Saal, 1985). Although some believe such screening to be premature (e.g., Spencer & Carpenter, 1985), if widely adopted over the next several years, it could substantially increase amniocentesis utilization by women 30–34 years of age, and indeed by those under 30 as well. Further, utilization would be more effective because women recommended for counseling would be at significantly increased risk. Still, models II and III presented in Table 4 assume utilization levels of 25% and 50% respectively, for women 30–34 years of age; this will require just such an additional screening breakthrough, when contrasted with Ohio's 1983 utilization ratio of 1.7%.

FUTURE DEVELOPMENTS

An interesting finding was presented as a poster at the recent aneuploid symposium in Washington, D.C. (March, 1985). In Italy, Bricarelli and co-workers studied 267 persons with Down syndrome who were karyotyped, along with their parents, to determine the origin of the extra chromosome. Their work extended previous findings because they analyzed parental age distributions in both those individuals in whom the extra chromosome was maternally derived and in whom it was paternally derived. When the extra chromosome was maternally derived, a strong maternal age effect but no paternal age effect was observed, very much as expected. When the extra chromosome was paternally derived, no paternal age effect was found, also as expected by most (the author included) who believe there is little or no paternal age effect. However, the data indicated a clear maternal age effect on those births with Down syndrome where the *father* contributed the extra chromosome.

The data are rather small in number, and have yet to be published, but if upheld, would provide strong evidence for another mechanism at work besides nondisjunction to produce the maternal age effect. The most likely post-meiotic age-related mechanism is generally seen to be the loss of capacity to differentially terminate, through spontaneous abortion, abnormal fetuses in older women. The differential loss of abnormal fetuses is well known and has been termed "terathanasia" by teratologist Joseph Warkany (1978), although he did not propose it to be age related. What must be learned is whether this mechanism is indeed age related. If it is, what then is the relative importance of increased nondisjunction vis-à-vis decreased natural terathanasia in producing the maternal age effect? This question of "relaxed selection" in older women has been discussed by Ayme and Lippman-Hand (1982), Ferguson-Smith and Yates (1984), Hook (1983), and others, but no definitive conclusion has yet been reached.

If the prevention of births of children with Down syndrome is the goal, then supplementation of the loss of natural terathanasia seems prudent, and is already available through prenatal chromosome diagnosis and therapeutic termination of affected fetuses. In this regard, perhaps chorionic villus sampling as a new procedure for prenatal chromosomal diagnosis will find an even better reception among older women than amniocentesis has found to date.

REFERENCES

Ayme, S., & Lippman-Hand, A. (1982). Maternal age effect in aneuploidy: Does altered embryonic selection play a role? *American Journal of Human Genetics, 34,* 558–565.

Baumgarten, A., Schoenfeld, M., Mahoney, M. J., Greenstein, R. M., & Saal, H. M. (1985). Prospective screening for Down syndrome using maternal serum AFP. *Lancet, 1,* 1280–1281.

Bell, J. A., Pearn, J., Cohen, G., Ford, J., Halliday, J., Martin, N., Mulcahy, M., Purvis-Smith, S., & Sutherland, G. (1985). Utilization of prenatal cytogenetic diagnosis in women of advanced maternal age in Australia, 1979–1982. *Prenatal Diagnosis, 5,* 53–58.

Bo, J-O., & Pedersen, M. (1982). The frequency of amniocentesis in pregnant women over the age of 35 years in Storstrom. A retrospective investigation of all pregnant women over the age of 35 years from 1.X.1978 to 1.X.1980. *Ugeskr Laeger, 144,* 2218–2219.

Diernaes, E., & Filtenborg, J. (1982). Prenatal diagnosis in the County of Vejle in the period 1978–80. *Ugeskr Laeger, 144,* 2211–2215.

Ferguson-Smith, M., & Yates, J. (1984). Maternal age specific rates for chromosome aberrations and factors influencing them: Report of a collaborative European study on 52,965 amniocenteses. *Prenatal Diagnosis, 4,* 5–44.

Goodwin, B. A., & Huether, C. A. (in press). Revised estimates and projections of Down syndrome births in the United States, and the effect of amniocentesis utilization, 1970–2002. *Prenatal Diagnosis.*

Hook, E. B. (1983). Down syndrome rates and relaxed selection at other maternal ages. American Journal of Human Genetics, 34, 1307–1313.

Hook, E. B., & Chambers, G. M. (1977). Estimated rates of Down's syndrome in live births by one year maternal age intervals for mothers aged 20–29 in a New York

Study: Implications of the risk figures for genetic counseling and cost-benefit analysis of prenatal diagnosis programs. *Birth Defects, 13,* 123–141.

Hook, E. B., & Fabia, J. J. (1978). Frequency of Down syndrome in live births by single-year maternal age interval: Results of a Massachusetts study. *Teratology, 17,* 223–228.

Hook, E. B., & Lindsjo, A. (1978). Down's syndrome in live births by single-year maternal age interval in a Swedish study. *American Journal of Human Genetics, 30,* 19–27.

Huether, C. A., & Gummere, G. R. (1981). Influence of demographic factors on annual Down's syndrome births in Ohio, 1970–1979, and the United States, 1920–1979. *American Journal of Epidemiology, 115,* 846–860.

Johnson, K. M., Huether, C. A., Hook, E. B., Crowe, C. A., Reeder, B. A., Sommer, A., McCorquodale, M. M., & Cross, P. K. (1985). False positive reporting of Down syndrome on Ohio and New York birth certificates. *Genetic Epidemiology, 2,* 123–131.

Koulischer, L., & Gillerot, Y. (1980). Down's syndrome in Wallonia (South Belgium), 1971–1978: Cytogenetics and incidence. *Human Genetics, 54,* 243–250.

Kuroki, Y., Yamomoto, Y., Matusi, I., & Kurita, T. (1977). Down's syndrome and maternal age in Japan 1950–1973. *Clinical Genetics, 12,* 43–46.

Lowry, R. B., Jones, D. C., Renwick, D. H. G., & Trimble, B. K. (1976). Down's syndrome in British Columbia, 1952–1973: Incidence and mean maternal age. *Teratology, 14,* 29.

Merkatz, I. R., Nitowsky, H. M., Macri, J. N., & Johnson, W. E. (1984). An association between low maternal serum alpha-fetoprotein and fetal chromosomal abnormalities. *American Journal of Obstetrics and Gynecology, 148,* 886–894.

Mikkelsen, M., Fischer, G., Stene, J., Stene, E., & Peterson, E. (1976). Incidence study of Down's syndrome in Copenhagen, 1960–1971: With chromosome investigation. *Annals of Human Genetics, 40,* 177–182.

Naber, J. M., Huether, C. A., & Goodwin, B. A. (in press). Temporal changes in Ohio amniocentesis utilization during the first twelve years (1972–1983) and frequency of chromosome abnormalities observed. *Prenatal Diagnosis.*

Owens, J. R., Harris, F., Walker, S., McAllister, E., & West, L. (1983). The incidence of Down's syndrome over a 19-year period with special reference to maternal age. *Journal of Medical Genetics, 20,* 90–93.

Spencer, K., & Carpenter, P. (1985). Screening for Down's syndrome using serum alpha-fetoprotein: A retrospective study indicating caution. *British Medical Journal, 290,* 1940–1943.

Sutherland, G. R., Clisby, S. R., Bloor, G., & Carter, R. F. (1979). Down's syndrome in South Australia. *Medical Journal of Australia, 2,* 58–61.

Tanaka, R. (1969). Incidence and distribution of Down's syndrome in Iwate district, Japan. *Saishin Igaku, 24,* 318–321.

Warkany, J. (1978). Terathanasia. *Teratology, 17,* 187–192.

Chapter 5

Health Concerns in Persons with Down Syndrome

Siegfried M. Pueschel

In past decades, most individuals with Down syndrome were usually not afforded adequate medical care and appropriate educational services. Many children with Down syndrome were institutionalized and they were often deprived of all but the most elementary medical services (e.g., immunizations were incomplete, nutrition was substandard, infections were rampant, and congenital heart disease and other medical problems were rarely treated appropriately). This resulted in a high mortality rate: only 50% of children with Down syndrome survived their first decade of life. Fortunately, there have been major improvements in health care provision during the last 20 years.

HEALTH MAINTENANCE

What is health maintenance? Briefly defined, health maintenance is the active pursuit of optimal well-being in a person. In order to provide health maintenance to individuals with Down syndrome, a number of factors need to be taken into consideration:

1. "Routine" health services such as immunizations and well-child care are of critical importance. Although such services are obvious and taken for granted in any other child, they must be part of a comprehensive health maintenance program for the child with Down syndrome. (In this chapter, these "routine" health care aspects are mentioned briefly without going into detail.)
2. Since congenital anomalies of various systems occur at a higher frequency, and certain medical disorders are more often observed in persons with Down syndrome, specific examinations and screening tests need to be carried out so that they can be identified and treated appropriately before

significant harm to the health of the individual occurs. Some of these specific medical concerns are described in a life cycle approach: for example, a search for congenital anomalies should take place in the newborn period, the detection of visual and hearing deficits needs to be pursued primarily in early childhood, sexual maturation is a topic of adolescence, and the accelerated aging process is observed during the adult years. Obviously, there are some medical conditions such as thyroid disorders, immunological deficiencies, and others that can occur at any time during the life of the person with Down syndrome.

3. Comprehensive health maintenance should focus on the "whole person." Hence, not only the physical well-being should be taken into account, but also the mental and social well-being and other factors in the life of the person that may have a direct or indirect effect on his or her health need the attention of the caregiving professionals.

4. In order to be successful, comprehensive health maintenance requires active participation of the person with Down syndrome, his or her parents, health care providers, and other professionals from the behavioral sciences.

Within the framework of this chapter, it is not possible to cover all medical concerns of the person with Down syndrome and to focus on the many aspects relating to health maintenance in an encyclopedic fashion. Since only the most important factors concerning the health and well-being of the individual with Down syndrome are covered, the reader is referred to other texts (Pueschel & Rynders, 1982; Smith & Berg, 1976) for a more detailed discussion.

HEALTH CONCERNS DURING INFANCY

The Significance of Appropriate Counseling

Parents who are told that their child has Down syndrome frequently experience profound emotional distress. Acute anxiety, desperation, disbelief, and confusion can become manifest in the grieving parents. What was expected as a joyous event, namely, the birth of a healthy infant, can become a catastrophe with profound psychological threads.

Although there is no completely satisfactory way of counseling parents during this initial, extremely traumatic experience, the physician's positive approach, tact, compassion, and truthfulness can have a vital influence on the parents' subsequent adjustment. The physician's style and manner of counseling is of utmost importance in as much as it sets the tone for the atmosphere that will prevail in future years. Using proper terminology and informing both parents together in a sensitive and honest way as soon as the diagnosis has been made are important ingredients of the initial counseling. The critical role of parenthood should be stressed—the chance for the infant to be nurtured and loved by caring parents. In emphasizing that the infant with Down syndrome is, first and foremost, a human being with inherent rights, the physician shows genuine concern, and thus helps the parents see the infant as significant.

Although the counseling process will have a profound impact upon parents, it cannot be an end in itself. Unless subsequent support and guidance are forthcoming, the counseling will have failed in its main objective of ensuring a realistic and positive future for the child (Pueschel & Murphy, 1975).

Neonatal Concerns

Due to the increased frequency of specific congenital anomalies in infants with Down syndrome, there are a number of neonatal concerns that require immediate attention. Some of these conditions may be life-threatening and need to be corrected immediately, whereas others may become apparent during the first few weeks and months subsequent to the child's birth.

Gastrointestinal Anomalies   Of primary importance are congenital anomalies of the gastrointestinal tract. Tracheoesophageal fistulas, duodenal atresia or stenosis, annular pancreas, aganglionic megacolon, and imperforate anus are known to occur more often in infants with Down syndrome than in other children. If nutrients and fluid cannot be absorbed by the infant because of tracheoesophageal abnormalities or duodenal atresia, the infant will starve to death if not operated on promptly.

According to an Australian study (Lynn, 1979), the incidence of duodenal obstruction occurs in 1 of 4,100 live births in the general population, while in Down syndrome it has been reported to be 4 in 100 live births and higher. A study done by Knox and Bensel (1972) showed the incidence of all types of gastrointestinal malformation in Down syndrome to be 12%. Of their 110 infants with Down syndrome, 3 had imperforate anus, another 3 had pyloric stenosis, 2 had aganglionic megacolon, 2 had duodenal atresia/stenosis, 1 had tracheoesophageal fistula, 1 had annular pancreas, 1 had Meckel diverticulum, and 1 had atrophy of the small intestine. Such congenital anomalies of the gastrointestinal tract can and should be corrected surgically. No form of treatment should be withheld from any child with Down syndrome that would be given unhesitatingly to a child without this chromosomal disorder.

Congenital Heart Disease   Congenital heart disease is observed in 30% to 45% of children with Down syndrome. Because of persistence of fetal circulation during the newborn period, clinical manifestations of significant congenital heart disease may not be apparent in the first few days or even weeks of life. Yet it is important that congenital heart disease in infants with Down syndrome be diagnosed as early as possible since some children may develop cardiac failure with concomitant life-threatening complications. Therefore, an electrocardiogram, chest radiograph, and, at times, an echocar-

Table 1. Frequency (%) of various anatomical defects in Down syndrome children with congenital heart disease

Studies conducted	Atrioventricular canal		Ventricular septal defect	Tetralogy of Fallot	Patent ductus arteriosus	Atrial septal defect	Other
	Complete	Partial					
Rowe and Uchida, 1961	36		33	1	10	9	11
Cullum and Liebman, 1969	21		43		10	17	9
Shaher et al., 1972	18		28	5	24	12	13
Tandon and Edwards, 1973	34	16	29	15	2	2	2
Greenwood and Nadas, 1976	23	26	29	8	7	3	4
Park et al., 1977	33	10	32	6	4	10	
Katlic et al., 1977	40		27	8	12	11	2
Buckley, 1983	26	26	28	7	2	11	

From Pueschel, S. M., & Rynders, J. (1982). *Down syndrome: Advances in biomedicine and the behavioral sciences* (p. 205). Cambridge, MA: Ware Press (Now Academic Guild Publishers); reprinted by permission.

diogram and consultation with a pediatric cardiologist are indicated in many newborns with Down syndrome.

The frequency of specific congenital heart defects in children with Down syndrome varies considerably, as seen in Table 1. Most infants with congenital heart disease have an atrioventricular canal; the second most common congenital heart defect is a ventricular septal defect, followed by patent ductus arteriosus, atrial septal defect, and tetralogy of Fallot. A number of other cardiovascular abnormalities have been described by Rosenquist, Sweeney, Amsel, and McAllister (1974) and Rowe and Uchida (1961).

The management of congenital heart disease in children with Down syndrome has changed significantly over the past 20 years. Previously, many cardiologists and cardiac surgeons were reluctant to recommend or perform cardiac surgery in children with Down syndrome. These physicians felt that children with Down syndrome were so severely intellectually handicapped that surgical intervention would not benefit them. Other arguments against cardiac surgery included the children's reduced life expectancy, their unemployability, and financial considerations. However, recent technological advances in cardiovascular surgery and society's altered viewpoint concerning persons with handicaps brought about a marked improvement in the management of congenital heart disease in children with Down syndrome. Physicians caring for these children have recognized that they can lead a meaningful life and deserve to be treated as are other children who do not have this chromosomal disorder. Therefore, appropriate medical management, including administration of digitalis and diuretics, if indicated, and prompt surgical repair of the heart defect at the optimal time will improve the quality of life of the individual with Down syndrome.

Congenital Cataracts Congenital cataracts occur in approximately 3% of children with Down syndrome. It is of utmost importance to identify children with dense congenital cataracts, which must be extracted, followed by appropriate corrections with glasses in order to assure adequate vision.

Since many children with Down syndrome have various ophthalmological disorders including blepharitis, strabismus, nystagmus, hypoplasia of the iris, refractive errors, and retinal problems, it is paramount that they be examined by a competent pediatric ophthalmologist who is able and willing to care for young children with Down syndrome. Mumma (1984) reported that 77% of children with Down syndrome have significant refractive errors, most often myopia; 49% have strabismus; 35% have congenital nystagmus, which could be horizontal, vertical, or rotary in nature; and 20% have blocked tear ducts.

Normal visual acuity is important for any child. However, for the child with mental retardation, an additional handicap of sensory impairment may further limit the child's functioning, and this may prevent him or her from participating in significant learning processes. Therefore, regular ophthalmological follow-up is of importance for children with Down syndrome.

Newborn and Well-Baby Care

As with any other children, infants with Down syndrome need a thorough physical examination in the newborn period, with particular focus on those systems and organs that are frequently affected in children with that disorder. The newborn examination should also include a neurological and neurobehavioral assessment. It is well known that children with significant congenital heart disease and severe hypotonia may have more developmental delay than those children who have normal cardiovascular function and relatively good muscle tone (see Figure 1).

Routine screening tests in the newborn period such as screening for phenylketonuria, galactosemia, and hypothyroidism (in some states, other screening tests for maple syrup urine disease, homocystinuria, etc. are added) should be carried out as they are for other children (Bennett, 1977). Although any of the aforementioned metabolic disorders, with the exception of those affecting the thyroid gland, are very rare, these problems, if detected, can be treated effectively. Congenital hypothyroidism has recently been reported to occur more often in infants with Down syndrome than in the general population (Fort et al., 1984).

Another aspect of routine infant care encompasses regular well-baby checkups, when physical growth, developmental progress, and general well-being of the child can be assessed and discussed with the parents. During these well-baby visits, the pediatrician or other health care provider is also

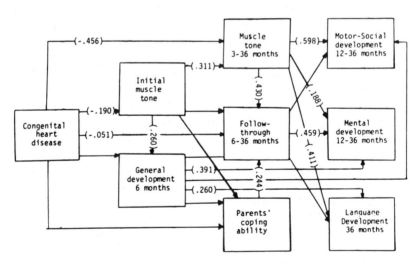

Figure 1. Overall path diagram relating potential causal factors to behavioral outcomes (numerals in parentheses represent the path coefficients). (From: Reed, R. B., Pueschel, S. M., Schnell, R. R., & Cronk, C. E. [1980]. Interrelationships of biological, environmental and competency variables in young children with Down syndrome. *Applied Research in Mental Retardation, 1,* 169. Copyright © 1981 by Pergamon Press, Ltd.; reprinted by permission.)

concerned with nutritional aspects, and a review of respiratory, cardiovascular, gastrointestinal, genitourinary, and neuromuscular systems should take place. The physician should discuss important aspects relating to the social milieu, the child's environment, and other concerns that may affect the physical and emotional well-being of the child.

As with any child, it is during the first few years of life when preventive medicine can be most effective. Parents should be informed of accident prevention, safety in the home, and avoidance of lead poisoning and other environmental hazards that may compromise the child's health.

Ongoing professional support and assistance in the adjustment process are also important for the child's developmental progress. Moreover, early intervention services, environmental enrichment, and other educational involvements that will foster the child's developmental progress need to be discussed. Also, screening for specific disorders more commonly observed in Down syndrome must be considered.

Another important aspect of preventive medicine relates to the immunization of infants. The child with Down syndrome needs the same protection against such diseases as tetanus, diphtheria, pertussis, poliomyelitis, mumps, rubeola, rubella, and Hemophilus influenza B (see Table 2) as do other children. Some children with Down syndrome who frequently have lower

Table 2. Recommended schedule for active immunization of infants and children

Recommended age	Vaccine(s)	Comments
2 months	Diphtheria, Pertussis, Tetanus, Oral Polio	Can be initiated earlier in areas of high endemicity
4 months	Diphtheria, Pertussis, Tetanus, Oral Polio	2-month interval desired for Oral Polio vaccine to avoid interference
6 months	Diphtheria, Pertussis, Tetanus, Oral Polio	Oral Polio vaccine optional for areas where polio might be imported (e.g., some areas of southwestern United States)
12 months	Tuberculin test	May be given simultaneously with MMR at 15 months
15 months	Measles, Mumps, Rubella (MMR)	MMR preferred
18 months	Diphtheria, Pertussis, Tetanus, Oral Polio	Consider as part of primary series
24 months	Hemophilus influenzae type B	
4–6 years	Diphtheria, Pertussis, Tetanus, Oral Polio	
14–16 years	Diphtheria, Tetanus	Repeat every 10 years for lifetime

Adapted from American Academy of Pediatrics. (1982). *Report of the committee on infectious diseases* (19th ed., p. 7). Evanston, IL: Author; reprinted by permission.

respiratory infections may benefit from additional vaccines against influenza virus and pneumococcal disease.

HEALTH CONCERNS DURING CHILDHOOD

Some of the general health care issues discussed in the previous section (infancy period), such as immunization and prevention of accidents, are also of significance throughout childhood. Similarly, certain medical concerns, such as infections, nutrition, and immunological considerations, which are described in the following section, are also important issues during infancy. Obviously, there is no clear-cut distinction of certain health aspects between infancy and later childhood.

Nutritional Considerations

Every person requires a balanced diet and an adequate qualitative and quantitative intake of nutrients, and the child with Down syndrome is no exception. At times, the question arises as to whether the child with Down syndrome requires additional vitamins, minerals, and other nutrients to augment his or her development. There are some reports in the literature that claim that "supplemental nutrients" and large doses of vitamins may benefit the child with Down syndrome (Harrell, Capp, Davis, Peerless, & Ravitz 1981; Turkel, 1975). Yet, other investigators who have pursued this issue scientifically found that supplemental minerals and vitamins (often provided in excess) do not enhance intellectual development in children with Down syndrome (Bennett, McClelland, Kriegsmann, Brazee Andrus, & Sells, 1983; Ellis & Tomporowski, 1983; Smith, Spiker, Peterson, Cicchetti, & Justine, 1984; Weathers, 1983). Although some authors have reported that the child with Down syndrome is deficient in certain trace elements and vitamins (Barlow, Sylvester, & Dickerson, 1981; Matin, Sylvester, Edwards, & Dickerson, 1984; Milunsky, Hackley, & Halsted, 1970), this is a controversial subject and recent investigations using modern methodology have cast doubt on results from some previous reports.

Sometimes feeding problems may be encountered in infants with Down syndrome, which may result in poor weight gain. However, increased weight often becomes apparent in many youngsters with Down syndrome as they grow older, in particular during the adolescent years. Therefore, it is important to educate parents concerning an appropriate caloric intake concomitant with physical exercise, in order to avoid undernutrition or excessive weight gain. Good eating habits, a balanced diet, avoidance of high caloric foods, and regular physical activities can prevent the child from becoming obese.

Infectious Diseases

Reports from the literature indicate that infectious diseases were responsible for the previously observed increased mortality in Down syndrome. Deaton (1973) reported that 30% of deaths of institutionalized persons with Down syndrome were due to infections. Increased immunoglobulins, in particular IgG, have been found in persons with Down syndrome (Rundle, Clothier, & Sudell, 1971; Skanse & Laurell, 1962), which were thought to be caused by an increased rate of infections.

There are numerous reports in the literature discussing a high prevalence of respiratory infections in children with Down syndrome. Although children with significant congenital heart disease and nutritional deficiencies generally have more respiratory infections, the author has found that the vast majority of children with Down syndrome who do not have congenital heart disease and who are provided with optimal health maintenance do not have more respiratory infections than children of equivalent age who do not have Down syndrome. Similarly, otitis media has been thought to occur more frequently in children with Down syndrome. Yet Pueschel (1984) showed that young children with Down syndrome have otitis media approximately as often as a control population, although fluid accumulation in the middle ear is a common finding in children with Down syndrome. Skin infections are more often observed in adolescents with Down syndrome; in particular, pyogenic skin infections at the thighs, buttocks, and the perianal area are common. Regular hygiene, frequent sitz baths, and topical (rarely systemic) antibiotic treatment are recommended.

Because some reports found an increased frequency of infectious disorders in persons with Down syndrome, some researchers investigated their immune system (Ablin, 1978; Jacobs, Burdash, Manos, & Duncan, 1978). Levin, Nir, and Mogilner (1975) noted the T cell functions of neonates with Down syndrome to be impaired. These investigators observed a decreased release of leukocyte migration-inhibition factors in response to phytohemagglutinine. B lymphocytes, however, were found to be normal in number and class. Whittingham, Pitt, Sharma, and Mackay (1977) did not find an increased percentage of IgG-bearing B cells in individuals with Down syndrome. They reported that the cutaneous delayed hypersensitivity is abnormal and up to 57% of persons with Down syndrome show some degree of anergy. Whittingham and co-investigators thought that the immune system in persons with Down syndrome is stressed and eventually begins to fail. Hann, Deakon, and London (1979) felt that the finding of a lower number of B lymphocytes, particularly IgM-bearing lymphocytes, might explain the decreased IgM concentration noted in some older individuals with Down syndrome. Gershwin, Crinella, Castles, and Trent (1977) observed decreased thymidine uptake and decreased deoxyribonucleic acid polymerase activity of lymphocytes in persons with Down syndrome in response to phytohemagglutinine stimulation, suggesting T cell hyporesponsiveness. These authors described a "loose association" between reduction in T cells and HLA-B8. It appears that T cell and probably B cell functions in individuals with Down syndrome are abnormal, and that some of these immunological aberrations may cause some children with Down syndrome to be more susceptible to infectious disorders.

Hearing Impairment

Previous investigations (Fulton & Lloyd, 1968; Glovsky, 1966; Rigrodsky, Prunty, & Glovsky, 1961) reported hearing impairment in 15% to 50% of persons with Down syndrome. In the last decade, newly developed assessment techniques have permitted investigators to evaluate children's hearing abilities in more varied ways. Brooks, Wooley, and Kanjilal (1972) employed impedance tympanometry and found that only 23% of patients with Down syndrome had normal hearing. Schwartz and Schwartz (1978) examined 39 home-reared children with Down syndrome, using pneumo-ostoscopy and acoustic impedance techniques, and noted that more than 60% of the children had middle ear effusion. Similarly, Balkany, Downs, Jafek, and Krajicek (1979), employing otoscopy, audiometry, and impedance tympanometry, found 78% of persons with Down syndrome to display some hearing loss. The vast majority had a conductive hearing impairment and the degree of hearing loss was mild to moderate, ranging from 15 to 40 dB. It was also reported that some children with Down syndrome had significant middle ear abnormalities, including fixation and superstructure deformity of the stapes and dehiscence of the Fallopian canal (Balkany, Mischke, & Downs, 1979).

There are numerous factors that are responsible for increased fluid accumulation in the middle ear with resulting hearing impairment in children with Down syndrome. Insufficient muscle control in the hypopharynx has been described, which affects Eustachian tube function and does not allow the pressure in the middle ear to equalize. A blocked Eustachian tube then often results in negative middle ear pressure, which gives way to secretion of a mucoid fluid from the lining of the middle ear space. If the fluid remains in the middle ear long enough, it may have a permanent effect on hearing.

The etiology of middle ear problems in children with Down syndrome has also been discussed by Schwartz and Schwartz (1978). These authors maintained that the tensor veli palatini muscle is part of the generalized muscular hypotonia and is contributing to Eustachian tube dysfunction, and that, in addition, the abnormal immune response in children with Down syndrome may contribute to the observed middle ear pathology.

Although treatment approaches to middle ear effusions vary considerably, it is generally accepted that conservative treatment is attempted before more aggressive therapeutic steps are considered. Decongestants usually are not effective, however, antibiotic treatment for long time periods have been found to be helpful. If there is no response to conservative treatment, the fluid can be removed surgically by the placement of ventilation tubes into the middle ear.

Since the significance of hearing impairment in young children with Down syndrome lies in its effect on all phases of psychological and emotional development, proper assessment of audiological functions and remediation, if a hearing loss is uncovered, are of paramount importance. It has been well documented that even a mild conductive hearing deficit can lead to a reduced rate of language development and secondary interpersonal problems.

Dental Considerations

In children with Down syndrome, the eruption of primary and secondary dentition is usually delayed and an abnormal sequence of tooth eruption occurs more frequently (Schulze, 1970; Shapiro, 1970). According to Roche and Barkla (1964), partial odontia is observed in children with Down syndrome at least four to five times more often than in a control group of children. There is also an increased incidence (35%–55%) of microdontia (Kisling, 1966; Spitzer & Mann, 1950). Previous reports indicated a high rate of periodontal disease in persons with Down syndrome (Cohen, Winer, Schwartz, & Sklar, 1961). Also, Cutress (1971) found a relatively high frequency of periodontal disease in institutionalized persons with Down syndorme; however, a relatively low prevalence of periodontal disorders was noted among individuals with this chromosomal disorder residing in the community. According to Cutress (1971), both a factor inherent in trisomy 21 and an environmental factor are responsible for the increased susceptibility to periodontal disease.

Cohen et al. (1961) have suggested that persons with Down syndrome are less susceptible to dental caries. However, when correction factors are utilized to account for the discrepancy between chronological age and post-eruptive tooth age, the difference of the caries rate between subjects with or without Down syndrome disappears or is greatly decreased in most instances (Orner, 1974).

Regular dental examinations, appropriate dental hygiene, fluoride treatments, restorative care, if needed, and good dietary habits will help prevent dental caries and periodontal disease in children with Down syndrome.

Thyroid Dysfunction

There are numerous reports in the literature of thyroid dysfunction in Down syndrome. The prevalence of thyroid problems has been reported to vary from 3% to 50%, depending on: the type of study, whether children were examined clinically, whether specific thyroid function studies were carried out, and the particular age group studied. If more refined thyroid studies are employed or if an older population of persons with Down syndrome is tested, a higher prevalence of thyroid disorders will be found. The studies of Pueschel and Pezzullo (1985) provided evidence that thyroid disorders are more frequently observed in individuals with Down syndrome (see Table 3). Although autoimmune phenomena might play a role in the development of thyroid dysfunction in individuals with Down syndrome, the underlying pathogenic mechanisms are not well understood.

Table 3. Number of patients with abnormal and normal TSH and/or T_4 values, contrasting ATA and/or AMA results

	Increased titers of ATA & AMA	Increased titers of ATA	Increased titers of AMA	No ATA and no AMA	Total
Increased TSH and decreased T_4	1	0	7	2	10
Increased TSH and normal T_4	2	0	4	15	21
Normal TSH and increased T_4	3	0	1	3	7
Normal TSH and decreased T_4	0	0	1	2	3
Normal TSH and normal T_4	8	5	15	82	110
Total	14	5	28	104	151

While much of the literature that has accumulated during the past decades on thyroid function of persons with Down syndrome indicates that the majority of children with this chromosome disorder are euthyroid, it is important to identify youngsters with thyroid disorders since hypothyroidism may compromise normal central nervous system function (Pueschel & Pezzullo, 1985). Because clinical symptoms of hypothyroidism are sometimes interpreted as being part of the "Down syndrome Gestalt," thyroid function studies should be obtained at regular intervals including T_4, TSH, and others if indicated. If a person with Down syndrome is found to be hypothyroid, prompt thyroid treatment should be instituted. Optimal thyroid function will then allow normal learning processes to take place.

Skeletal Problems

Skeletal abnormalities in persons with Down syndrome are common and may be found in many parts of the body. They include hypoplasia of maxillary and sphenoid bones, rib abnormalities, absence of ribs, structurally altered pelvis with reduced acetabular angles, hip dislocation, and patella subluxation.

Another skeletal abnormality that has been discussed more frequently in recent years involves the upper cervical spine segment. Because of the increased laxity of the transverse ligaments between the atlas and the odontoid process, atlantoaxial instability has been observed in many children with Down syndrome (Pueschel, Scola, Perry, & Pezzullo, 1981). By definition, atlantoaxial instability is present when the shortest distance between the posterior-inferior aspect of the anterior arch of the atlas and the adjacent anterior surface of the odontoid process is 5 mm or more. Atlantoaxial instability is found in 12%–20% of persons with Down syndrome. The majority of these individuals do not display symptoms (Pueschel, 1983). A follow-up study of 37 children with Down syndrome who have asymptomatic atlantoaxial instability (Pueschel, unpublished observations) did not detect any significant changes in their neurological functions over a 5-year period.

In contrast to the asymptomatic condition, only 1%–2% of individuals with Down syndrome have symptomatic atlantoaxial subluxation. In these individuals, the joint interval between the anterior arch of the atlas and the odontoid process is usually more than 6 mm; the majority of them have a joint interval of approximately 10 mm. Many persons with symptomatic atlantoaxial subluxation display pyramidal tract signs including hyperreflexia, a positive Babinski sign, ankle clonus, muscle weakness, abnormal gait, and difficulties with walking. Some individuals also complain of neck discomfort, limited neck mobility, and may exhibit a head tilt resembling torticollis. It is generally agreed that persons with symptomatic atlantoaxial subluxation should undergo surgery whereby pre-operative reduction of the subluxation is followed by spinal fusion using wire and autogenous bone graft.

Children with asymptomatic atlantoaxial instability usually do not require surgery. However, these children should not engage in contact sports, somersaults, trampoline exercise, diving, and a number of other activities that could potentially lead to cervical spine injury.

It is of importance that atlantoaxial instability in individuals with Down syndrome be identified early because of its relatively high prevalence and its potential for remediation. Therefore, the author recommends that cervical spine radiographs be obtained in all persons with Down syndrome aged 2 years and older. The majority of these individuals may have difficulty verbalizing specific complaints relating to neck discomfort and neuromotor difficulties. Sometimes, their motor dysfunction and broad-based gait may conceal significant neurological concerns. Therefore, it is important to diagnose children with atlantoaxial subluxation, since a delay in recognizing this condition may result in irreversible spinal cord damage.

Maturation During Adolescence

Adolescence is frequently a challenge for both the young person with Down syndrome and his or her family. While this may be a very troublesome time period for those of normal intellectual abilities, in adolescents with Down syndrome these problems are frequently intensified. Adolescents with Down syndrome have many physical attributes of "normal" youngsters, but often do not possess the intellectual or behavioral capabilities to cope with either the demands of the environment or their own desire for independence. They are faced with preparing for vocational competence as well as developing an array of social skills needed to function in society.

In studies of adolescent development in males with Down syndrome (Pueschel, Orson, Boylan, & Pezzullo 1985), the subjects' secondary sex characteristics were found to be similar to that of youngsters who did not have this chromosomal disorder. However, the axillary hair development and the emergence of facial hair, particularly mustache development, were delayed in the study population when compared with "normal" subjects. There was no statistically significant difference between the size of the genitalia of adolescents with Down syndrome and that of normal controls. Concerning hormone measurements, the serum follicle stimulating hormone, luteinizing hormone, and testosterone levels in the study cohort increased with advancing age up to 18 years, which is similar to those hormonal changes observed in normal adolescents (Pueschel et al., 1985).

Although the subjects with Down syndrome displayed normal sequential development of primary and secondary sex characteristics and their pituitary-gonadal axis appeared to be intact, there were still many unanswered questions about the adolescents' sexual function, libido, sperm production, and fertility. Since most individuals with Down syndrome now live in the community, with all its risks, opportunities, and freedoms, it is paramount that further studies concerning sexual development be pursued.

With regard to sexual maturation of females with Down syndrome, studies revealed that the average onset of menstruation in the majority of females with Down syndrome was 12 years, 6 months, while the average menarche of nonhandicapped females was 12 years, 1 month. Most of the girls with Down syndrome had regular menstrual cycles. The length of the menstrual cycle varied between 22 and 33 days with a mean of 27 days. On the average, menstrual flow lasted about 4 days. Two-thirds of the adolescent girls with Down syndrome had concomitant symptoms such as behavior changes, headaches, and abdominal bloating. Most of them did not require help with menstrual hygiene (Scola & Pueschel, 1985).

Ovulatory patterns of women with Down syndrome were studied by Tricomi, Valenti, and Hall (1964). These investigators found that 38.5% of the women showed a definite pattern of ovulation, 15.4% probably ovulated, another 15.4% possibly ovulated, and 30.7% had no evidence of ovulation. Reports from the literature indicate that there have been 30 pregnancies in 26 women with Down syndrome, suggesting adequate ovarian function in at least some of the females with Down syndrome (Bovicelli, Orsini, Rizzo, Montacuti, & Bacchetta, 1982).

In the author's investigations of parental perceptions of social interactions, interest in the opposite sex, and sexual functions in persons with Down syndrome, he found that more than half of the study population showed interest in the opposite sex and were attending social gatherings. Many of the youngsters with Down syndrome had expressed a desire to marry; however, only a few had an interest in sexual relationships.

HEALTH CONCERNS IN ADULTS WITH DOWN SYNDROME

Appropriate nutrition, regular exercise, prevention of infectious diseases, testing for thyroid disorders, identification of skeletal abnormalities, routine dental examinations, and other health maintenance concerns just discussed are as important in adults as in younger individuals with Down syndrome. Three conditions need particular mention:

1. A high frequency (30%–60%) of acquired cataracts have been reported in adults with Down syndrome. Most cataractous changes, however, rarely become dense enough to warrant surgical intervention.
2. Hypothyroidism is more often observed in adults with Down syndrome than in younger children. Therefore, thyroid function tests should be carried out in these individuals at regular intervals, at least yearly.
3. Mitral valve prolapse and aortic regurgitation have been found to be more prevalent in adults with Down syndrome, necessitating regular cardiac examinations.

Another condition that deserves special attention in the adult with Down syndrome is related to the aging process. For more than a century, it has been known that persons with Down syndrome age more rapidly than those who do not have this chromosome disorder. In the last 20 years, there have been many reports in the literature indicating a high prevalence of Alzheimer disease in adults with Down syndrome. Malamud (1964) reported that almost 100% of the autopsies of 35 persons with Down syndrome 40 years and older had Alzheimer disease, in contrast to only 14% of a comparable mentally retarded non–Down syndrome group. Also, Burger and Vogel (1973) acknowledged full development of Alzheimer morphology in individuals with Down syndrome. They found senile plaques beginning even in the second and third decades of life. They also noted neurofibrillary changes, senile plaques, and granulovacular degenerations in the hippocampal region in persons with Down syndrome.

Although neuropathological specimens from autopsies indicate that persons with Down syndrome have the neurohistological substrate of Alzheimer disease, one cannot state categorically that Alzheimer disease is present in all persons with Down syndrome beyond the age of 30 or 40. There are reports from institutions for persons with mental retardation that some elderly persons with Down syndrome are as normal as their juniors and hardly ever exhibit the personality changes or psychological problems observed in Alzheimer disease. Ellis, McCulloch, and Corley (1974) indicated that the detection of dementia in the presence of longstanding mental retardation may be difficult. In spite of these difficulties, some observations of early signs of Alzheimer disease have been reported in persons with Down syndrome. Francis (1970) noted an increase in self-oriented behavior and a decrease in attention to external events in persons with Down syndrome. In another study, Owens, Dawson, and Losin (1971) found significant differences between a group of 35- to 50-year-olds and a group of 20- to 25-year-olds with Down syndrome. The older group gave poorer responses for identification of authority and displayed a positive Babinski sign. Also, Dalton, Crapper, and Schlotterer (1974) found evidence of memory loss in a group of persons with Down syndrome between the age of 44 and 58 years that was similar to that exhibited by nonretarded persons with Alzheimer disease. Dalton and Crapper (1977) extended their studies over a 3-year period, during which 4 of the 11 older individuals with Down syndrome deteriorated to a point at which they could not learn a simple discrimination task. They also found that 5 of 11 older subjects with Down syndrome actually improved on their memory test over the 3-year period.

In a prospective study, Dalton (1982) examined 49 persons with Down syndrome who were 40 years of age and older. Dalton reported a prevalence rate of 22% of memory loss in these individuals. From these and other data that he had obtained previously, he determined that the average rate of onset of memory failure was 49.1 years, with a standard deviation of 6 years. Dalton concluded that there was no simple relation between age and onset of memory changes in Down syndrome. He found many persons with Down syndrome over the age of 40 who did not show any evidence of memory change and cited three persons who were 62, 63, and 71 years of age, respectively, who did not display any deterioration of mental abilities.

Another clinical study of dementia in Down syndrome was carried out by Thase, Liss, Smeltzer, and Maloon (1982). These investigators observed that persons with Down syndrome had significantly greater impairment on measures of orientation, attention span, digit span recall, visual memory, and object identification. They were also more likely to have pathological reflexes when compared with age- and IQ-matched controls.

It has been suggested that there is a genetic interrelation between Alzheimer disease and Down syndrome. An excess of persons with Down syndrome was found in families who had a proband with Alzheimer disease, and an increased prevalence of Alzheimer disease has been noted in families who have a child with Down syndrome.

An interesting hypothesis that attempts to explain the accelerated aging process in persons with Down syndrome has been developed by Lott (1982). This author stated that increased superoxide dismutase activity in cells of individuals with Down syndrome leads to higher intracellular concentrations of peroxide and superoxide, which are potentially capable of pathologically interacting with many structural elements of the cell, thus leading to early aging. As did many other investigators, Sinet (1982) found an excess of superoxide dismutase in persons with trisomy 21, which, according to Sinet, could lead to oxidative damage and other cell dysfunction, resulting in rapid aging with brain lesions similar to those observed in Alzheimer disease. Other authors have studied cortical cholinergic innervation in relation to Alzheimer disease in Down syndrome. Bartus, Dean, Beer, and Lippa (1982) presented biochemical, electrophysiological, and pharmacological evidence for cholinergic dysfunction in age-related memory disturbance. Also Coyle, Price, and DeLong (1983) found that acetylcholine-releasing neurons selectively degenerate.

Although there is ample evidence that persons with Down syndrome age earlier and that many of these individuals have neuropathological findings that resemble Alzheimer disease, there is an urgent need for further studies. Investigations should focus on the elucidation of pathogenetic mechanisms and therapeutic strategies that could prevent the neuronal insult that may lead to Alzheimer disease in persons with Down syndrome.

SUMMARY

This chapter has emphasized the importance of optimal health maintenance by fostering the well-being of persons with Down syndrome in all areas of human functioning. If provided with appropriate health services, individuals with Down syndrome can live a more meaningful life and can contribute more fully to society.

REFERENCES

Ablin, J. R. (1978). Immunity in Down's syndrome. *European Journal of Pediatrics, 27,* 149–152.

American Academy of Pediatrics. (1982). *Report of the committee on infectious diseases* (19th ed., p. 7). Evanston, IL: Author.

Balkany, T. J., Downs, M. P., Jafek, B. W., & Krajicek, M. J. (1979). Hearing loss in Down syndrome: A treatable handicap more common than generally recognized. *Clinical Pediatrics, 18,* 116–118.

Balkany, T. J., Mischke, R. E., & Downs, M. P. (1979). Ossicular abnormalities in Down syndrome. *Otolaryngology and Head and Neck Surgery, 87,* 372–384.

Barlow, P. J., Sylvester, P. E., & Dickerson, J. W. T. (1981). Hair trace metal levels in Down syndrome patients. *Journal of Mental Deficiency Research, 25,* 161–168.

Bartus, R. T., Dean, R. L., III, Beer, B., & Lippa, A. S. The cholinergic hypothesis of geriatric memory dysfunction. *Science, 217,* 408–417.

Bennett, A. J. E. (1977). New England Regional Newborn Screening Program. *New England Journal of Medicine, 297,* 1178–1179.

Bennett, F. C., McClelland, S., Kriegsmann, E. A., Brazee Andrus, L., & Sells, C. J. (1983). Vitamin and mineral supplementation in Down's syndrome. *Pediatrics, 72,* 707–713.

Berg, J. M., Crome, L., & France, N. E. (1960). Congenital cardiac malformations in mongolism. *British Heart Journal, 22,* 331–346.

Bovicelli, L., Orsini, L. F., Rizzo, N., Montacuti, V., & Bacchetta, M. (1982). Reproduction in Down syndrome. *Obstetrics & Gynecology, 59,* 135–175.

Brooks, D. N., Wooley, H., & Kanjilal, G. C. (1972). Hearing loss and middle ear disorders in patients with Down's syndrome (mongolism). *Journal of Mental Deficiency Research, 16,* 21–29.

Burger, P. C., & Vogel, F. S. (1973). The development of the pathologic changes of Alzheimer's disease and senile dementia in patients with Down's syndrome. *American Journal of Pathology, 73,* 457–475.

Buckley, L. P. (1983). Congenital heart disease in infants with Down syndrome. In S. M. Pueschel (Ed.), *A study of the young child with Down syndrome.* New York: Human Science Press.

Cohen, M. M., Winer, R. A., Schwartz, S. I., & Sklar, G. (1961). Oral aspects of mongolism. *Oral Surgery, 14,* 92–98.

Coyle, J. T., Price, D. L., & DeLong, M. R. (1983). Alzheimer's disease: A disorder of cortical cholinergic innervation. *Science, 219,* 1184–1190.

Cullum, L., & Liebman, J. (1969). The association of congenital heart disease with Down's syndrome (mongolism). *American Journal of Cardiology, 24,* 354–357.

Cummings, G. R. (1962). Cardiopatia en pacients con anomalias cromosomales [Cardiac disease in patients with chromosomal anomalies]. *Memorias dol IV Congresso Mundial de Cardiologia* (1962, October; Mexico).

Cutress, T. W. (1971). Periodontal disease and oral hygiene in trisomy 21. *Archives of Oral Biology, 16,* 1345–1350.

Dalton, A. J. (1982, August). *A prospective study of Alzheimer's disease in Down's syndrome.* Paper presented at a meeting of the International Association of the Scientific Study of Mental Deficiency, Toronto.

Dalton, A. J., & Crapper, D. R. (1977). Down's syndrome and aging of the brain. In P. Mittler (Ed.), *Research to practice in mental retardation: Biomedical aspects* (Vol. 3, pp. 391–400). Baltimore: University Park Press.

Dalton, A. J., Crapper, D. R., & Schlotterer, G. R. (1974). Alzheimer's disease in Down's syndrome; visual retention deficits. *Cortex, 10,* 366–377.

Deaton, J. G. (1973). The mortality rate and abuses of death among institutionalized mongols in Texas. *Journal of Mental Deficiency Research, 17,* 117–123.

Ellis, W. G., McCulloch, J. R., & Corley, C. L. (1974). Presenile dementia in Down's syndrome: Ultrastructural identity with Alzheimer's disease. *Neurology, 24,* 101–106.

Ellis, N. R., & Tomporowski, P. D. (1983). Vitamin/mineral supplements and intelligence of institutionalized mentally retarded adults. *American Journal of Mental Deficiency, 88,* 211–214.

Evans, P. R. (1950). Cardiac anomalies in mongolism. *British Heart Journal, 12,* 258–262.

Fabia, J., & Drolette, M. (1970). Life tables up to the age of 10 for mongols with and without congenital heart disease. *Journal of Mental Deficiency Research, 14,* 235–242.

Fort, P., Lifshitz, F., Bellisario, R., Davis, J., Lanes, R., Pugliese, M., Richman, R., Post, E. M., & David, R. (1984). Abnormalities of thyroid function in children with Down syndrome. *The Journal of Pediatrics, 104,* 545–549.

Francis, S. H. (1970). Behavior of low-grade institutionalized mongoloids: Changes with age. *American Journal of Mental Deficiency, 75,* 92–101.

Fulton, R. T., & Lloyd, L. L. (1968). Hearing impairment in a population of children with Down syndrome. *American Journal of Mental Deficiency, 73,* 298–302.

Gershwin, M. E., Crinella, F. M., Castles, J. J., & Trent, J. K. (1977). Immunologic characteristics of Down's syndrome. *Journal of Mental Deficiency Research, 21,* 237–249.

Glovsky, L. (1966). Audiological assessment of a mongoloid population. *Training School Bulletin, 63,* 27–36.

Granata, G., Bencini, A., & Parenzan, L. (1952). Contributo alla conoscenza della malformazioni cardiache congenite nei saggetti mongoloid: [Contributions to the knowledge of cardiac congenital malformations in mongoloid children]. *Pediatria (Napoli), 60,* 281.

Greenwood, R. D., & Nadas, A. (1976). The clinical course of cardiac disease in Down's syndrome. *Pediatrics, 58,* 893–897.

Hann, H. L., Deakon, J. C., & London, W. T. (1979). Lymphocyte surface markers and serum immunoglobulins in persons with Down's syndrome. *American Journal of Mental Deficiency, 84,* 245–251.

Harrell, R. F., Capp, R. H., Davis, D. R., Peerless, J., & Ravitz, L. R. (1981). Can nutritional supplements help mentally retarded children? An exploratory study. *Proceedings of the National Academy of Science (USA), 78,* 574–578.

Ito, T. (1968). Cardiovascular malformations in association with chromosomal aberrations. In H. Watson (Ed.), *Pediatric cardiology.* St. Louis: C. V. Mosby.

Jacobs, P. F., Burdash, N. M., Manos, J. P., & Duncan, R. C. (1978). Immunologic parameters in Down's syndrome. *Annals of Clinical and Laboratory Science, 8,* 17–22.

Katlic, M. R., Clark, E. B., Neill, C., & Haller, A. (1977). Surgical management of congenital heart disease in Down's syndrome. *Journal of Thoracic Cardiovascular Surgery, 74,* 204–209.

Kisling, E. (1966). *Cranial morphology in Down's syndrome. A comparative roentgenocephalometric study in adult males.* Copenhagen: Munksgaard.

Knox, G. E., & Bensel, R. W. (1972). Gastrointestinal malformations in Down's syndrome. *Minnesota Medicine, 55,* 542–544.

Levin, S., Nir, E., & Mogilner, B. M. (1975). T-system immune-deficiency in Down syndrome. *Pediatrics, 56,* 123–126.

Liu, M., & Corlett, K. (1959). A study of congenital heart defects in mongolism. *Archives of Diseases in Children, 34,* 410–419.

Lott, I. T. (1982). Down's syndrome, aging, and Alzheimer's disease: A clinical review. *Annals of the New York Academy of Science, 396,* 15–27.

Lynn, H. B. (1979). Duodenal obstruction: Atresia, stenosis, and annular pancreas. In M. M. Ravitch, K. J. Welch, C. D. Benson, & E. Aberdeen (Eds.), *Pediatric Surgery.* Chicago: Yearbook Medical Publishers.

Malamud, N. (1964). Neuropathology. In H. A. Stevens & R. Herber (Eds.), *Mental retardation: A review of research.* Chicago: The University of Chicago Press.

Matin, M. A., Sylvester, P. E., Edwards, D., & Dickerson, J. W. T. (1984). Vitamin and zinc status in Down syndrome. *Journal of Mental Deficiency Research, 25,* 121–126.

Milunsky, A., Hackley, B. M., & Halstead, J. A. (1970). Plasma, erythrocyte, and leucocyte zinc levels in Down's syndrome. *Journal of Mental Deficiency Research, 74,* 99–105.

Mumma, P. (1984). *Ophthalmological concerns in Down syndrome.* Paper presented at the meeting of the National Down Syndrome Congress, San Antonio, TX.

Orner, G. (1974). Post-eruptive tooth age in children with Down's syndrome and their sibs. *Journal of Dental Research, 54,* 581–589.

Owens, D., Dawson, J. C., & Losin, S. (1971). Alzheimer's disease in Down's syndrome. *American Journal of Mental Deficiency, 75,* 606–612.

Park, S. C., Matthews, R. A., Zuberbuhler, J. R., Rowe, R. D., et al. (1977). Down syndrome with congenital heart malformation. *American Journal of Diseases of Children, 131,* 29–33.

Pueschel, S. M. (1983). Atlanto-axial subluxation in Down syndrome. *Lancet, i,* 980.

Pueschel, S. M. (1984). *The young child with Down syndrome.* New York: Human Sciences Press.

Pueschel, S. M., & Murphy, A. (1975). Counseling parents of infants with Down's syndrome. *Postgraduate Medicine, 58,* 90–95.

Pueschel, S M., Orson, J. M., Boylan, J. M., & Pezzullo, J. C. (1985). Adolescent development in males with Down syndrome. *American Journal of Diseases of Children, 139,* 236–238.

Pueschel, S. M., & Pezzullo, J. C. (1985). Thyroid dysfunction in Down syndrome. *American Journal of Diseases of Children, 139,* 636–639.

Pueschel, S. M., & Rynders, J. (1982). *Down syndrome: Advances in biomedicine and the behavioral sciences.* Cambridge, MA: Ware Press.

Pueschel, S. M., Scola, F. H., Perry, C. D., & Pezzullo, J. C. (1981). Atlanto-axial subluxation in children with Down syndrome. *Pediatric Radiology, 10,* 129–132.

Reed, R. B., Pueschel, S. M., Schnell, R. R., & Cronk, C. E. (1980). Interrelationships of biological, environmental, and competency variables in young children with Down syndrome. *Applied Research in Mental Retardation, 1,* 161–174.

Rigrodsky, S., Prunty, F., & Glovsky, L. (1961). A study of the incidence, types, and associated etiologies of hearing loss in an institutionalized mentally retarded population. *Training School Bulletin, 58,* 30–44.

Roche, A. F., & Barkla, D. H. (1964). The eruption of deciduous teeth in mongols. *Journal of Mental Deficiency Research, 8,* 54–58.

Rosenquist, G. C., Sweeney, L. J., Amsel, J., & McAllister, H. A. (1974). Enlargement of the membranous ventricular septum: An internal stigma of Down's syndrome. *Journal of Pediatrics, 85,* 490–493.

Rowe, R. D., & Uchida, L. A. (1961). Cardiac malformation in mongolism: A prospective study of 184 mongoloid children. *American Journal of Medicine, 31,* 726–735.

Rundle, A. T., Clothier, B., & Sudell, B. (1971). Serum IgD levels and infection in Down's syndrome. *Clinica Chimica Acta, 35,* 389–393.

Schulze, C. (1970). Developmental abnormalities of teeth and jaws. In R. J. Gorlin & H. Goldman (Eds.), *Thomas' oral pathology.* St. Louis: C. V. Mosby.

Schwartz, D. M., & Schwartz, R. H. (1978). Acoustic impedance and otoscopic findings in young children with Down syndrome. *Archives of Otolaryngology, 104,* 652–656.

Scola, P. S., & Pueschel, S. M. (1985). [Adolescent development in girls with Down syndrome.] Unpublished data.

Shapiro, B. L. (1970). Prenatal dental anomalies in mongolism: Comments on the basis and implications of variability. *Annals of the New York Academy of Science, 171,* 562–569.

Sinet, P. M. (1982). Metabolism of oxygen derivatives in Down's syndrome. *Annals of the New York Academy of Science, 396,* 83–94.

Skanse, B., & Farrell, C. B. (1962). The immune globulins in mongolism. *Acta Medica Scandinavica, 172,* 63–65.

Smith, G. F., & Berg, J. M. (1976). *Down's anomaly* (2nd ed.). New York: Churchill Livingstone.

Smith, G. F., Spiker, D., Peterson, C. P., Cicchetti, D., & Justine, P. (1984). Use of megadoses of vitamins with minerals in Down syndrome. *The Journal of Pediatrics, 105,* 228–234.

Spitzer, R., & Mann, J. (1950). Congenital malformations in the teeth and eyes of mental defectives. *Journal of Mental Science, 96,* 681–687.

Tandon, R., & Edwards, J. E. (1973). Cardiac malformation associated with Down's syndrome. *Circulation, 47,* 1349–1355.

Thase, M. E., Liss, L., Smeltzer, D., & Maloon, J. (1982). Clinical evaluation of dementia in Down's syndrome: A preliminary report. *Journal of Mental Deficiency Research, 26,* 239–244.

Tricomi, V., Valenti, C., & Hall, J. E. (1964). Ovulatory patterns in Down's syndrome. *American Journal of Obstetrics and Gynecology, 89,* 651–656.

Turkel, H. (1975). Medical amelioration of Down's syndrome incorporating the orthomolecular approach. *The Journal of Orthomolecular Psychiatry, 4,* 102–115.

Weathers, C. (1983). Effects of nutritional supplementation on IQ and certain other variables associated with Down syndrome. *American Journal of Mental Deficiency, 88,* 214–217.

Whittingham, S., Pitt, D. B., Sharma, D. L., & Mackay, I. R. (1977). Stress deficiency of the T-lymphocyte system exemplified by Down syndrome. *Lancet, i,* 163–166.

RESPONSE

Interrelation of Alzheimer Disease and Down Syndrome

Miriam Schweber

There have been reports from a variety of disciplines on interrelations between Alzheimer disease and Down syndrome. Because the brain abnormalities of Alzheimer disease have been found through autopsy in older persons with Down syndrome, many neuropathologists have simply stated that all persons with Down syndrome develop Alzheimer disease with age. But primary care providers have long been aware that the majority of adults with Down syndrome live out their lives with no apparent changes in personality or behavior. This discrepancy between laboratory and clinical observations has been difficult to understand. The crucial issues are the existence and prevalence of Alzheimer disease in persons with Down syndrome.

EVIDENCE OF ASSOCIATION

Neuropathological changes similar to those of Alzheimer disease have been reported in the brains of autopsied persons with Down syndrome repeatedly. The author has recently compiled such information on more than 200 reports of adults with Down syndrome over the age of 35 years, on more than 500 reports of persons with Down syndrome aged 35 years and younger, and on more than 1,200 reports of other mentally retarded persons of all ages (Schweber, 1986a). Of the 203 autopsies performed on persons with Down syndrome over age 36, each reported the typical structural abnormalities in the brain associated with Alzheimer disease; claimed exceptions are not defensible. Some persons with Down syndrome under age 36 also have been found to have similar changes with a strong age dependence in the incidence.

Generous support for the preparation of this chapter has been provided by the Retirement Research Foundation.

The identities extend to both light and electron microscopic levels of resolution, the anatomical distribution of aberrant formations, and the degree and pattern of neuronal loss.

At the biochemical level, changes in the concentration of specific compounds have been found in recent years in persons with Alzheimer disease as compared to unaffected individuals. Similar changes have been detected in older, but not younger, individuals with Down syndrome. Of particular interest are the marked changes in enzymes involved in cholinergic neurotransmission, because of the central role this system occupies in cognition and memory (Bartus, Dean, Beer, & Zippa, 1982), and the correlation of losses of these enzymes to the symptomology of Alzheimer disease (McGeer, McGeer, Suzuki, Dolman, & Nagai, 1984; Wilcock, Esiri, Bowen, & Smith, 1982). In this system, decreases parallel to those found in Alzheimer disease have been detected in older persons with Down syndrome in the crucial enzymes acetylcholine esterase and choline acetyltransferase (Yates et al., 1985; Yates, Harmar, et al., 1983; Yates, Simpson, et al., 1983; Yates, Simpson, Maloney, Gordon, & Reid, 1980). The declines of the enzyme concentrations are similarly distributed, but the degree of effect is generally more severe in Down syndrome than Alzheimer disease. Patterns of decreases parallel to those of Alzheimer disease have also been found in the brain in components of other neurotransmitter systems in adults with Down syndrome. Similar changes have been reported for the catecholamines dopamine and noradrenaline, plus their breakdown products, homovanillic acid and 3-methoxy-4-hydroxyphenylglycol (Mann, Lincoln, Yates, Stamp, & Toper, 1980; Nyberg, Carlsson, & Winblad, 1982; Yates, Harmar, et al., 1983; Yates, Ritchie, Simpson, Maloney, & Gordon, 1981; Yates, Simpson, et al., 1983). In the serotonin system, similar alterations have been traced in serotonin and its breakdown product, 5-hydroxyindolacetic acid (Nyberg et al., 1982). Those substances not affected in Alzheimer disease have also been found to be normal in persons with Down syndrome, such as substance P, which affects the presynaptic release of acetylcholine (Yates, Harmar, et al., 1983).

Other biochemical alterations similar to those occurring with Alzheimer disease have been found in the autopsied brains of adults with Down syndrome. These included markedly decreased glucose metabolism (Cutler, Heston, Davies, Haxby, & Schapiro, 1985), the accumulation and localized deposit of aluminum (Perl, 1983) and silicon (Nikaido, Austin, Trueb, & Rinehart, 1972), and the development of amyloidosis (Glenner, 1983). Virtually identical abnormal proteins have been isolated from the brains of adults with Down syndrome and adults with Alzheimer disease (Glenner & Wong, 1984; Masters et al., 1985). Such results serve to verify the similarities in reactivity of brain components found with immunological techniques (Selkoe, 1983).

Further biochemical implications can be drawn from the recent derivation of mice made trisomic for the equivalent of human chromosome 21

(Epstein, Cox, & Epstein, 1985). Studies on such mice have shown many of the same biochemical alterations found in persons with Alzheimer disease and older persons with Down syndrome (Ozand et al., 1984; Singer, Tiemeyer, Hedreen, Gearhart, & Coyle, 1984). The only exception to the identity of biochemical alterations for persons with Alzheimer disease and adults with Down syndrome has been the report of decreased superoxide dismutase in persons with Alzheimer disease versus increased levels in persons with Down syndrome (Delahunty, Kling, & McCormack, 1982). The gene for this enzyme is located on the long arm of chromosome 21; hence, persons with Down syndrome of all ages produce $3\times$ instead of the normal $2\times$ level (Epstein, Epstein, Cox, & Weil, 1981; Franke, 1981). Since the gross chromosomal aberrations of Down syndrome have not been detected for Alzheimer disease (Buckton, Whalley, Lee, & Christie, 1983; Fischman, 1983), there is no reason to expect that persons with Alzheimer disease would have three copies of the gene. Thus, the increase in the enzyme level in Down syndrome compared to the decrease in Alzheimer disease may not be of significance for possible interrelationships. The same situation may apply for phosphofructokinase, whose gene locus is also on the long arm of chromosome 21 (Sorbi & Blas, 1983).

A genetic association between Alzheimer disease and Down syndrome has been claimed because of the finding of an increased incidence of Down syndrome among families traced through Alzheimer disease cases in two separate studies, one in Minnesota (Heston, 1983), and the other in North Carolina (Heyman et al., 1983). In both cases, increments were only found if both second and third degree relatives were included. The incidence of a specific translocation involving chromosomes 15 and 21 among persons with Down syndrome in such families appears highly significant (Schweber, 1985). Translocation Down syndrome constitutes only 3%–5% of all Down syndrome occurrences (Hamerton, 1981; Hook, 1981; Mikkelsen, 1982) and the specific type found in families with Alzheimer disease occurs in only one-fifth of that 3%–5% (Hamerton, 1981). Furthermore, the frequency of translocation Down syndrome decreases with maternal age (Hook, 1981, 1984). Thus, if the increased incidence of Down syndrome in families with Alzheimer disease is ascribed to undetected maternal age effects, the abnormal proportion of the translocation Down syndrome becomes even more striking.

DOUBTS OF ASSOCIATION

The frequency of Down syndrome is known to be affected by parental age and birth order (Hook, 1981; Mikkelsen, 1982). The lack of such effects for Alzheimer disease has been adduced as evidence for a lack of relationship between Alzheimer disease and Down syndrome (Whalley, 1982). However, birth order and parental age affect the rate of nondisjunction that produces trisomy 21. They have no effect on translocation Down syndrome and thus, are only integral to the etiology of trisomy 21, not of Down syndrome per se. Their presence or absence is irrelevant to the basic question of the relation of Alzheimer disease and Down syndrome.

A more serious objection is the lack of correspondence between the neuropathological findings in older persons with Down syndrome and the rate of diagnosis of dementia (i.e., the discrepancy between laboratory results and clinical observations). In the author's compilation of information, all of the adults with Down syndrome over age 36 who came to autopsy had been shown to have the neuropathology of Alzheimer disease, yet only about one-fourth of them were designated as having dementia. Almost all of these individuals also exhibited epilepsy or late onset seizures. An additional approximate one-fourth were denoted as having seizures but not recorded as having dementia. Seizures can be a symptom of the late stages of Alzheimer disease (Reisberg, 1983). Although it is possible that examination for symptoms of dementia was not rigorously conducted for patients with seizures, the point remains that three-fourths of the autopsied adults with Down syndrome were not characterized as having dementia. Yet all had been shown to have the brain neuropathology of Alzheimer disease, and presumably had abnormal biochemical changes as well.

This disproportionality has led to suggestions that what develops in Down syndrome may not be Alzheimer disease at all, but some form of mimicking condition (Ropper & Williams, 1982). The identity of both the anatomical and biochemical results has made such a hypothesis unlikely (Williams & Matthysse, 1986). There are no reasons to suppose that the autopsy results indicating that all adults with Down syndrome over age 36 have the brain neuropathological changes of Alzheimer disease are biased in any way since the studies included institutionalized as well as noninstitutionalized adults from all over the world; for dementia, the rates have been calculated only from random studies (Schweber, 1986a). For the one-fourth of older persons with Down syndrome who were designated as having dementia, the diagnosis of Alzheimer disease was usually applied and seemed justifiable. The question is whether the three-fourths who were noted to be relatively unaffected clinically should be said to have Alzheimer disease. Such a diagnosis would not be acceptable for the non–Down syndrome population, especially as low levels of the anatomical aberrations seen in Alzheimer disease occur as a natural part of the aging process. How this issue is approached is crucial for the direction of medical treatment, for familial and social attitudes, and for public health management.

Several possible explanations of this situation have been suggested. First, it is argued that since most of the frequency estimates of dementia have been done by retrospective examination of the records of institutionalized patients, gross underestimation of the dementia rate is possible (Miniszek, 1983; Thase, Liss, Smeltzer, & Maloon, 1982). This effect would be enhanced because Down syndrome imposes an attenuated life span (Balarajan, Donnan & Adelstein, 1982; Thase, 1982); that is, older persons with Down syndrome may die *with* Alzheimer disease much more frequently than *of* it. Survival rates for Down syndrome have increased markedly in recent years but are still much less than the general population. Second, there is a problem in measuring mental function in adults with mental retardation (Berry, Groeneweg, Gibson, & Brown, 1985; Francis, 1970; Nakamura, 1961) and then of defining and detecting the early stages of possible loss (Lott & Lai, 1982; Wiesniewski, Dalton, Crapper-McLachlan, Wen, & Wisniewski, 1985). Studies that have prospectively measured mental processes as a function of age in Down syndrome have found measurable subtle decreases in various factors, including short-term memory and visual retention frequency. Some authors have regarded these as evidence of early stages of dementia (Dalton, Crapper, & Schlotterer, 1974; Miniszek, 1983; Rollins, 1946; Thase, Rigner, Smeltzer, & Liss, 1984), some felt that the changes did not justify such diagnoses (Dalton & Crapper, 1977; Owens, Dawson, & Losin, 1971), and some simply ascribed them to premature aging (Wisniewski, Howe, Williams, & Wisniewski, 1978; Wisniewski & Wisniewski, 1983). Yet it is well known that decline in mental processes also occurs with aging in normal individuals. It does not seem that the relatively subtle changes that have so far been reported for older persons with Down syndrome should be taken as evidence of the early stages of Alzheimer disease.

DISCUSSION

Among institutionalized individuals with Down syndrome, the diagnosis of dementia is based on marked personality change, incontinence, apathy, withdrawal, etc. For the non–Down syndrome population, such symptoms are classed as the terminal stages of Alzheimer disease. Descriptions of the early stages of Alzheimer disease seem to involve losses of advanced cognitive abilities that Down syndrome persons may never have possessed. Thus, in one categorization of six stages of Alzheimer disease, the fourth stage describes losses in orientation as to time and place and the ability to count backward from 40 by 4s, with almost total maintenance of social skills (Reisberg, 1983). This conclusion is buttressed by brain weight analyses from the survey of autopsied Down syndrome cases (Schweber, 1986b). There is a marked decrease in the mean brain weight of persons with Down syndrome over the age of 40; the decrease is more severe for demented than for nondemented older persons with Down syndrome. This implies that dementing processes in persons with Down syndrome are related or even due to loss of brain tissue.

The survey results further indicated that the rate of diagnosed dementia does not increase linearly with age in Down syndrome, but behaves as a decay function; that is, the chances of a person with Down syndrome becoming demented do not increase with age but are the same for each 10-year interval after age 40 (Schweber, 1986a). This again implies that the onset of dementia in Down syndrome is due to a specific neuropathological process, and is not an inevitable result of normal aging in persons with Down syndrome. If true, this implies that a cause could be identified, and if that is so, prevention might become possible.

CONCLUSIONS

On the one hand are the laboratory findings, which argue that all older persons with Down syndrome have Alzheimer disease based on anatomical and bio-chemical grounds (i.e., the universal autopsy anatomical identity, and the findings that the patterns of biochemical alterations in Alzheimer disease occur with aging in persons with Down syndrome). On the other hand are the clinical observations that up to three-fourths of the older persons with Down syndrome who came to autopsy never developed significant mental problems with age. One way of reconciling these positions is to consider that Alzheimer disease is simply expressed differently in persons with Down syndrome than in persons who do not have the chromosome disorder.

Such a model provides a variety of testable hypotheses. It further stresses the need for appropriate medical treatment for adults with Down syndrome. It is unacceptable to label older persons with Down syndrome who exhibit behavioral symptoms as having Alzheimer disease automatically, unless other types of treatable dementing etiologies have been rigorously excluded. In particular, dementia from thyroid imbalance must be considered, given the high rate of thyroid problems among persons with Down syndrome. The misdiagnosis of one of the treatable dementias as Alzheimer disease is as tragic for a person with Down syndrome as for a person without it. It also seems important that treatment strategies being tested on Alzheimer disease dementia are extended to the demented group with Down syndrome to see if alleviation is possible.

The model presented here suggests that the development of Alzheimer disease with age in persons with Down syndrome need not be reflected at the behavioral level. If the imposition of dementia in adults with Down syndrome is due to a pathological process, as suggested by the incidence rates and the brain weight losses, then a specific etiology must be involved. If that is the case, it should be possible to identify that cause and, perhaps, to prevent it. With improved treatment, especially early infant stimulation and appropriate special education, it may be possible to increase the ability of the brain in individuals with Down syndrome to withstand the losses involved in the dementia of "active" Alzheimer disease. Preventing the expression of the behavioral level of Alzheimer disease in all adults with Down syndrome will require much effort and the accumulation of much more knowledge than is presently possessed.

REFERENCES

Balarajan, R., Donnan, S., & Adelstein, A. (1982). Mortality and cause of death in Down's syndrome. *Journal of Epidemiology and Community Health, 36,* 127–129.
Bartus, R., Dean, R., Beer, B., & Zippa, A. (1982). The cholinergic hypothesis of geriatric memory dysfunction. *Science, 217,* 408–417.
Berry, P., Groeneweg, G., Gibson, D., & Brown, R. (1985). Mental development of adults with Down syndrome. *American Journal of Mental Deficiency, 89,* 252–256.
Buckton, K., Whalley, L., Lee, M., & Christie, J. (1983). Chromosome changes in Alzheimer's presenile dementia. *Journal of Medical Genetics, 20,* 46–51.
Cutler, N., Heston, L., Davies, P., Haxby, J., & Schapiro, M. (1985). Alzheimer's disease and Down's syndrome: New insights. *Annals of Internal Medicine, 103,* 566–578.
Dalton, A., & Crapper, D. (1977). Down's syndrome and aging of the brain. In P. Mittler (Ed.), *Research to practice in mental retardation: Biomedical aspects* (Vol. 3, pp. 391–400). Baltimore: University Park Press.
Dalton, A., Crapper, D., & Schlotterer, G. (1974). Alzheimer's disease in Down's syndrome: Visual retention deficits. *Cortex, 10,* 366–377.
Delahunty, D., Kling, A., & McCormack, M. (1982). Oxygen metabolism in Alzheimer's disease (AD). *American Journal of Human Genetics, 34,* 49A.
Epstein, C., Cox, D., & Epstein, L. (1985). Mouse trisomy 16; An animal model of human trisomy 21 (Down syndrome). *Annals of the New York Academy of Science, 450,* 157–168.
Epstein, C., Epstein, L., Cox, D., & Weil, J. (1981). Functional implications of gene dosage effects in trisomy 21. In G. Burgio, M. Fraccaro, L. Tiepolo, & U. Wolf (Eds.), *Trisomy 21* (Suppl. 2 to Human Genetics, pp. 155–172). New York: Springer-Verlag.
Fischman, H. (1983). Chromosomal factors. In B. Reisberg (Ed.), *Alzheimer's disease* (pp. 161–170). New York: Free Press.
Francis, S. (1970). Behavior of low-grade institutionalized mongoloids: Changes with age. *American Journal of Mental Deficiency, 75,* 92–101.
Franke, U. (1981). Gene dosage studies in Down's syndrome. A review. In F. de la Cruz and P. Gerald (Eds.), *Trisomy 21 (Down syndrome): Research perspectives* (pp. 237–251). Baltimore: University Park Press.
Glenner, G. (1983). Alzheimer's disease: Multiple cerebral amyloidosis. In R. Katzman (Ed.), *Biological aspects of Alzheimer's disease. (Banbury Report, #15,* pp. 137–144). Cold Spring Harbor, NY: Cold Spring Harbor Laboratory.
Glenner, G. & Wong, C. (1984). Alzheimer's disease and Down's syndrome; sharing of a unique cerebrovascular amyloid fibril protein. *Biochemistry and Biophysics Research Communications, 122,* 1131–1135.
Hamerton, J. (1981). Frequency of mosaicism, translocation, and other variants of trisomy 21. In F. de la Cruz and P. Gerald (Eds.), *Trisomy 21 (Down syndrome): Research perspectives* (pp. 99–110). Baltimore: University Park Press.
Heston, L. (1983). Dementia of the Alzheimer type. In R. Katzman (Ed.), *Biological aspects of Alzheimer's disease* (Banbury Report #15, pp. 183–192). Cold Spring Harbor, NY: Cold Spring Harbor Laboratory.

Heyman, A., Wilkinson, W., Hurwitz, B., Schmechel, D., Sigmon, A., Weinberg, T., Helms, M., & Swift, M. (1983). Alzheimer's disease: Genetic aspects and associated clinical disorders. *Annals of Neurology, 14*, 507–515.

Hook, E. (1981). Down's syndrome: Its frequency in human populations and some factors pertinent to variation in rates. In F. de la Cruz and P. Gerald (Eds.), *Trisomy 21 (Down syndrome): Research perspectives* (pp. 3–69). Baltimore: University Park Press.

Hook, E. (1984). Parental age and unbalanced Robertsonian translocations associated with Down syndrome and Patau syndrome: Comparison with maternal and paternal age effects for 47, + 21 and 47, + 13. *Annals of Human Genetics, 48*, 313–325.

Lott, I., & Lai, F. (1982). Dementia in Down's syndrome; observations from a neurology clinic. *Applied Research in Mental Retardation, 3*, 233–239.

Mann, D., Lincoln, J., Yates, P., Stamp, J., & Toper, S. (1980). Changes in monoamine containing neurones in the human CNS in senile dementia. *British Journal of Psychiatry, 136*, 533–541.

Mann, D., Yates, P., & Marcyniuk, B. (1984). Relationship between pigment accumulation and age in Alzheimer's disease and Down syndrome. *Acta Neuropathologica (Berl.), 63*, 72–77.

Masters, C., Simms, G., Weinman, N., Multhaup, G., McDonald, B., & Beyreuther, K. (1985). Amyloid plaque core protein in Alzheimer disease and Down syndrome. *Proceedings of the National Academy of Science (USA), 82*, 4245–4249.

McGeer, P., McGeer, E., Suzuki, J., Dolman, C., & Nagai, T. (1984). Aging, Alzheimer's disease, and the cholinergic system of the basal forebrain. *Neurology, 34*, 741–745.

Mikkelsen, M. (1982). Down syndrome: Current stage of cytogenetic epidemiology. In B. Bonné-Tamir, B. Cohen, & R. Goodman (Eds.), *Human Genetics: Part B. Medical aspects* (pp. 297–309). New York: Alan R. Liss.

Miniszek, N. (1983). Development of Alzheimer's disease in Down syndrome individuals. *American Journal of Mental Deficiency, 87*, 377–385.

Nakamura, H. (1961). Nature of institutionalized adult mongoloid intelligence. *American Journal of Mental Deficiency, 66*, 456–458.

Nikaido, T., Austin, J., Trueb, L., & Rinehart, R. (1972). Studies in aging of the brain. II. Microchemical analyses of the nervous system in Alzheimer patients. *Archives of Neurology, 27*, 549–554.

Nyberg, P., Carlsson, A., & Winblad, S. (1982). Brain monoamines in cases with Down's syndrome with and without dementia. *Journal of Neurological Transmission, 55*, 289–299.

Owens, D., Dawson, J., & Losin, S. (1971). Alzheimer's disease in Down's syndrome. *American Journal of Mental Deficiency, 765*, 606–612.

Ozand, P., Hawkins, R., Collins, R., Reed, W., Baab, P., & Oster-Granite, M. (1984). Neurochemical changes in murine trisomy 16: Delay in cholinergic and catecholaminergic systems. *Journal of Neurochemistry, 43*, 401–408.

Perl, D. (1983). Aluminum and Alzheimer's disease: Intraneuronal x-ray spectrometry studies. In R. Katzman (Ed.), *Biological aspects of Alzheimer's disease* (Banbury Report #15, pp. 425–431). Cold Spring Harbor, NY: Cold Spring Harbor Laboratory.

Reisberg, B. (1983). Clinical presentation, diagnosis, and symptomatology of age-associated cognitive decline and Alzheimer's disease. In B. Reisberg (Ed.), *Alzheimer's disease* (pp. 173–187). New York: Free Press.

Rollins, H. (1946). Personality in mongolism with special reference to the incidence of catatonic psychosis. *American Journal of Mental Deficiency, 51*, 219–237.

Ropper, A. & Williams, R. (1982). Relationship between plaques, tangles, and dementia in Down syndrome. *Neurology, 30,* 639–644.

Schweber, M. (1985). A possible unitary genetic hypothesis for Down syndrome and Alzheimer's disease. *Annals of the New York Academy of Science, 450,* 223–238.

Schweber, M. (1986a). Alzheimer's expression in Down syndrome: Neuropathology, seizures, and dementia. Manuscript submitted for publication.

Schweber, M. (1986b). Alzheimer's expression in Down syndrome: Age, sex, and symptom effects on brain weight. Manuscript submitted for publication.

Selkoe, D. (1983).General discussion. In R. Katzman (Ed.), *Biological aspects of Alzheimer's disease* (Banbury Report #15, pp. 201). Cold Spring Harbor, NY: Cold Spring Harbor Laboratory.

Singer, H., Tiemeyer, M., Hedreen, J., Gearhart, J., & Coyle, J. (1984). Morphologic and neurochemical studies of embryonic brain development in murine trisomy 16. *Development of Brain Research, 15,* 155–166.

Sorbi, S. & Blas, J. (1983). Fibroblast phosphofructokinase in Alzheimer's disease and Down's syndrome. In R. Katzman (Ed.), *Biological aspects of Alzheimer's disease* (Banbury Report #15, pp. 297–308). Cold Spring Harbor, NY: Cold Spring Harbor Laboratory.

Thase, M. (1982). Longevity and mortality in Down's syndrome. *Journal of Mental Deficiency Research, 26,* 177–182.

Thase, M., Liss, L., Smeltzer, D., & Maloon, J. (1982). Clinical evaluation of dementia in Down's syndrome: A preliminary report. *Journal of Mental Deficiency Research, 26,* 239–244.

Thase, M., Rigner, R., Smeltzer, D., & Liss, L. (1984). Age-related neuropsychological deficits in Down's syndrome. *Biological Psychology, 199,* 571–585.

Whalley, L. (1982). The dementia of Down's syndrome and its relevance to aetiological studies of Alzheimer's disease. *Annals of the New York Academy of Science, 396,* 39–54.

Wilcock, G., Esiri, M., Bowen, D., & Smith, C. (1982). Correlation of cortical choline acetyltransferase activity with the severity of dementia and histological abnormalities. *Journal of Neurological Science, 57,* 407–417.

Williams, R., & Matthysse, S. (in press). Age related changes in Down syndrome brain and the cellular pathology of Alzheimer disease. *Progress in Brain Research.*

Wisniewski, K., Dalton, A., Crapper-McLachlan, M., Wen, G., & Wisniewski, H. (1985). Alzheimer disease in Down syndrome: Clinico-pathological studies. *Neurology, 35,* 957–961.

Wisniewski, K., Howe, J., Williams, D., & Wisniewski, H. (1978). Precocious aging and dementia in patients with Down's syndrome. *Biological Psychiatry, 13,* 619–628.

Wisniewski, K., & Wisniewski, H. (1983). Age-associated changes and dementia in Down's syndrome. In B. Reisberg (Ed.), *Alzheimer's disease* (pp. 319–325). New York: Free Press.

Yates, C., Fink, G., Bennie, J., Gordon, A., Simpson, J., & Eskay, R. (1985). Neurotensin immunoreactivity in post-mortem brain is increased in Down's syndrome but not in Alzheimer-type dementia. *Neurological Science, 67,* 327–335.

Yates, C., Harmar, A., Rosie, R., Sheward, J., Sanchez, K., De Levy, G., Simpson, J., Maloney, A., Gordon, A., & Fink, G. (1983). Thyrotropin-releasing hormone, luteinizing hormone-releasing hormone and substance P immunoreactivity in post-mortem brain from cases of Alzheimer-type dementia and Down's syndrome. *Brain Research, 258,* 45–52.

Yates, C., Ritchie, I., Simpson, J., Maloney, A., & Gordon, A. (1981). Noradrenaline in Alzheimer-type dementia and Down syndrome. *Lancet, i,* 39–40.

Yates, C., Simpson, J., Gordon, A., Maloney, A., Allison, Y., Ritchie, I., & Urquhart, A. (1983). Catecholamines and cholinergic enzymes in presenile and senile Alzheimer-type dementia and Down's syndrome. *Brain Research, 280,* 119–126.

Yates, C., Simpson, J. Maloney, A., Gordon, A., & Reid, A. (1980). Alzheimer-like cholinergic deficiency in Down syndrome. *Lancet, ii,* 979.

SECTION II

EDUCATION

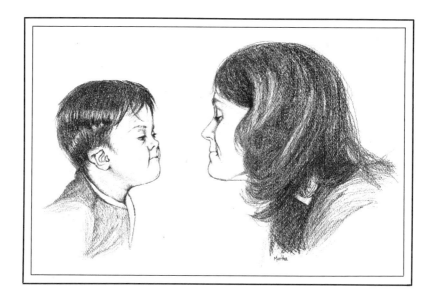

Introduction

John E. Rynders

✦✦✦

In 1975, with the passage of PL 94-142, the Education for All Handicapped Children Act, the right to a free, public education was guaranteed to every school-age child in the United States. No longer could children be excluded because of a disability, or because someone thought that having Down syndrome signaled the automatic imposition of a ceiling on learning prospects.

The eight chapters and responses in this section show clearly that children with Down syndrome often exhibit educational accomplishments that exceed many persons' expectations. Chapter 9 points to the universal need of children with Down syndrome for proper speech and language stimulation, and documents childrens' responsiveness, particularly in the early period of life, to good communication intervention. Chapter 6 discusses the young child's home and preschool, and presents a strong case for the importance and effectiveness of early education. The remaining chapters and responses discuss a period of life in which a great deal of research evidence on the effects of schooling should be available—the elementary and secondary years—but, as the authors point out, there are very large gaps in that knowledge base. In fact, after reading this section, one cannot help but be struck by a paradox: namely, that contemporary evidence of educational achievement is meager in the age period in which education is often regarded as most important. Possibly, researchers have not wanted to show which children with mental disabilities in their studies have one specific condition or another. Or perhaps educators have moved from discrete categorizations of children-by-condition, in an attempt to foster heterogeneity (i.e., mainstreaming) in the fullest way possible. But, by doing so, researchers cannot document whether children with Down syndrome are even physically present in a particular study; nor, if they are there, can it be described how their performance compares with that of other children with mental disabilities who do not have Down syndrome. To make matters worse, there are so few studies of academic learning involving children with Down syndrome at the elementary and secondary level that this linchpin aspect of the knowledge base is shaky at best. For example, the author can find just one study done during the school years showing that children with Down syndrome, if given a sound experimental program, can learn to read proficiently (Brown, Jones, Troccolo, Heiser, et al., 1972); and only one study during those years showed that they can learn to do mathematics proficiently, as a result of a good experimental program (Dalton, Rubino, & Hislop, 1973). Yet, most people are aware of numerous individual children with Down syndrome who read fluently and with good comprehension at a reasonable grade level, and who handle everyday computational and other arithmetic demands capably. In the area of young adults learning to live independently, the knowledge base is even poorer: all of the studies are done with institutionalized populations or with persons who have been released from an institution, even though many young adults with Down syndrome live in community settings, have always done so, and probably always will.

Obviously, educators and researchers must seek funding for a number of national studies, both descriptive as well as experimental, that will ultimately provide findings that allow parents, educators, and organizations such as the National Down Syndrome Congress to advocate more effectively for school-age children and young adults with Down syndrome. Until then, this section provides a review of the state-of-the-art in education that parents and educators will find stimulating, useful, and practical, as well as representative of the "cutting edge" in research and instruction today. Moreover, these eight chapters and responses document clearly that the child with Down syndrome has his or her "foot in the school door" to *stay*.

REFERENCES

Brown, L., Jones, S., Troccolo, E., Heiser, C., et al. (1972). Teaching functional reading to young trainable students: Toward longitudinal objectives. *Journal of Special Education, 3,* 237–246.

Dalton, A., Rubino, C., & Hislop, M. (1973). Some effects of token rewards on school achievement of children with Down's syndrome. *Journal of Applied Behavior Analysis, 6,* 251–259.

Chapter 6

Early Intervention for Children with Down Syndrome

Marci J. Hanson

✦✦✦

Travis is 9 years old. He plays on his school's soccer team and participates in regular school programs and receives additional educational assistance through a resource room. He is the top reader in the slow reader group. Travis has Down syndrome. At the time of his birth, his congenital heart condition was considered inoperable and he was given less than 2 years to live. Few believed that he could benefit from any special health or educational services. Most professionals counseled that loving care by the family was the only treatment. However, his parents and a persistent social worker believed otherwise. Travis was enrolled in a home-based early intervention program at 4 months of age. Three years later, surgery was performed and his heart condition was corrected. His mother ascribes his adjustment and developmental achievements to the following conditions: 1) the fact that he was fully accepted into his family and treated normally—being given the same love and expectations as his siblings; 2) early educational services which helped the parents know how to work with their child—what kind of activities could help the child and how to observe the child; and 3) the support of family and friends, and a positive faith and attitude about the child.

The complexity of child development is such that the relative contributions of each of these factors to developmental outcome cannot be determined. Nor does this information on early development allow one to forecast Travis's development and life-style for the years to come. However, this case study raises a number of important questions regarding early intervention efforts with children with Down syndrome:

What was the effect of early intervention?
What components were most important, perhaps crucial?

Did early intervention contribute to the family's positive acceptance and adjustment to the birth of a child with Down syndrome?

Are other individuals with Down syndrome similarly affected by their early intervention experiences?

Several issues raised by this case study are explored in this chapter. Specifically, the identification of goals or content for early intervention efforts are discussed and methods for implementing these procedures are reviewed, with the intent of formulating recommendations for early intervention programs for infants with Down syndrome.

RATIONALE FOR EARLY INTERVENTION

Four areas from the literature are examined in order to identify and define appropriate goals and methods for early intervention. These topics are: family service needs, a transactional model of development, the relation between development and learning, and past research on early intervention effects with infants who have Down syndrome.

Family Service Needs

The birth of a child brings new joys, stresses, and changes to a family, but the birth of a child with a disability may produce additional stress and place unusual demands on the parents.

The needs of the family are at a peak at the time of the child's birth—a crucial time when early parent-infant attachments are forming. Parents are faced not only with the knowledge that their infant's condition is abnormal, but find also that they have a child who may be somewhat unresponsive and difficult to care for and who may have significant health care concerns (Hanson, 1984).

Solnit and Stark (1961) discussed the feelings that parents may experience at the time their child with a disability is born, likening their reactions to the mourning process, in that the parent mourns the loss of the expected normal child. But unlike adjustment to a death in the family, the presence of a disabling condition presents a continuing need for adaptations and adjustments throughout the life cycle. A number of moving and informative accounts have described these adjustments, including the joys, needs, and stresses involved in them (Featherstone, 1980; Paul, 1981; Seligman, 1983; Turnbull & Turnbull, 1985). These accounts also highlighted the need for a wide range of support and service resources—medical, educational, psychological, financial—and the necessity for early and continued assistance and coordination of services across agencies.

The study of family adjustment helps to focus attention on the range of long-term early intervention needs across disciplines. However, for the purposes of this chapter, "early intervention" is restricted to the broad parameters of the educational and support services provided for the child and his or her family within the first 3 years of the child's life.

Transactional Model of Development

Developmental theorists have emphasized the importance of the early years and the plasticity of mental development during this period of life (Hunt, 1961). Studies on the effects of early experiences—both nurturing and traumatic—have focused attention on the interaction of biological and environmental factors as determinants of developmental outcome. The model most appealing for explaining developmental outcome for individuals with disabilities (e.g., Down syndrome) is a transactional model, as articulated by Sameroff and Chandler (1975). Briefly, this model stresses the active role of the child in interacting with her or his world, described as the child's "perpetual state of active reorganization" (p. 235). It highlights the "continual and progressive interplay between the organism and its environment."

Of concern in the study of disabilities such as Down syndrome are the secondary problems that may develop as a result of environmental responses to the child's disability. This model (Sameroff & Chandler, 1975), posits that not only do caregiver and child actively influence one another from the beginning of the child's life, but that other environmental factors (e.g., family, agencies, society) also impinge on and influence the interaction. Further, these interactions are not static across time, but rather are continuously being modified. Therefore, the individual at one point in time may be very different from the individual at other points in time, as based on the dynamic interplay between the individual and the environment.

Applied specifically to the child with Down syndrome, this model (Sameroff & Chandler, 1975) suggests that developmental predictions cannot be made from a purely medical or main-effects model. The diagnosis of Down syndrome (genotype) at birth—the presence of a biologically based disability resulting from a chromosomal aberration—fails to explain or predict the child's future development (phenotype), in part because the individual's interaction with the environment is not a static phenomenon, but a constantly changing one. This notion mitigates a totally environmental explanation of subsequent outcome.

Consider a case in which the early helplessness and incompetence of a young child gratifies the parent's need for caregiving and a dependency relationship with the child. As the child gains competence and independence, what formerly may have been a satisfactory relationship between both parties becomes fraught with stress unless the parent's needs shift with regard to the relationship with the child. Most parents and children go through these stages and struggles in relationships, and most are resolved naturally and smoothly. When this is not the case, however, this lack of "match" may adversely affect the child's development. This example is used to underscore the fact that an adaptive response by the parent (or child) at one stage of development may be maladaptive at another stage because of the constantly changing, reorganizing nature of the interplay between the child and parent.

The environment in a larger sense—society—must also be taken into account. For years, persons with Down syndrome were believed to be severely retarded, and hence were relegated from birth to life in an institution. Today, an individual with Down syndrome is usually more integrated into and accepted by society. This broader acceptance has been demonstrated by the featuring of children with Down syndrome in several television programs, such as *Quincy, The Fall Guy,* and *Dallas.* Were this topic not reasonably acceptable to society, Down syndrome would not be discussed so openly. Society's mores influence the quantity and quality of opportunities for the individual to learn and develop. These mores may influence, for instance, the parents' expectations for and acceptance of their child.

"Environment" in the transactional model assumes that a complex, dynamic set of events influence the individual. Conversely, the individual influences society. For example, as individuals with Down syndrome are more commonly seen interacting competently in society, the view of others toward them changes favorably. Thus, the transactional model provides a framework for tracing the course of development and also for conceptualizing intervention strategies designed to alter that course.

Relation Between Development and Learning

Intervention strategies at any age level are dictated to a large degree by one's theoretical stance on the relation between development and learning. This argument is particularly cogent in infancy, as this period is often viewed from a purely biologically based, developmentally bound course. For the purposes of this discussion, development, on the one hand, is defined as change attributed to a stage of growth or maturation based on genetic determinance and physiological structures. The degree to which the environment is seen as influential in this process depends on one's theoretical views. Learning, on the other hand, typically refers to the acquiring of knowledge or a skill through practice or experience.

Due to the rapid and dramatic changes during infancy, concerns with regard to both normal and atypical infants have focused almost exclusively on developmental issues. This orientation is also reflected in early intervention programs, which are often referred to as "infant stimulation" or "infant development programs." The major goal of most of these programs, whether the theoretical stance is to "stimulate the senses" or is that of an ardent behavioral approach, is usually to enhance or accelerate the child's development. Typically, the teacher or therapist implements a curriculum based on a predetermined set of goals or objectives founded on the normal developmental sequence.

However, in order to define an optimal early intervention regimen, it is necessary to move beyond a purely developmental approach to an examination of the relation between development and learning and the nature of the infant's contributions to these processes. In this regard, Vygotsky (1978) reviewed three major theoretical positions and postulated a fourth. Briefly, the three theoretical positions he reviewed are: 1) a view of the processes of child development as independent of learning, 2) a view of learning as development, and 3) a perspective that combines the first two views and postulates that maturation depends on the development of the nervous system but that learning is also a developmental process. The first position, that learning and development are independent, assumes that learning always comes after development and that it never plays a role in development. The second position, that learning is development, essentially defines development as the accumulation of all responses. (The previous discussion of a transactional model of development calls these positions into question.) The third position combines the first two seemingly opposite positions and allows that the maturational process makes the learning process possible, and, in turn, the learning process then facilitates the developmental process.

Vygotsky (1978) rejected all three positions and stated that learning and development are interrelated from the first day of the child's life. Further, in his discussion of school-age learning, he introduced the concept of "the zone of proximal development" (p. 85). This "zone" is defined as the difference between the child's actual level of development and the level of potential development, utilizing adult or peer guidance. Such a zone reveals functions that are in the process of developing, rather than just those that have matured. Vygotsky maintained that developmental processes do not coincide with learning but lag behind the learning processes. Though Vygotsky specifically related this notion to "school-age learning" and made a distinction between nonstructured education in the early years and systematic instruction in later years, the concept appears equally valid at other ages, particularly for work with children who have disabilities for whom specialized training may be needed. Interestingly, his notions are much akin to the more recent work of Feuerstein (1979a, 1979b) and his Active Modification theory, which has been applied with children who have cognitive delays. Feuerstein advocated a process approach to assessment and intervention, emphasizing the importance of interactions between teacher and child and the process of continuously modifying the demands of the task situation according to the child's responses. His concern was in measuring the modifiability of child behavior through active, mediated learning experiences.

The relation between learning and development assumes even greater importance as one attempts to intervene in the lives of children who, through disability, are developmentally delayed. Down syndrome, of course, is characterized by developmental retardation. Many investigations have identified delays for individuals with Down syndrome across the mental, motor, and social developmental domains (Carr, 1970; Cicchetti & Sroufe, 1976; Dameron, 1963; Dicks-Mireaux, 1966, 1972; Share, Koch, Webb, & Graliker, 1964). Though this evidence documents delays in the development of children with Down syndrome, a question remains as to whether their development proceeds in the normal developmental pattern or sequence. Several investigators have shown, using various measures to document the normal developmental course, that infants with Down syndrome demonstrated similar developmental sequences as compared to normally developing infants, but that they typically developed at a slower rate (Berry, Gunn, & Andrews, 1980—attachment behaviors as measured in a Strange Situation paradigm; Cicchetti & Sroufe, 1976—affective and cognitive measures; Cicchetti & Sroufe, 1978—measures of fear reactions; Mans, Cicchetti, & Sroufe, 1978—self-recognition measures; Miranda & Fantz, 1973—visual preference measures; Miranda & Fantz, 1974—recognition memory measures; Rothbart & Hanson, 1983—temperament measures of smiling and laughing behavior; Serafica & Cicchetti, 1976—attachment and exploration behavioral measures). Morss (1983), however, maintained that in his tests of cognitive development, the development of infants with Down syndrome was not just slower, but was different as compared to normal infants.

Other studies have suggested differences in the styles in which infants with Down syndrome approach and gather information. For instance, children with Down syndrome have been observed to show lower persistence, approach, and threshold for stimulation (Bridges & Cicchetti, 1982); more interpersonal looking behavior to the mother during a play session, and less referential looking and visual exploration of the environment (Gunn, Berry, & Andrews, 1982); fewer referential looks to the mother during communication (Jones, 1977); greater impulsive responding (less ability to delay touch of a forbidden object) and fewer kinds of strategy behavior (verbal, nonverbal, social, object, and other directed) (Kopp, Krakow, & Johnson, 1983); differences in qualititative aspects of sustained attention such as less time-oriented socially as giving or seeking assistance from mother, less visual exploration of room and others, more time unoccupied or engaged in stereotypic activity, and less shift of activities spontaneously (Krakow & Kopp, 1982); and greater distress and latency in approaching intense or novel stimuli, and longer periods of orienting to stimuli (Rothbart & Hanson, 1983). Though studies reported group differences (normally developing versus Down syndrome), great individual differences within groups were noted as well. If, as Kopp et al. (1983) suggested, the source of lags may lie in the differential experiences of infants, then early intervention regimens may be of crucial importance in modifying the learning styles and developmental patterns of these infants.

Research on Early Intervention
with Infants who have Down Syndrome

A variety of studies have addressed the effectiveness of early educational experiences for infants with Down syndrome. Ample evidence exists that the provision of these early intervention services can positively alter the developmental course of these infants and toddlers.

Clunies-Ross (1979) studied 36 children ranging in age from 3 to 37 months. The children received a combination home- and center-based program and training in language, social, self-care, cognitive, fine perceptual motor, and gross motor development. The children were involved in the program for between 4 months and 2 years. Parents of these children attended a course in child development and child management where they learned to implement home training programs. Assessments of these children, utilizing the Early Intervention Developmental Profile, indicated that the children progressed developmentally over the course of the treatment and that their rate of progress was inversely related to the age at which they began the program.

Hanson and Schwarz (1978) compared the developmental achievements of 12 children who were participants in an intensive home-based program with developmental data on children with Down syndrome who were home-reared but who had not received early intervention. Children were identified and enrolled in the program as soon after birth as possible (at an average age of 14 weeks). The duration of their participation ranged from 15 to 30 months. Intervention procedures centered on teaching parents how to implement educational programs for their children across areas of development. Families were visited in their homes on a bi-weekly basis and specific teaching programs were planned with the parents. Findings showed that the children receiving home intervention exhibited developmental achievements across domains beyond levels expected for the comparison group. The cognitive development of these infants was also compared to a group of infants with Down syndrome who did not receive early intervention (Carr, 1970). Again, these infants scored higher as measured by the Bayley Scales of Infant Development than did the comparison group (Hanson, 1981).

Similarly, Ludlow and Allen (1979) studied three groups of children with Down syndrome: children in an intervention nursery school where parents received counseling (N=75), children being home-reared but receiving no special services (N=80), and children placed in residential care before their second birthday (N=43). The children in the intervention group attended a developmental clinic with their mothers twice per week where they received assistance in all areas of development. These children received at least 2 years of this service before their fifth birthday. Though all groups showed a developmental decline over the first few years, children in the first group—the early intervention group—outperformed the others on the Griffiths Mental Development Scales, the Stanford-Binet, Personal Social Development Scale, and speech development measures. Later, children in that group were more often placed in ordinary school placements than were those from the other two groups.

Connolly and Russell (1976) demonstrated that 40 children who received center-based early intervention services attained gross motor, fine motor, feeding, and social skills at earlier ages than a comparison group of children who did not receive these services. The authors also suggested that the age of entry into the program was of importance in that those children who began after 6 months of age showed more evidence of delays. Further, they reported evidence of improved family relationships due to program participation. In a follow-up study (Connolly, Morgan, Russell, & Richardson, 1980), 20 children from the original study who had received family-based early intervention were compared with 53 noninstitutionalized children who had not received early intervention. At 3–6 years of age, the former group showed higher intellectual and social quotients and earlier acquisition of motor and self-help skills than did the latter.

Results of a study by Bidder, Bryant, and Gray (1975) also confirmed that children participating in a parent-implemented intervention program made greater gains than those who did not have a treatment program. In that study, mothers of 16 children (ranging in age from 12 to 33 months) with Down syndrome were divided into two groups. One group received 12 sessions of behavior modification training and group counseling over a 6-month period, whereas the control group received no special assistance. The children in the treatment group showed clear gains, particularly in the language development area, and the mothers were reported to have gained more competence and confidence in their management of the children. Similar effects were noted by Aronson and Fallstrom (1977) in their study of 16 children in a Swedish residential care facility. Children ranged in age from 21 to 69 months, and were divided into a training group and a control group matched for age and sex. Training lasted for nearly 18 months and consisted of developmental exercises across areas of development which were implemented twice weekly. The group of children in a preschool training group showed a greater increase in mental age than the control group, as measured on the Griffiths Mental Developmental Scales.

Further, Project EDGE at the University of Minnesota focused on the use of maternal tutoring through structured play to develop receptive and expressive language skills in young children with Down syndrome. Subjects were divided into experimental and control groups. The experimental group mothers received training on instructional methods and materials, followed by home visits and monthly group meetings. At 3 years of age, the group of children who received the maternal-implemented intervention scored higher than the control group on measures of intellectual and receptive language development (Rynders & Horrobin, 1980). At the end of the 5-year program, the 35 children who were enrolled (17 experimental and 18 control) were again tested on language and cognitive measures. Statistical analyses revealed no significant group differences in specified target variables (concept utilization and/or expressive language), although there were significant differences in IQ favoring the experimental group. Rynders and Horrobin concluded that their findings on intellectual development highlight the importance and general effectiveness of early education for children with Down syndrome, but that their cognitive achievement results do not support the use of their curriculum, which emphasized linguistic development.

Many other studies have addressed the effects of early intervention with populations of children that have included children with Down syndrome. Similarly, the results of these investigations have demonstrated positive early intervention effects (Bricker & Dow, 1980; Fredericks, Baldwin, Moore, Templeman, & Anderson, 1980; Hanson, 1985).

The results of these investigations provide general support for the provision of early intervention services for infants with Down syndrome. Although, overall, these early intervention services appear to be valuable to the infants and families who participated, the challenge remains to ferret out those factors that are responsible for the desired changes. In each study, a comprehensive intervention approach was taken. However, when examined closely, a few common variables can be identified, despite the fact that these investigations were done at different sites, using different interventions and evaluation tools. First, and perhaps most important, these programs typically involved the child's parent actively, often in a teaching role. Second, most programs offered a structured or systematic approach to the child's training, with specified goals or objectives and procedures for implementation. Third, most were aimed at making the child more competent across areas of development—although some investigations highlighted a particular area such as language.

While findings related to the effectiveness of early intervention with this population of children are encouraging, appropriate caution should be observed in interpreting the outcomes of these studies. Some studies do not employ control or comparison groups; in instances where comparisons are made, often control and experimental group subjects are not matched and/or assessed at the same point in time. Questions also persist as to the maintenance of the developmental gains reported. Thus, a need remains for carefully controlled long-term studies in this area.

This need also presents a research dilemma. Given the probable positive impact of early intervention, most researchers cannot ethically support the use of control groups which receive no treatment. Additionally, it is difficult to establish such groups in that parents are actively seeking information from other parents and professionals and are unlikely to be willing to just care for their children and have them assessed periodically. Further, the issue of effectiveness of early intervention must be viewed from a much broader perspective than merely examining the intellectual changes. Such questions include:

Are parents more accepting and pleased with their children when they receive early services?
Are they less likely to institutionalize their children?
Are families happier?
Are children who participate in early educational services more likely to "graduate" into less restrictive educational environments?
Are they more likely to interact with peers in a mutually satisfying manner?
Do the children behave more "normally" and are they more accepted by the population at large?

It appears that these very difficult-to-answer questions are at the crux of the evaluation of early intervention efforts. However, the anecdotal evidence to date and the few research studies in this area support the provision of early intervention services for young children with Down syndrome.

FACTORS OF EARLY INTERVENTION

Family Variables

Early intervention attempts have focused traditionally on making the child more competent by accelerating the child's development. The emphasis has been on remediating the effects of the child's disability, an approach that stresses one aspect of the child's contribution to the interaction—the disability. This approach is not uncommon in special education, where practices have tended to focus on the disability itself and its effects. The literature in developmental psychology, however, has typically looked at the influence of the parent on the developing child, that is, until the last 2 decades when Bell's (1968) landmark article served to shift attention to the child's contributions in the interaction as well.

Early interventionists must re-examine their area of emphasis and consider the effects of both parent and child on one another and on the dynamics of the family system. Given that environmental interventions via specific early education programs, such as those previously reviewed, have produced beneficial results for infant participants, it is logical to continue that goal. But what about the role of the parent? A wide range of models and roles that parents play in early intervention efforts, roles ranging from teacher to advocate (Lillie & Trohanis, 1976; Tjossem, 1976; Vincent & Broome, 1977), have been identified. However, attention to family coping styles and early parent-infant relationships is warranted.

In addition to his or her unique personality, the parent brings a variety of characteristics to this interaction: views on child rearing, knowledge of the child's disability, attitude about the disability, expectations for the child, concept of child development, and individual support systems and resources. Given the difficulty in modifying certain characteristics of the child, such as hypotonicity, responsivity, soothability, and rhythmicity, one likely place to intervene is through support for the parent.

Consider the case of Martha. Martha is white, married, and in the upper middle–class socioeconomic group. She has successfully parented a son and she has many friends and support resources. In short, she has a lot going for her. Recently, however, Martha gave birth to a child with Down syndrome and is having tremendous difficulties interacting with the infant. Far from joyous, the mother-child interactions, particularly feeding, are fraught with tension and failure. In helping this mother and infant, one arena for intervention is the feeding situation itself. Speech and occupational therapists assist Martha in positioning and handling the child therapeutically and in working to normalize his oral-motor muscle tone. However, by far the most successful interventions have focused on Martha. Feeding is particularly troubling for her because the infant must undergo surgery and she feels a tremendous need to "fatten him up" so that he will be ready for surgery. Further, she sees her inability to feed him as evidence that she is an incompetent mother with this child. This is exacerbated by the fact that, because her husband is much older than she is, she anticipates being left alone to care for this difficult child.

This mother and child have been active participants in the early intervention program of the author and her colleagues, and the initial tensions and asynchronies are beginning to vanish. Their interventions, although they have included the child, have centered on the mother. Specifically, they have helped Martha reinterpret her behaviors in order to see her competencies and those of her child, to have a more realistic and accurate view of Down syndrome, and to relax and enjoy the many positive characteristics of her son. Had they focused only on helping Martha teach her child to eat from a spoon more effectively, her anxieties may have actually increased and the feeding situation might have worsened. Thus, the view of parent involvement in an early intervention program is much more complex than identifying various roles (e.g., teacher) in which parents may function. Rather, families should be supported around the individual and unique needs and wishes they present.

This emphasis on early interaction is supported from a variety of sources previously reviewed in this chapter—family service needs, a transactional model of development, and a knowledge of early child development. Attention to the early parent-child environment may highlight intervention strategies and needs. Several studies, for instance, have examined early parent–

handicapped infant interactional patterns and found relations between the mother's degree of cognitive child stimulation and the mental development of the child with Down syndrome (Crawley & Spiker, 1983), and between the mother's responsivity and infant competence (Brooks-Gunn & Lewis, 1984). Further, though most studies find few group differences in mother-infant interactions when mothers of infants with Down syndrome are compared with mothers of normally developing infants (Hanson, 1984), several researchers have noted that the early maternal linguistic input and parent-infant communication interaction may be different on certain dimensions (Berger & Cunningham, 1983; Buckhalt, Rutherford, & Goldberg, 1978; Buium, Rynders, & Turnure, 1974; Cardoso-Martins & Mervis, 1985; Jones, 1977; Petersen & Sherrod, 1982). These studies underscore the relation between parenting and infant behavior, and identify the interactional arena as a major target for early intervention when dysfunction occurs.

Identifying Early Intervention Goals

Developmental and Functional Goals   Just as the parents bring important characteristics to the interaction, so does the infant: temperament, appearance, responsivity, and the disability itself. Some of these characteristics can be modified, others are not likely to be. Early teaching is aimed typically at helping the infant become more developmentally competent. Through treatment approaches, infants can be taught to sit, stand, walk, play with objects, and say words. These skills not only help the child interact more competently with the environment, they also may affect the parents' expectations and attitudes regarding the child. Likewise, the degree to which the characteristic is malleable or modifiable may affect the parents' feelings of competency in the parenting role.

A major emphasis in early intervention, thus, is in facilitating child change. It may be useful at this point to differentiate between the types or levels of goals: developmental and functional. In infancy, particularly when studying the child with Down syndrome, these types of goals may not be mutually exclusive. Developmental teaching goals may include the full range of developmental skills demonstrated across behavioral domains in infancy: sitting, standing, walking, grasping, releasing, solving simple problems, recognizing and discriminating familiar persons and things, participating in simple games, using single words, gesturing, and imitating. These skills allow infants to interact more competently with and relate better to their environment. Since a major part of that environment is people, chiefly the child's parents, emphasis should be placed on the social and communicative skills early in life and on skills that allow the child to maneuver around and manipulate his or her environment. The normally developing infant generates new learning opportunities through this exploration. These opportunities, however, may be denied the child with a disability unless he or she is helped to develop these skills.

Goals should also include skills that are functional for the child. Many of the developmental milestones that are typically taught in early intervention programs, such as feeding and walking or other forms of locomotion, obviously meet this criterion. However, attention in recent years has been given also to a broader range of skills such as "survival skills," which children may need in order to participate fully in their next educational experience, which could be a preschool program with nondisabled peers (Vincent et al., 1980). Included are skills such as waiting for a turn, sitting quietly, and following teacher directions. These skills may help the child in the long run to achieve more independence and to be integrated more readily into society.

Further, the identification of functional skills serves to focus the attention of parents and teachers on teaching skills that are useful for the child and are not taught in isolation. For example, "placing pegs in a pegboard" is an item found on most infant development tests, and also is included in most infant development curricula. One must examine, however, the need for this experience. Placing of pegs can be taught in a rich, socially interactive game-like style involving parent and child and it may enhance eye-hand coordination, turn-taking, and feelings of competency or success; or, "placing a peg" can be taught as an isolated skill in which it may serve little function in the child's overall development and ability to interact with the world.

Family Considerations Clinical observations show that the most important goal of early intervention and support services is assisting the family to accept the child as a contributing member and to treat the child the same as other members. This acceptance implies both that exceptional considerations are not implemented (the family does not revolve around the child) and that the child is respected and allowed to take the same risks and face the same or similar demands as those experienced by other family members. This notion of treating the child first and foremost as a child has important implications for early intervention with infants who have disabilities and for their families.

Integration Research on the effects of early mainstreaming or integration efforts and the spirit of Public Law 94-142, the Education for All Handicapped Children Act, highlight the need for improved integration efforts. Benefits to children with and without disabilities have been documented from these efforts (e.g., Guralnick, 1977, 1978). While most early intervention programs do not have access to groups of nondisabled children and, thus, do not have the opportunity to provide an integrated environment, they can nevertheless assist children and parents in developing the resources they need to find integrated settings as children move to subsequent educational environments. Even during infancy, program providers can help ensure that parents and their infants with Down syndrome have access to and participate with families with nondisabled children.

Health Concerns   Given what is known about Down syndrome and related health concerns, it is incumbent upon infant intervention specialists to incorporate this knowledge into early education programs. This includes providing information about such issues as early and continued screening for visual and auditory problems and assisting parents to seek appropriate medical care so as to check for disorders such as atlantoaxial instability and thyroid problems, for which children with Down syndrome are at increased risk.

Summary   Thus, the task of identifying early intervention goals is complex and multifaceted. It draws from practical concerns, developmental needs, and previous intervention research on infants and toddlers with Down syndrome. Decisions regarding the content of early intervention programs must include developmental concerns and functional concerns, and must also recognize related needs such as health concerns while at the same time recognizing that the child is a member of a family.

FOCUS OF EARLY INTERVENTION

Process of Learning

The author's previous discussion of the relation between development and learning raises many questions regarding the focus of early intervention. One such question is whether early intervention efforts should concentrate on the products of learning (e.g., teaching developmental milestones) or the process of learning (e.g., self-initiation), or both.

Research on early learning processes has established that response-contingent experiences are essential to learning, cognitive development, and motivation for the young infant. More specifically, studies have found that infants who received response-contingent training learned target responses as contrasted with a group of infants who received noncontingent feedback and failed to learn the targeted responses (Watson, 1971, 1972; Watson & Ramey, 1972). Further, infants who received the contingent learning experiences demonstrated affective responses believed to be indicative of "contingency awareness" (Watson, 1966). The role of response-contingent experiences in early development has been documented similarly by other researchers who considered these experiences essential for the development of "feelings of efficacy" (White, 1959), social competence (Goldberg, 1977; Watson, 1972), and cognitive ability (Lewis & Goldberg, 1969). Furthermore, investigations have established that early contingency learning experiences may enhance retention and learning of other responses (Finkelstein & Ramey, 1977; Rovee & Fagan, 1976). This work has led researchers (Brinker & Lewis, 1982a; Hanson & Hanline, 1985) to explore early intervention procedures to facilitate learning processes in young children with disabilities through response-contingent experiences.

The importance of a response-contingent environment on the infant's development must not be underestimated. Consider the child whose cues or signals are difficult for the parent to interpret, or the child who is passive and nondemanding and considered a "good baby," or the child whose affective responses (e.g., smiles) are "dampened" or less intense than those of the normal child. Research studies (e.g., Emde, Kligman, Reich, & Wade, 1978) and clinical experience have shown that these phrases are often attached to descriptions of young children with Down syndrome. Still other research studies have indicated that infants with Down syndrome may differ in their communicative skills from normally developing infants (Greenwald & Leonard, 1979; Jones, 1977; Leifer & Lewis, 1984; Mahoney, Glover, & Finger, 1981). These characteristics may place children at increased risk for having a less responsive environment than desirable without some sort of intervention. Taken to the extreme, infants who do not have the motor, social, or sensory skills to interact with the environment or who rarely have the opportunity to exercise control over their environment due to social deprivation factors may withdraw increasingly and be at risk for developing "learned helplessness," as characterized by Seligman (1975). However, the provision of a response-contingent environment provides the infant with both the opportunity and motivation to explore. Through these experiences, infants are allowed to initiate interactions, receive feedback from the environment, and acquire an expectancy that they are able to control the environment. Again, the emphasis in this process-oriented learning is on the infant as an active learner or initiator, rather than on an environment that is entirely adult regulated.

This body of literature suggests that early intervention strategies should focus increasingly on the process of learning so that children will learn how to learn. This focus, however, does not minimize the importance of teaching children certain skills (e.g., walking, eating with utensils, manipulating objects) so that they can interact more competently with the world around them. Hence, early intervention efforts should be concerned with both the products and process of learning.

Cross-Discipline Approach

Denhoff (1981) noted, with regard to early intervention, that there is "a refocusing of the traditional medical role away from a disease model to a more comprehensive one" (p. 33). A comprehensive approach encourages collaborative efforts between all infant care and service providers. Further, it recognizes the parent as an equal partner on the team of collaborators.

Because of the extensive, cross-disciplinary needs of infants with Down syndrome and their families, early intervention programs typically employ professionals from the health care, psychological services, and education fields. Though staffing patterns vary considerably across programs and funding restrictions preclude the diversity or amount of professional time that may be necessary for an optimal program, early intervention programs typically operate in an interdisciplinary spirit. More recently, a great deal of attention has been given to implementing a transdisciplinary model. This model is characterized by Lyon and Lyon (1980) as incorporating joint team effort, staff development, and role release. Team members, thus, work together to assess children across developmental domains, develop intervention plans together, and train one another in various aspects of their areas of expertise. This ensures that each member recognizes and treats the "whole child."

Collaborative efforts must occur both within the program, through a team approach to delivery of services, and across programs. The latter coordination among agencies ensures a more efficient and less costly service delivery model, as well as a model that more closely meets family needs. Particularly during infancy, the need for these coordinated, cross-disciplinary efforts is great.

Structuring the Environment

Another challenge for the infant development specialist is to design a learning environment that, on the one hand, is structured to enhance learning in certain areas, and, on the other hand, fosters children's spontaneous and continued interactions with the environment. While children need to learn to comply with a number of adult directives for the sake of safety and socialization, the interventionist must strike a delicate balance between this structured compliance and allowing and encouraging children's spontaneity.

Cognitively, infancy is a period in which the child moves from a sensory and reflexive being to a being who can act on objects and infer causality from observing the effects of events. During this period, the child learns imitation and simple problem solving. Further, play develops and becomes "ritualized" and symbolic in that the child engages in "make believe" representations of previous events.

The question of whether children with Down syndrome develop cognitively in the same sequence and pattern as do normally developing children remains only partially addressed. The bulk of the evidence indicates similar developmental patterns (e.g., Cicchetti & Sroufe, 1976), though some studies show differences (Morss, 1983). Just as with normally developing children, however, the cognitive developmental levels of children with Down syndrome are linked to levels of play (Hill & McCune-Nicolich, 1981) and linguistic competence (Greenwald & Leonard, 1979; Mahoney et al., 1981).

Regardless of whether children with Down syndrome differ from nondisabled children in terms of cognitive development, environmental manipulations by caregivers may enhance their development. However, this intervention should not be confused with overstructuring the environment. Many early education programs for children with disabilities "train" children to respond correctly in highly specific ways under highly specific situations. With too much structure, children often fail to generate any original responses or generalize responses to other situations.

Some of the most exciting moments the author has experienced in working with children in early education programs have come from a child's creative response to an environmental situation or event. She recalls a time when two children were waiting in a clinic room; their parents were talking with the author and her colleagues. The children made themselves into "sandwiches" by placing couch cushions above and under their bodies. Another example is the young child who was roughhousing. When the author said, "You're acting like a little monkey," he emphatically stated, "I'm not a monkey, I'm a boy." Both of these responses were made by a child who as a young infant was one of the least alert and responsive babies. Further, the child's mother was one of the most demanding and didactic of the parents with whom the author worked. However, she was also a tremendous observer of her child and believed strongly in treating him the same as other children. In actuality, like a good teacher, she knew when to structure and when not to structure a situation, and when to make demands and when to allow the child to initiate and respond without adult intervention. In short, she was directive but also warm and supportive; these important characteristics are discussed by Crawley and Spiker (1983).

A "good teacher" must know how to construct a learning task (e.g., reading) when the child won't learn just by watching, and yet he or she must also learn when to modify, restructure, and/or not intervene in rich, naturally occurring situations. This crucial balance is difficult to achieve but must be an overriding goal of intervention efforts.

SUMMARY

It is evident that any early intervention program must be of high quality, multifaceted, and flexible. Furthermore, these efforts must apply principles gleaned from one's knowledge of child development, such as the notion of the infant as active, competent, and social, and the importance of viewing the infant as an interacting member of a family. Given the diverse needs of infants with disabilities, these efforts are likely to succeed only if a collaborative cross-discipline approach is implemented.

Ramey, Beckman-Bell, and Gowan (1980) have suggested four guidelines or principles for facilitating the development of at-risk and handicapped infants. They include:

1. Recognizing the infant's active role
2. Using the infant's repertoire

3. Using natural reinforcers
4. Using daily routines as educational settings

To these Hanson (1984, pp. 197–198) has added the following:

1. Assessing the strengths, resources, and needs of the family
2. Identifying the infant's unique signaling system
3. Assisting parents to read and understand their infant's cues
4. Recognizing that early learning is largely social in nature
5. Providing contingent responses to the infant's behavior
6. Furnishing continuous follow-up and support to parents in their interactions with their infants as the developmental and interactional needs change over time

The importance of the early years to subsequent development is well documented. The foundations for social relationships, basic skills, and learning processes are established during this crucial time. A statement from the mother of a child with Down syndrome best summarizes the effects of early intervention:

> We have learned the answers to three important questions that we asked and that we have been asked many times: (1) What does a baby do? (2) what can you do with a handicapped baby? (3) how do you get a baby to do things? We have learned there is a great deal of work involved with a handicapped child, but also the rewards are well worth it.
>
> This program has helped us first to get to know Tony better and to know him as an individual with a great deal of potential. I think it has helped me personally to know that I am capable of helping both my child and other children. Most of all it has helped us to hang in there and not give up on Tony or give up hope. (Hanson, 1977, p. 5)

REFERENCES

Aronson, M., & Fallstrom, K. (1977). Immediate and long-term effects of developmental training in children with Down's syndrome. *Developmental Medicine and Child Neurology, 19*, 489–494.
Bell, R. Q. (1968). A reinterpretation of the direct effects of studies of socialization. *Psychological Review, 75*, 81–95.
Berger, J., & Cunningham, C. C. (1983). Development of early vocal behaviors and interactions in Down's syndrome and nonhandicapped infant-mother pairs. *Developmental Psychology, 19*(3), 322–331.
Berry, P., Gunn, P., & Andrews, R. (1980). Behavior of Down syndrome infants in a strange situation. *American Journal of Mental Deficiency, 85*(3), 213–218.
Bidder, R. T., Bryant, G., & Gray, O. P. (1975). Benefits to Down's syndrome children through training their mothers. *Archives of Disease in Childhood, 50*, 383–386.
Bricker, D. D., & Dow, M. G. (1980). Early intervention with the young severely handicapped child. *Journal of the Association for the Severely Handicapped, 5*(2), 130–142.

Bridges, F. A., & Cicchetti, D. (1982). Mothers' ratings of the temperament characteristics of Down syndrome infants. *Developmental Psychology, 18*(2), 238–244.

Brinker, R. P., & Lewis, M. (1982a). Discovering the competent handicapped infant: A process to assessment and intervention. *Topics in Early Childhood Special Education, 2*(2), 1–16.

Brinker, R. P., & Lewis, M. (1982b). Making the world work with microcomputers: A learning prosthesis for handicapped infants. *Exceptional Children, 49*(2), 163–170.

Brooks-Gunn, J., & Lewis, M. (1984). Maternal responsivity in interactions with handicapped infants. *Child Development, 55*, 782–793.

Buckhalt, J. A., Rutherford, R. B., & Goldberg, K. E. (1978). Verbal and nonverbal interaction of mothers with their Down's syndrome and nonretarded infants. *American Journal of Mental Deficiency, 82*(4), 337–343.

Buium, N., Rynders, J., & Turnure, J. (1974). Early maternal linguistic environment of normal and Down's syndrome language-learning children. *American Journal of Mental Deficiency, 79*(1), 52–58.

Cardoso-Martins, C., & Mervis, C. B. (1985). Maternal speech to prelinguistic children with Down syndrome. *American Journal of Mental Deficiency, 89*(5), 451–458.

Carr, J. (1970). Mental and motor development in young mongol children. *Journal of Deficiency Research, 14*, 205–220.

Cicchetti, D., & Sroufe, L. A. (1976). The relationship between affective and cognitive development in Down's syndrome infants. *Child Development, 47*, 920–929.

Cicchetti, D., & Sroufe, L. A. (1978). An organizational view of affect: Illustration from the study of Down's syndrome infants. In M. Lewis & L. A. Rosenblum (Eds.), *The development of affect* (pp. 309–350). New York: Plenum.

Clunies-Ross, G. G. (1979). Accelerating the development of Down's syndrome infants and young children. *The Journal of Special Education, 13*(2), 169–177.

Connolly, B., Morgan, S., Russell, F. F., & Richardson, B. (1980). Early intervention with Down syndrome children. *Physical Therapy, 60*(11), 1405–1408.

Connolly, B., & Russell, F. (1976). Interdisciplinary early intervention program. *Physical Therapy, 56*(2), 155–158.

Crawley, S. B., & Spiker, D. (1983). Mother-child interactions involving two-year-olds with Down syndrome: A look at individual differences. *Child Development, 54*, 1312–1323.

Dameron, L. E. (1963). Development of intelligence of infants with mongolism. *Child Development, 34*, 733–738.

Denhoff, E. (1981). Current status of infant stimulation or enrichment programs for children with developmental disabilities. *Pediatrics, 67*(1), 32–46.

Dicks-Mireaux, M. J. (1966). Development of intelligence of children with Down's syndrome: Preliminary report. *Journal of Mental Deficiency Research, 10*, 89–93.

Dicks-Mireaux, M. J. (1972). Mental development of infants with Down's syndrome. *American Journal Of Mental Deficiency, 77*(1), 26–32.

Emde, R. N., Kligman, D. H., Reich, J. H., & Wade, T. D. (1978). Emotional expression in infancy: I. Initial Studies of social signaling and an emergent model. In M. Lewis & L. A. Rosenblum, (Eds.), *The development of affect* (pp. 351–360). New York: Plenum.

Featherstone, H. (1980). *A difference in the family: Living with a disabled child*. New York: Basic Books.

Feuerstein, R. (1979a). *The dynamic assessment of retarded performers*. Baltimore: University Park Press.

Feuerstein, R. (1979b). *Instrumental enrichment: An intervention program for cognitive modifiability.* Baltimore: University Park Press.

Finkelstein, N. W., & Ramey, C. T. (1977). Learning to control the environment in infancy. *Child Development, 48,* 806–819.

Fredericks, B., Baldwin, V., Moore, W., Templeman, T., & Anderson, R. (1980). The Teaching Research data-based classroom model. *Journal of the Association for the Severely Handicapped, 5*(3), 211–223.

Goldberg, S. (1977). Social competence in infancy: A model of parent-infant interaction. *Merrill-Palmer Quarterly, 23,* 163–177.

Greenwald, C. A., & Leonard, L. B. (1979). Communicative and sensorimotor development of Down's syndrome children. *American Journal of Mental Deficiency, 84*(3), 296–303.

Gunn, P., Berry, P., & Andrews, R. J. (1982). Looking behavior of Down syndrome infants. *American Journal of Mental Deficiency, 87*(3), 344–347.

Guralnick, M. J. (1977). Nonhandicapped peers as educational and therapeutic resources. In P. Mittler (Ed.), *Research to practice in mental retardation: Vol. 1. Care and intervention* (pp. 165–170). Baltimore: University Park Press.

Guralnick, M. J. (1978). *Early intervention and the integration of handicapped and nonhandicapped children.* Baltimore: University Park Press.

Hanson, M. J. (1977). *Teaching your Down's syndrome infant: A guide for parents.* Austin, TX: PRO-ED.

Hanson, M. J. (1981). Down's syndrome children: Characteristics and intervention research. In M. Lewis & L. A. Rosenblum (Eds.), *The uncommon child* (pp. 83–114). New York: Plenum.

Hanson, M. J. (1984). *Atypical infant development.* Austin, TX: PRO-ED.

Hanson, M. J. (1985). An analysis of the effects of early intervention services for infants and toddlers with moderate and severe handicaps. *Topics in Early Childhood Special Education, 5*(2), 36–51.

Hanson, M. J., & Hanline, M. F. (1985). An analysis of response-contingent learning experiences for young children with severe handicaps. *The Journal of the Association for Persons with Severe Handicaps, 10*(1), 31–40.

Hanson, M. J., & Schwarz, R. H. (1978). Results of a longitudinal intervention program for Down's syndrome infants and their families. *Education and Training of the Mentally Retarded, 13*(4), 403–407.

Hayden, A. H., & Dmitriev, V. (1975). The multidisciplinary preschool program for Down's syndrome children at the University of Washington Model Preschool Center. In B. Z. Friedlander, B. M. Sterritt, & G. E. Kirk (Eds.), *Exceptional infant: Assessment and intervention* (Vol. 3). NY: Brunner/Mazel.

Hayden, A. H., & Haring, N. G. (1976). Programs for Down's syndrome children at the University of Washington. In T. D. Tjossem (Ed.), *Intervention strategies for high-risk infants and young children.* Baltimore: University Park Press.

Hill, P. M., & McCune-Nicolich, L. (1981). Pretend play and patterns of cognition in Down's syndrome children. *Child Development, 52,* 611–617.

Hunt, J. M. (1961). *Intelligence and experience.* New York: Ronald Press.

Jones, O. H. M. (1977). Mother-child communication with pre-linguistic Down's syndrome and normal infants. In H. R. Schaffer (Ed.), *Studies in mother-infant interaction,* (pp. 379–401). New York: Academic Press.

Kopp, C. B., Krakow, J. B., & Johnson, K. L. (1983). Strategy production by young Down syndrome children. *American Journal of Mental Deficiency, 88*(2), 164–169.

Krakow, J. B., & Kopp, C. B. (1982). Sustained attention in young Down syndrome children. *Topics in Early Childhood Special Education, 2*(2), 32–42.

Leifer, J. S., & Lewis, M. (1984). Acquisition of conversational response skills by young Down syndrome and nonretarded young children. *American Journal of Mental Deficiency, 88*(6), 610–618.

Lewis, M., & Goldberg, S. (1969). Perceptual-cognitive development in infancy: A generalized expectancy model as a function of the mother-infant interaction. *Merrill-Palmer Quarterly, 15,* 81–100.

Lillie, D. L., & Trohanis, P. L. (Eds.). (1976). *Teaching parents to teach.* New York: Walker & Co.

Ludlow, J. R., & Allen, L. M. (1979). The effect of early intervention and preschool stimulus on the development of the Down's syndrome child. *Journal of Mental Deficiency Research, 23,* 29–44.

Lyon, S., & Lyon, G. (1980). Team functioning and staff development: A role release approach to providing integrated educational services for severely handicapped students. *Journal of the Association for the Severely Handicapped, 5*(3), 250–263.

Mahoney, G., Glover, A., & Finger, I. (1981). Relationship between language and sensorimotor development of Down syndrome and nonretarded children. *American Journal of Mental Deficiency, 86*(1), 21–27.

Mahoney, G., & Snow, K. (1983). The relationship of sensorimotor functioning to children's response to early language training. *Mental Retardation, 21*(6), 248–254.

Mans, L., Cicchetti, D., & Sroufe, L. A. (1978). Mirror reactions of Down's syndrome infants and toddlers: Cognitive underpinnings of self-recognition. *Child Development, 49,* 1247–1250.

Miranda, S. B., & Fantz, R. L. (1973). Visual preferences of Down's syndrome and normal infants. *Child Development, 44,* 555–561.

Miranda, S. B., & Fantz, R. L. (1974). Recognition memory in Down's syndrome and normal infants. *Child Development, 45,* 651–660.

Morss, J. R. (1983). Cognitive development in the Down's syndrome infant: Slow or different? *British Journal of Educational Psychology, 53,* 40–47.

Paul, J. L. (1981). *Understanding and working with parents of children with special needs.* New York: Holt, Rinehart & Winston.

Petersen, G. A., & Sherrod, K. B. (1982). Relationship of maternal language to language development and language delay of children. *American Journal of Mental Deficiency, 86*(4), 391–398.

Ramey, C. T., Beckman-Bell, P., & Gowan, J. (1980). Infant characteristics and infant-caregiver interactions. In J. J. Gallagher (Ed.), *New Directions for Exceptional Children: Parents and Families of Handicapped Children* (No. 4, pp. 59–84). San Francisco: Jossey-Bass.

Rothbart, M. K., & Hanson, M. J. (1983). A caregiver report comparison of temperamental characteristics of Down syndrome and normal infants. *Developmental Psychology, 19,* 766–769.

Rovee, C. K., & Fagan, J. W. (1976). Extended conditioning and 24-hour retention in infants. *Experimental Child Psychology, 21,* 1–11.

Rynders, J. E., & Horrobin, J. M. (1980). Educational provisions for young children with Down's syndrome. In J.Gottlieb (Ed.), *Educating mentally retarded persons in the mainstream.* Baltimore: University Park Press.

Sameroff, A. J., & Chandler, M. J. (1975). Reproductive risk and the continuum of caretaking causality. In F. D. Horowitz, (Ed.), *Review of child development research* (Vol. 4, pp. 187–244). Chicago: University of Chicago Press.

Seligman, M. (1975). *Helplessness: On depression, development, and death.* San Francisco: W. H. Freeman.

Seligman, M. (Ed.). (1983). *The family with a handicapped child: Understanding and treatment.* New York: Grune & Stratton.

Serafica, F. C., & Cicchetti, D. (1976). Down's sydrome children in a strange situation: Attachment and exploration behaviors. *Merrill-Palmer Quarterly, 22*(2), 137–150.

Share, J., Koch, R., Webb, A., & Graliker, B. (1964). The longitudinal development of infants and young children with Down's syndrome (mongolism). *American Journal of Mental Deficiency, 68*, 685–692.

Solnit, A. J., & Stark, M. H. (1961). Mourning and the birth of the defective child. *Psychoanalytic Study of the Child, 16*, 523–537.

Tjossem, T. D. (Ed.). (1976). *Intervention strategies for high-risk infants and young children.* Baltimore: University Park Press.

Turnbull, H. R., & Turnbull, A. P. (1985). *Parents speak out: Then and now.* Columbus, OH: Charles E. Merrill.

Vincent, L. J., & Broome, K. (1977). A public school service delivery model for handicapped children between birth and five years of age. In E. Sontag, J. Smith, & N. Certo (Eds.), *Educational programming for the severely and profoundly handicapped* (pp. 177–185). Reston, VA: The Council for Exceptional Children.

Vincent, L. J., Salisbury, C., Walter, G., Brown, P., Gruenewald, L. J., & Powers, M. (1980). Program evaluation and curriculum development in early childhood/special education: Criteria of the next environment. In W. Sailor, B. Wilcox, & L. Brown (Eds.), *Methods of instruction for severely handicapped students* (pp. 303–328). Baltimore: Paul H. Brookes Publishing Co.

Vygotsky, L. S. (1978). *Mind in society.* (M. Cole, V. John-Steiner, S. Scribner, & E. Souberman; Eds.; Trans.). Cambridge, MA: Harvard University Press.

Watson, J. S. (1966). The development and generalization of "contingency awareness" in early infancy: Some hypotheses. *Merrill-Palmer Quarterly, 12*, 123–135.

Watson, J. S. (1971). Cognitive-perceptual development in infancy: Setting for the seventies. *Merrill-Palmer Quarterly, 17*, 139–152.

Watson, J. S. (1972). Smiling, cooing, and "the game." *Merrill-Palmer Quarterly, 18*, 323–339.

Watson, J. S., & Ramey, C. T. (1972). Reactions to response-contingent stimulation in early infancy. *Merrill-Palmer Quarterly, 18*, 219–227.

White, R. W. (1959). Motivation reconsidered: The concept of competence. *Psychological Review, 66*, 297–333.

Response

Further Notes
on Early Intervention

Diane Bricker

In writing this response, the author set two goals: to react to the content of Chapter 6, and to amplify or expand areas that she believed would benefit from additional discussion. In large measure, the issues raised by Hanson in Chapter 6 can be better understood in the context of their historical development. Thus, when appropriate, an effort has been made to provide a brief description of salient antecedent events that may assist the reader in appreciating the current status of many critical issues in the area of early intervention.

ISSUES ADDRESSED

Hanson's review of family service needs led her to conclude that early intervention programs should be prepared to deliver a range of services because the needs of participating families can be vastly different. In the late 1960s, initial discussions and efforts focusing on early intervention programs reflected a very different attitude of program staff toward child and family needs. At that time, the child was the focus of attention and if family members were involved, that involvement was generally minimal and directed by the professional staff. As Hanson made clear, our current information suggests that early intervention programs need to provide a range of services for involved family members if these programs are to serve properly the children who participate in them.

The predominant model currently employed for the delivery of early intervention services uses a transactional or interactional approach. As pointed out by Hanson, adoption of this model is appropriate for early interventionists because the "main effects" model has little relevance for persons with Down syndrome. The model suggests an emphasis on environmental manipulation since the biological base of the organism is not currently modifiable (e.g., we cannot manipulate the nervous system). A second important feature of the model is the dynamic nature of growth and development over time and the implications for responsive systems to react productively to successive changes in the child. Hanson rightly pointed out that a productive strategy used by a mother with a 9-month-old infant may be inappropriate to use with a 3-year-old child. She argued that interventionists should be aware of the interactional contribution of biology and environment, and the dynamic nature of such interactions.

In the section on the relation between development and learning, Hanson described four models that juxtapose these two basic processes in different ways. The theoretical position she advocated is the one articulated by Vygotsky (1978), who has argued that development and learning are inextricably interrelated. Although Vygotsky's position currently appears more defensible, it may be instructive to ask what effect the nature of such debates has had or should have on early intervention programs. Is program operation affected if learning and development are seen as separable or seen as inseparable? If the content of instruction and the methods of instruction are affected by such debate, then it would seem advisable for early interventionists to become knowledgeable about and enmeshed in such controversy. If programs are not significantly affected, then interventionists' time might be spent more profitably in discussing other issues.

The fourth area she discussed was research focused on infants with Down syndrome. This section addressed that part of the literature that has examined the effectiveness of early intervention. Hanson's evaluation of the efficacy studies indicated that such services appear to be valuable to participating infants and their families. Her statements concerning the impact of early intervention were thoughtfully chosen and reflected the nature of current intervention research. To date, most intervention research conducted with handicapped infants and young children is open to serious criticism (see, for example, Bricker, Bailey, & Bruder, 1984; Dunst & Rheingrover, 1981; Odom & Fewell, 1983; Strain, 1984; White, Mastropieri, & Casto, 1984) in terms of sample size, control procedures, and design and analysis strategies. If one relies on traditional empirical methodology, much of this criticism is legitimate. Often, intervention researchers are faced with a myriad of problems that require serious compromise when using traditional evaluation approaches. The goal of obtaining large subject pools, adequate controls, and uncontaminated test procedures may be unrealistic. Thus, for early interventionists and critics alike, the question becomes: Given current resources and design and analysis limitations, what strategies can be undertaken that will generate believable data on the impact of early programming on the Down syndrome infant? (More is said about this issue later.)

MAJOR THEMES

Four major themes presented by Hanson are discussed in this section: quality versus quantity differences, program structures, inclusion of the family, and attention to the individuality of children.

A major theme that occurs throughout Chapter 6, as well as in the literature on children with Down syndrome, is the quality versus quantity issue. That is, do children with Down syndrome differ from the non–Down syndrome population because as a group they learn and acquire skills more slowly, or do their behavioral repertoires show qualitative differences? More specifically, during infancy and childhood, are the fine motor, gross motor, social, cognitive, and communication behaviors of children with Down syndrome simply delayed (i.e., develop later in time), or are they different (i.e., not behaviorally the same as those of nonhandicapped children)? For example, do children with Down syndrome who begin walking independently at 24 months instead of 12 months show a qualitative difference in the way in which they learn to walk, and the manner in which they do walk, or is their learning and behavior qualitatively the same, only slower to develop?

At first glance, this quantity-quality issue may seem of little relevance for interventionists; however, this may not be so. Many current curricula in use are based on a developmental perspective. Training sequences reflect patterns and sequences of behavior most often displayed by children of the same age (i.e., norms). If children with Down syndrome are only delayed in their development, employing such curricular approaches would appear to be appropriate. If, however, children with Down syndrome deviate from the norm in terms of the manner in which they acquire or manifest skills, following a normal developmental sequence may not be effective or even appropriate.

The qualitative versus the quantitative issue also has relevance for parents. Historically, parents have been criticized for their handling of their handicapped children (e.g., parents are criticized as being rejecting, overprotective, resentful). A number of studies have examined the interactions between infants with Down syndrome and their mothers (see, for example, Berger & Cunningham, 1981; Jones, 1980; Mahoney, Finger, & Powell, 1985; Petersen & Sherrod, 1982). Many of these investigators have suggested that the reactions and interactions of mothers and their infants with Down syndrome are different from those seen between mothers and nonhandicapped infants. Although rarely overtly stated, the implications appear to be that the interactional style of the infants with Down syndrome and their parents is somehow deviant, and that some action should be taken to see that parents begin to act more like parents of non–Down syndrome infants. Although their assumptions may be accurate, it is possible that parental responses are different because infants with Down syndrome are different; rather than being inappropriate, parental responses may be appropriate and adaptive. Thus, again, it may be that resolution of the quantitative versus qualitative difference has important implications for interventionists.

A second major theme pervading Chapter 6 was the need for structure when intervening with children and parents. The literature on early intervention programs indicates that questionable benefit is derived from programs or interventions that are not thoughtfully planned and executed. Indeed, to be effective, programs require an underlying structure from which to develop goals and objectives, and to select assessment and curricular materials. By structure, the author is not referring to a rigid set of operational parameters, but rather to a sense of purpose and organization that permits staff to intervene appropriately and purposefully with participating children and families.

A third theme well represented in Hanson's chapter was the inclusion of family members in early intervention efforts. As mentioned earlier, the contemporary view of the role of the parents and family in intervention is significantly different from that found in initial program efforts. The field has moved from a focus on the infant/child, to a focus on the parents, to a focus on the family. That focus includes attempting to determine the handicapped infant/child's impact on the family and what resources the family has to effectively manage that impact. The data appear to indicate that children with handicaps who are successfully maintained in the family and the community reside in families where adequate internal and external support systems exist. Those families that remain together today may be those that can develop and maintain effective internal and external support systems (Parke & Tinsley, 1982).

Interestingly, the data reported in the literature on the impact of handicapped children on their families raise an issue similar to the quantitative versus qualitative issue. That is, does the advent of a child with a handicap cause undue stress on families? Initially, there appeared to be a consensus among professionals that every family with a handicapped member would suffer great stress produced by guilt and other "unsavory" feelings generated by the handicapped member. No one appeared to believe that these families could possibly be happy or well adjusted. More recent findings suggest that the advent of the child with a handicap may or may not produce a negative impact on the parents and family. Family interactions are more a function of the family's inherent strengths rather than the advent of a handicapped member. Recent data suggest that problems encountered by many families have more to do with management of time and workload than stress or grief over the advent of a handicapped member (Bristol & Gallagher, in press).

A fourth theme that Hanson noted was the recognition of the individuality of child, parents, and family. A myth has pervaded the Down syndrome literature about the similarity of individuals who have this genetic disorder. Parents and interventionists contend that children with Down syndrome are not similar; nevertheless, research literature continues to perpetuate this myth. If one believes that the genetic pedigree is the most salient factor in an individual's growth and development, it would seem to follow that individuals with the same genetic disorder would be similar. However, if one believes that growth and development are determined by the dynamic interaction between the individual's genetic/biological status and the environment, then one would expect individuals to be as varied as their environments. To continue to assess the impact of procedures on groups of individuals with Down syndrome and their parents as if they are a uniform population will not advance the behavioral or biological sciences. Rather, grouping constellations of individuals using a variety of relevant variables should permit the more precise determination of the impact on parents and children.

UNADDRESSED ISSUES

Several important issues not directly addressed in Hanson's chapter require mention. First, intervention efforts often must counter the expectation of a "quick fix." Inappropriate expectations of consumers (e.g., parents) can be heightened by interventionists who promise that their intervention strategy will make the person with a disability function normally. The age of the persons involved in early intervention programs makes this field particularly ripe for unrealistic promises about a child's future behavior. A review of intervention strategies proffered over the years suggests a clear tendency toward the development and perpetuation of fads. An interventionist or an approach (e.g., hammock spinning) may be advertised as a quick and sure way to eliminate a child's difficulties. Parents hoping to have a normal child are susceptible to such claims and, consequently, may waste valuable time and other resources by, for example, pumping vitamins into their children or carrying out elaborate patterning procedures that have no empirical evidence of effectiveness.

The euphoria of the 1960s and early 1970s associated with early intervention programs should be tempered today by more realistic views of what can be accomplished. Since the 1960s, a pool of sound educational policy and practice has been developing, but it has been learned that early intervention offers no quick cure for the child with a moderate or serious disability. Time and systematic effort are required to build increasing competence in the young child with Down sydrome as well as in children with other significant disabilities.

A second area not addressed in Chapter 6 is the growing effort to integrate persons with Down syndrome into community life. Where the author lives, it is not unusual to encounter a child or an adult with Down syndrome in stores, theaters, parks, or schools. However, she is still sometimes surprised and delighted by the sight, for she remembers when this population was encountered almost exclusively in large state residential facilities. A number of factors—in particular, federal mandates—have contributed to this important change. For two reasons, the advent of early intervention programs has also contributed to the nurturance of persons with handicaps in their homes and communities. First, accessibility to early intervention programs has offered parents a reasonable placement alternative for their young child. Parents no longer have to institutionalize their child to receive services. Second, parents acquire early an expectation that their child should remain at home and participate in community programs. Further, many of these programs include nonhandicapped children, a situation that offers exciting opportunities for the integration of handicapped youngsters with their nonhandicapped peers. These early experiences no doubt set the stage for many parents to expect, and demand if necessary, that their child be treated as a valued member of the community, with the same opportunities as other children/adults to participate in all community programs. Clearly, further efforts are necessary, but significant progress has been made in the community integration of persons with Down syndrome.

Finally, issues concerning documenting the effectiveness of early intervention require mention. A major question posed since the 1970s is the impact of early intervention on persons with handicaps. The question has been difficult to address in scientifically defensible ways because of design, method, and measurement problems inherent in intervention research (Baer, 1981; Bricker, 1978).

Few investigations of early intervention programs have been able to use matched controls as a basis of comparison for assessing program efficacy. Most programs cannot ethically deny educational or intervention services to children with handicaps in order to establish nonintervention control groups. Designs employing nonintervention controls are, in most states, legally impossible. Once a child has been identified as having a handicap, some form of intervention is proffered in all but the most unusual cases and this is likely to become more compelling as current cases such as Baby Jane Doe are resolved. The alternative to a nonintervention control group design is a comparison of groups of children who receive different treatments or interventions. However, there are substantial design problems when one intervention program is compared to another (Bricker & Littman, 1982). Program and population variability (e.g., variable program goals and intervention approaches, diverse population etiologies) are two major design problems that make valid program comparisons difficult. In addition to the difficulty of determining comparability of programs and populations, a program comparison design may be confounded by the problem of attrition (e.g., families moving or seeking alternative programs). Finally, many field-based programs lack resources to conduct ongoing evaluations to build an adequate data base necessary for program comparisons.

Design problems are further compounded by the lack of measurement strategies that are appropriate for persons with handicaps yet contain some relevant benchmarks that provide information for objective evaluation. Use of standardized tests is highly unsatisfactory for the more severely disabled populations (Bagnato & Neisworth, 1980; Bricker, Sheehan, & Littman, 1981; Fewell, 1983; Sheehan & Gallagher, 1983). However, employing a completely idiosyncratic system is equally unsatisfying. For example, reporting that a program reached 50% of the educational objectives established for the enrolled children is difficult to interpret for many reasons, such as the nature of the objectives, the established criteria, and the size of the interval between steps. Since no standards or benchmarks are provided, the interpretation of such reported changes becomes meaningless. Most investigators are faced with the choice between two imperfect options which, in turn, reflects on the quality and sensitivity of the data collected to determine program impact on infants and young children with handicaps. More practical designs and appropriate measures are needed.

For example, such measures might yield information that indicate a family's initial level of comfort with and adjustment to their handicapped child and how this changes following intervention. Measures that provide an accurate picture of children's daily interactional skills with peers offer more useful and functional information than examining isolated social skills elicited under structured conditions. Discovering children's actual communicative competence as they need to obtain information or objects and convey messages through interacting with their social environment provides more functional data on linguistic abilities than measures of vocabulary size. The development of these and other such measures should produce outcome data reflecting functional changes in children and families that have significant meaning for the quality of family life and community involvement.

REFERENCES

Baer, D. (1981). The nature of intervention research. In R. Schiefelbusch & D. Bricker (Eds.), *Early language: Acquisition and intervention*. Baltimore: University Park Press.

Bagnato, S., & Neisworth, J. (1980). The intervention efficiency index: An approach to preschool program accountability. *Exceptional Children 46*, 264–269.

Bailey, E., & Bricker, D. (1984). The efficacy of early intervention for severely handicapped infants and young children. *Topics in Early Childhood Special Education, 4*(3), 30–51.

Berger, J., & Cunningham, C. (1981). The development of eye contact between mothers and normal vs. Down's syndrome infants. *Developmental Psychology, 17*, 678–689.

Bricker, D. (1978). A rationale for the integration of handicapped and nonhandicapped preschool children. In M. Guralnick (Ed.), *Early intervention and the integration of handicapped and nonhandicapped children*. Baltimore: University Park Press.

Bricker, D., Bailey, E., & Bruder, M. (1984). The efficacy of early intervention and the handicapped infant: A wise or wasted resource? In M. Wolraich & D. Routh (Eds.), *Advances in developmental and behavioral pediatrics* (Vol. V, pp. 372–423). Greenwich, CT: JAI Press.

Bricker, D., & Littman, D. (1982). Intervention and evaluation: The inseparable mix. *Topics in Early Childhood Special Education, 1*, 23–33.

Bricker, D., Sheehan, R., & Littman, D. (1981). *Early intervention: A plan for evaluating program impact*. Seattle: WESTAR.

Bristol, M., & Gallagher, J. (in press). Families of young handicapped children. In M. Wang, H. Walberg, & M. Reynolds, (Eds.), *The handbook of special education: Research and practice.* Oxford, England: Pergamon Press.

Dunst, C., & Rheingrover, R. (1981). An analysis of the efficacy of infant intervention programs with organically handicapped children. *Evaluation and Program Planning, 4,* 287–323.

Fewell, R. (1983). Assessing handicapped infants. In G. Garwood & R. Fewell (Eds.), *Educating handicapped infants* (pp. 257–297). Rockville, MD: Aspen Systems.

Jones, O. (1980). Prelinguistic communication skills in Down's syndrome and normal infants. In T. Field (Ed.), *High-risk infants and children* (pp. 205–225). New York: Academic Press.

Mahoney, G., Finger, I., & Powell, A. (1985). The relationship of maternal behavioral styles to the developmental status of organically impaired mentally retarded infants. *American Journal of Mental Deficiency, 90*(3), 296–302.

Odom, S., & Fewell, R. (1983). Program evaluation in early childhood special education: A meta evaluation. *Educational Evaluation and Policy Analysis, 5,* 445–460.

Parke, R., & Tinsley, B. (1982). The early environment of the at-risk infant. In D. Bricker (Ed.), *Intervention with at-risk and handicapped infants* (pp. 153–177). Baltimore: University Park Press.

Petersen, G., & Sherrod, K. (1982). Relationship of maternal language to language development and language delay of children. *American Journal of Mental Deficiency, 86,* 391–398.

Sheehan, R., & Gallagher, R. (1983). Conducting evaluations of infant intervention. In G. Garwood & R. Fewell (Eds.), *Educating handicapped infants* (pp. 495–524). Rockville, MD: Aspen Systems.

Strain, P. (1984). Efficacy research with young handicapped children: A critique of the status quo. *Journal of the Division for Early Childhood, 9*(1), 4–10.

Vygotsky, L. S. (1978). *Mind in society* (M. Cole, V. John-Steiner, S. Scribner, & E. Souberman; Eds.; Trans.). Cambridge, MA: Harvard University Press.

White, K., Mastropieri, M., & Casto, G. (1984). An analysis of special education early childhood projects approved by the Joint Dissemination Review Panel. *Journal of the Division for Early Childhood, 9*(1), 11–26.

Chapter 7

Integration of Children with Down Syndrome at the Elementary School Level
A Pilot Study

H. D. Bud Fredericks,
John Mushlitz, Jr., and Chris DeRoest

What is known about elementary school–age children with Down syndrome? What is their academic performance? Where are they educated? How are they educated? A review of the literature on academic performance, school placement, and integration reveals very little about the characteristics of children with Down syndrome at this age and little about their capabilities. The extant literature states that the educational capabilities of children with Down syndrome have been underestimated (Rynders, Spiker, & Horrobin, 1978). However, little has been reported that systematically describes their educational or academic capabilities.

Anecdotal reports of unexpectedly high academic achievement in individual children with Down syndrome are numerous. One need only refer to issues of the *Down Syndrome News* and *Exceptional Parent* to see such reports. Seagoe (1965) and Butterfield (1961) have reported exemplary academic performances in children with Down syndrome, on a single subject, case study basis.

A review of the literature in three academic areas, reading, writing, and mathematics, revealed the following. There were no reported studies of the teaching of writing to children with Down syndrome. In the area of reading, only one study focused on children with Down syndrome. Brown, Jones, Troccolo and Heiser (1972) taught basic labeling and phrases to two children with Down Syndrome: a girl, age 6, and a boy, age 5, each of whom had an

IQ of 49. The first part of this study taught the children not only to match the printed words to 12 3-dimensional objects, but also to recognize the printed word independently of the object. Both children acquired these skills. The second part of this study taught these same children adjective-noun phrases. Again, both children acquired these skills. Training time for each child was approximately 13 trials for the first part and 9 trials for the second part of the study. In the mathematics area, Dalton, Rubino, and Hislop (1973) conducted a study to teach arithmetic skills to 13 children with Down syndrome, ages 6–14, with IQs ranging from 30 to 64. Children were randomly assigned to token economy or no token economy groups. Instruction utilized DISTAR questions (Englemann & Carnine, 1969). At the end of the program every child but one in the token economy group made arithmetic achievement score gains, whereas only three of the no token economy group made similar gains. After 1 year, the token group showed a decline in the number of arithmetic questions passed, whereas the no token group showed no change in arithmetic scores.

Thus, it is evident that little information has been gathered systematically about the academic abilities of elementary school–age children with Down syndrome. This paucity of research is disturbing; but, as Rynders (1982) states, it "is probably due to the generally low expectations held for Down syndrome persons until recent times" (p. 425).

THE OREGON SURVEY OF ELEMENTARY EDUCATION

Background Information

This chapter is the first stage of an attempt to draw a profile of the educability of elementary school–age children with Down syndrome. It focuses on the extent to which they are integrated in one state, Oregon, and provides some preliminary data about their reading and math performance in that state.

Before discussing the results of the survey some basic facts about this population and their education in Oregon should be noted:

Eighteen years ago, 128 children with Down syndrome between the ages of 7 and 11 resided at Oregon's state institution for persons with mental retardation. Today, no children with Down syndrome in that age group reside in the state institution.

Fifteen years ago, no public school programs existed in Oregon at the elementary school level for children with Down syndrome. Eight years later, all children with Down syndrome attended publicly sponsored educational programs.

Ten years ago, there were two segregated schools in Oregon which housed children with Down syndrome. Today, there are none.

Thus, there has been progress. Indeed, within the past 20 years, Oregon has moved from a state that institutionalized a large portion of its population with Down syndrome to one that routinely integrates children with Down syndrome with nonhandicapped children. The amount of change that has occurred in Oregon should make it obvious that children with Down syndrome were not always accepted in public schools. In fact, as recently as 20 years ago, the number of children with Down syndrome in public school–sponsored programs in Oregon was less than five. As a matter of fact, in the past, children with Down syndrome were found primarily in schools sponsored by private groups such as the Associations for Retarded Children (now Citizens). With the advent of Public Law 94-142, public schools accepted the responsibility for the education of children with Down syndrome; but they have not, as yet, universally accepted that that education should take place in an integrated environment.

On a national basis, there is no body of reported data that describes where children with Down syndrome are being educated today at the elementary school level or to what degree they are integrated or mainstreamed. Stainback, Stainback, Strather, and Dedrick (1983) and Hamre-Nietupski and Neitupski (1981) advocated and provided procedures for the integration of those with severe handicaps, but others have questioned whether it is possible or desirable to integrate or mainstream those who are educably mentally retarded (Gottlieb & Leyser, 1981; MacMillan & Borthwick, 1980; Peck & Semmel, 1982).

Although children with Down syndrome in Oregon are in public schools and are to some degree integrated, as the data contained herein indicate, it must be recognized that that is not the usual pattern throughout the United States. In fact, it is unusual for a state to have a totally integrated system. Most states still have vestiges of self-contained educational programming. For instance, Freagon, Peters and Brandt (1984) reported that more than half of the population identified as severely handicapped in Illinois are served in segregated facilities. Of these, one-third are identified as being trainable mentally retarded. (In their study, there is no breakdown provided of children with Down syndrome versus other forms of mental retardation, but one might guess that children with Down syndrome are among the nonintegrated group.) In Missouri, as recently as 1982, more than 90% of the children with Down syndrome were being educated in segregated environments. There is no evidence to indicate that that segregated situation has changed appreciably across the United States between 1982 and 1986. Thus, throughout the United States, wide variance exists regarding the degree of integration that occurs as a matter of public policies and the implementation of those policies. The range is epitomized by a state such as Oregon, which has better than 98% of its elementary school–age population with Down syndrome being educated in integrated environments, to states such as Missouri, which has better than 90% of its elementary school–age population with Down syndrome being educated in segregated environments.

The question continues as to the value of integration for this population. As previously cited, the research literature does not provide a strong case for the academic accomplishments of children with Down syndrome. That is not to say that they do not have those abilities, but descriptive and experimental research has been lacking for a long time.

Although the case cannot be made definitively for the integration of children with Down syndrome based on their potential for academic learning, the case can be made that children with Down syndrome need and profit from the opportunity to function in the world of nonhandicapped persons. Indeed, one cannot learn how to socialize with nonhandicapped peers unless one has the opportunity to interact and socialize with them; one cannot learn the give-and-take of young children's play and verbalizations unless one has the opportunity to play and communicate with young children; one cannot learn how to cope with unpleasant interactions with peers unless one has been subjected to peers and has learned how to respond to them. The logical conclusion is that the child with Down syndrome needs the opportunity to interact with the nonhandicapped world as much as possible in order to learn how to do so.

Related Literature

Unfortunately, the mere placing of students with Down syndrome with non-handicapped students will not necessarily produce positive interactions between the two groups. There is evidence, however, that properly constructed experiences between those with handicaps and those without handicaps will produce positive results. Fredericks et al. (1978) demonstrated that structured integration resulted in greater social interactions of handicapped and nonhan-dicapped peers; and that, after such integration, there was some evidence of increased language usage and level of usage among the handicapped popula-tion. Of the six students in the study, two were students with Down syn-drome. Although this study was conducted with preschool children, one could hypothesize that the procedures used in this study of structured and reinforced interactions between handicapped preschool children and their peers could be utilized with equal effectiveness with elementary school–age children. Knox (1983) focused on elementary school–age children and reported changes in language fluency in six children with Down syndrome as a result of integra-tion on the playground.

Rynders, Johnson, Johnson, and Schmidt (1980) demonstrated the im-portance of providing structured interactions in a recreational setting. The subjects were 30 junior high school students, ages 13 to 15. Twelve of the students were children with Down syndrome; the other 18 were nonhandicap-ped students. The setting was a regular bowling alley. Comparing cooperative goal structuring with competitive or individual goal structuring, the investigators found that a cooperative goal structure promoted significantly more praise, encouragement, and support from nonhandicapped teenagers toward peers with Down syndrome than did the individualistic or competitive goal structure. Positive interactions occurred in the cooperative group despite the fact that the performance of the students with Down syndrome tended to pull down the overall group bowling achievement.

Results of the Survey

Consequently, there is evidence that properly structured integration activities increase positive interactions between children with Down syndrome and their nonhandicapped peers. The published research literature, unfortunately, does not provide many details of such effects with elementary school–age children with Down syndrome.

In 1985, a survey was conducted among 39 school districts in Oregon. Twenty-three (60%) responded in time to be included in the results of the survey. Because of the rural nature of much of Oregon, many of the responding school districts were county education service districts, serving a number of rural school districts. It should be emphasized that county education service districts, in some cases, also provide the special education programs for larger school districts for children with moderate and severe handicaps. Of those who responded to the survey, 14 of the 23 respondents were county education service district representatives. The two largest education service districts in the state did not respond, one neglecting to do so and the other refusing on the grounds that the director of special education did not think that children with Down syndrome should be singled out merely because "they have a common cosmetic characteristic." Releases were obtained from all parents so that the information could be shared by the school districts with the researchers.

Table 1 lists the districts whose representatives responded, shows their total population sizes, and indicates which of them are education service districts. The entire population of Oregon is approximately 2 million. The population represented by the respondents is approximately 35% of that population, distributed in a uniform manner throughout the state. As indicated, three of the education service districts serve counties with populations of less than 5,000. The three largest city school systems in the state were included. The two largest, (V and W in Table 1), however, utilize the education service district in their counties to provide services for those who are moderately and severely handicapped and so, relatively few persons are listed in the table.

Programs for persons with moderate and severe handicaps in Oregon are generally noncategorical. Three types of special education programs are identified as serving children with Down syndrome. One type is developmental disabilities classrooms (DDC), usually separate classrooms located in public school buildings. In most cases, children are placed age-appropriately in these

Table 1. Population of children with Down syndrome by age, sex, and school district

School district/ catchment area	Ages																					
	5		6		7		8		9		10		11		12		13		14		15	
	M	F	M	F	M	F	M	F	M	F	M	F	M	F	M	F	M	F	M	F	M	F
Less than 5,000																						
A[a]													0	1	0	1						
B[a]																			1	0	1	0
C[a]			1	0																		
5,000–20,000																						
D																						
E[a]					1	0	0	2			1	0					0	1				
F[a]					0	1	1	0			1	0										
G[a]							0	1					0	1	0	1						
H													0	1								
I[a]																						
J			1	0	0	1	1	0	0	1	1	1	1	0								
K					0	1			1	0	1	0		1	1	0						
L[a]					0	1					1	0				1						
M[a]											1	0					1	0				
N																						

20,000–50,000
O[a]
P[a]
Q[a]
R[a]
50,000–75,000
S
T[a]
Over 75,000
U
V
W
Totals
M = 40
F = 34

185

settings. In other words, a DDC serving elementary school–age children is located in an elementary school. There are some exceptions, most of which are found in rural areas. For example, a 14-year-old boy is served in an education service district program in one of the most rural counties in the state, which has only one DDC serving all ages (see Table 1).

Children with Down syndrome are also served in separate classrooms for the mentally handicapped (SCMH). These are usually categorized as educable mentally retarded classes. Resource rooms (RR) are the third type of special education program in which children with Down syndrome are placed. Although originally established for those with learning disabilities, in many school districts they now also serve those who are educable mentally retarded. The advantage of placement in a resource room, as cited by many school districts and many parents, is that a child with moderate handicaps can be placed in his or her home school. In many of the DDC classrooms, children are bused into central programs from a broad catchment area.

Table 1 shows the breakdown by sex, age, and size of school district where children with Down syndrome are placed. Seventy-four children with Down syndrome were identified for inclusion in the survey. Others were not included in these same school districts because of parents' refusals to sign releases of information. The exact number of such refusals was unknown at time of publication. Included in this survey are 40 males and 34 females, ranging in age from 5 to 15 years. All are located in elementary schools. Some question must be raised as to the age placement of the five children aged 13, 14, and 15. As previously indicated, the 14-year-old boy is in a rural school district where only one DDC serves all ages of students with moderate and severe handicaps. All of the 13-year-olds are also in DDCs. The 15-year-old is in a non-special education program (NSEP) in an elementary school.

The distribution of students by type of special education program is shown in Table 2. As shown, 45 students are served in developmental disabilities classrooms. Seventeen are served in separate classrooms for those with mental handicaps; eight are served in resource rooms; and four children are not placed in special education programs—one is in a very rural area and the other three are in school districts with populations between 5,000 and 20,000.

Tables 3 and 4 display the placements of children in integrated settings. All 74 children are integrated into some curricular areas. Children with Down syndrome are integrated into nonhandicapped settings encompassing 16 curricular areas. In Table 3, the number of children placed in each of these is shown together with the size of the school district and the type of special education placement. Table 4 shows integration based on the age of the children.

Twenty-seven of the children are integrated in lunch and recess. Other than lunch and recess, children are most often integrated into physical educa-

Table 2. Placement of students with Down syndrome in types of special education programs by size of school district

School district	DDC[a]	SCMH[b]	RR[c]	NSEP[d]
Less than 5,000	3	1	0	1
5,001–20,000	14	7	3	3
20,001–50,000	4	0	2	0
50,001–75,000	18	3	0	0
Over 75,000	6	6	3	0
Totals	45	17	8	4

[a]Developmental disabilities classroom.
[b]Separate classroom for the mentally handicapped.
[c]Resource room.
[d]Non-special education program.

tion (PE) classes; six children have placements in those activities. Thus, 33 of the 74 children are integrated in no settings other than lunch and/or recess and/or PE. As indicated by Table 3, the next most frequently integrated setting is music. Approximately 10% of the children are also integrated in reading, library, social studies, and science.

The mean number of hours of integration for all children daily is 2.02 hours, with a range of .45–4.5 hours daily. Children who are placed in resource rooms are integrated for an average of 2.64 hours, with a range of 1.0–4.5 hours daily. Those who are in classes for the mentally handicapped are integrated for an average of 2.2 hours a day, with a range of 1.0–4.0 hours daily, whereas those who are in developmental disabilities classes are integrated for an average of 1.42 hours per day, with a range of .45–3.0 hours daily.

Table 5 shows preliminary data regarding reading and math levels of a sample of children with Down syndrome. For purposes of obtaining these data, all children were listed on a master roster in the order in which the survey responses from the field were received. The age of each of these children was also shown on this master roster. The master roster was then divided into 11 separate rosters by age while preserving the same random order of placement on the roster. The plan was to select randomly an age-stratified sample of students and to survey the school districts again about the reading and math functioning levels of the students. For purposes of the stratification of ages, ages 5 and 6 were combined, as were ages 13, 14, and 15. Eight groups by ages were thus formulated. One child from each group was randomly selected except for ages 7 and 10, both of which had more than 10 children. From these two groups, two children were selected. Then, 12 numbers were placed in a box, numbered from 1 to 12. For each age group, a number was picked from the box and the child whose number on the roster

Table 3. Areas of integration of students with Down syndrome by size of district and type of educational placement

	Lunch	Recess	Physical education	Music	Art	Reading	Library	Computer	Social studies	Science	Writing	Language arts	Math	Study period	Kindergarten	Counseling
School district																
Less than 5,000	5	5	2	1	0	1	1	0	2	1	1	1	0	0	1	0
5,001–20,000	25	24	17	15	3	4	4	0	4	3	3	1	0	0	2	4
20,001–50,000	5	5	2	2	1	0	1	0	0	0	0	0	0	1	0	0
50,001–75,000	21	19	4	1	0	5	1	3	3	0	0	0	0	0	0	0
Over 75,000	14	15	7	1	0	0	1	0	0	3	1	0	1	1	0	0
Totals	70	68	32	20	4	10	8	3	9	7	5	2	1	2	3	4
Type of placement																
DDC[a]	44	41	12	7	3	5	6	3	2	1	1	0	0	1	1	1
SCMH[b]	15	16	12	6	1	2	2	0	2	2	0	1	0	0	1	3
RR[c]	8	8	5	4	0	0	0	0	4	3	1	0	1	0	0	0
NSEP[d]	3	3	3	3	0	3	0	0	1	1	3	1	0	1	0	0
Totals	70	68	32	20	4	10	8	3	9	7	5	2	1	2	3	4

[a]Developmental disabilities classroom.
[b]Separate classroom for the mentally handicapped.
[c]Resource room.
[d]Non-special education program.

Table 4. Areas of integration of students with Down syndrome by age of students

Age	N	Lunch	Recess	Physical education	Music	Art	Reading	Library	Computer	Social studies	Science	Writing	Language arts	Math	Study period	Kindergarten	Counseling
5	3	3	3	2	0	0	0	0	0	0	0	0	0	0	0	0	0
6	6	6	4	1	0	0	0	0	0	0	0	0	0	0	0	2	0
7	12	10	10	3	2	1	2	1	0	1	0	1	0	0	0	0	0
8	10	10	10	6	5	1	2	2	0	2	2	2	0	1	0	0	0
9	8	7	8	3	4	1	2	2	0	1	1	0	0	0	0	0	1
10	12	11	10	6	5	0	1	1	0	3	3	1	1	0	1	1	3
11	9	9	9	3	1	0	0	0	0	0	0	0	0	0	0	0	0
12	9	9	9	6	0	0	0	1	3	0	0	0	0	0	1	0	0
13	3	3	3	1	2	1	2	0	0	0	0	0	0	0	0	0	0
14	1	1	1	0	0	0	0	1	0	1	0	0	0	0	0	0	0
15	1	1	1	1	1	0	1	0	0	1	1	1	1	0	0	0	0
Totals	74	70	68	32	20	4	10	8	3	9	7	5	2	1	2	3	4

Table 5. Reading and math levels of a sample of students with Down syndrome (1.2 = 1st grade, 2nd month)

Student	Age	Level by grade	Placement
Reading			
1	6	0	DDC[a]
2	7	0	DDC
3	7	1.2	DDC
4	8	2.2	RR[b]
5	9	2.0	SCMH[c]
6	10	0	DDC
7	10	2.8	SCMH
8	11	3.2	RR
9	12	2.8	DDC
10	13	3.8	DDC
Math			
11	6	0	DDC
12	7	1.2	DDC
13	7	0	SCMH
14	8	0	DDC
15	9	2.4	RR
16	10	0	DDC
17	10	0	RR
18	11	1.5	SCMH
19	12	1.2	DDC
20	13	0	DDC

[a]Developmental disabilities classroom.
[b]Resource room.
[c]Separate classroom for the mentally handicapped.

matched the number selected was chosen for the survey. If the number selected was too high and no such number appeared on the roster, another number was selected until there was a matching number on the roster. Thus, 10 children were selected, and the school districts were called to obtain the reading and math functioning levels of the children so selected. These data were obtained in all cases from the teachers of the children (see Table 5).

Table 5 presents a very small amount of academic data. Obviously, a much larger sample needs to be gathered to determine if these data are representative. The reading data for nine students ages 7–13 indicate that seven of the nine have some reading ability; in most cases, however, the reading ability is substantially below grade level. Nevertheless, the data suggest that reading instruction should definitely be *tried* with all children with Down syndrome so as to provide them with as much reading ability as possible. The math data in Table 5 present a different picture. Of the nine students ages 7–13, only four demonstrate some math ability and this ability is obviously at a very basic level.

Limitations of the Survey

Looking across all of the findings presented adds to the general state of knowledge about children with Down syndrome. However, there are limitations that must be considered in the interpretation of these data. The overall survey attempted to portray the levels of integration of all children with Down syndrome at the elementary school–age level in the state of Oregon. Data were not available for all children. The authors estimate that the data presented here represent one-third of the state's elementary school–age population; however, that figure must be viewed cautiously because neither the exact number of parents who refused to sign the release, nor the exact number of children with Down syndrome in the nonresponding school districts is known.

Also, the data on integration cannot be generalized across states since Oregon has no segregated facilities for children with Down syndrome. Moreover, the administration of special education services in Oregon is somewhat unique, which may affect the delivery of services. DDCs are funded in part from the mental health division of the state; this agency also sets standards for those programs. One of those standards has been to make maximum use of integration opportunities.

One must also consider the possibility of author bias, although they do not believe it is affecting the results presented here. The authors of this chapter favor integration. They recognize that not all other professionals agree with them. Their belief is that an important goal in the education of children with handicaps is to teach them how to function in the world of the nonhandicapped.

SUMMARY AND CONCLUSIONS

The survey examined in this chapter begins a systematic investigation of the degree to which children with Down syndrome are integrated. It reveals that all children with the condition are integrated to some extent. However, 27 of 74 children are integrated only for lunch and/or recess. This represents minimal integration.

An examination of the data reveals some other interesting facts. There seems to be no difference in the degree of integration based on size of school district (Table 1). In addition, children from all types of special education placements are being integrated (Table 3). Children in resource rooms are, on the average, being integrated into regular programs for longer periods of time. The authors hypothesize that the higher functioning children have been placed in these resource rooms. Moreover, most children who are placed in resource rooms for part of their education generally spend most of their day in non-special education programs. However, it must be recognized that the hypothesis about higher functioning students being so placed must be tempered by the possibility that in smaller school districts, this is the only special education program available. In other cases, placement in these programs may have been a decision reached in order to reduce busing time for students or to maintain a student in his or her home school. Further investigation as to why students are placed in resource rooms needs to be done. Such an investigation is planned by the authors.

Table 3 presents some interesting information that warrants further investigation. At ages 5 and 6, integration does not exist for children outside of lunch, recess, and physical education except for two children integrated into kindergarten. If one examines the number of integrated settings of children from ages 7 through 12, however, a pattern is suggested. Excluding lunch and recess, children at age 7 are in an average of 1.16 other settings; at age 8, 2.3 other settings; at age 9, 1.87 other settings; at age 10, 2.16 other settings. At ages 11 and 12, the average number of integrated settings diminishes to .44 and 1.33, respectively. The number of students at each age level is small, so these figures may not represent a true trend. At the very least, however, these data suggest the need for further investigation.

Results of the survey presented in this chapter do not address the quality of integration that occurs. Quality is a major area in need of exploration. A number of questions must be asked. Are students gainfully employed when they are integrated? Are integrated settings bona fide learning experiences for them? Do children have the opportunity to interact with nonhandicapped peers in integrated settings, especially in those that present the opportunity for social interaction? Is there a relation between the amount and type of integration occurring, and social acceptance by nonhandicapped peers? What is the relation between the amount of integration that occurs during school hours and the amount that occurs after school? These questions are topics for additional studies by the authors which are currently in progress.

The data about academic abilities suggest that the type of special education placement does not dictate whether a student is taught academic subjects or has academic ability. Students in the sample came from a variety of academic settings and no relation could be discerned between special education placement and academic performance. One would have suspected that children placed in resource rooms would have greater academic abilities and that children placed in developmental disabilities classrooms would not have much academic ability. This suspected pattern was not realized. There were children in DDCs who were functioning academically as high as those children in RRs. However, it should be recognized that more children in DDCs were also functioning at a lower level, and that the overall sample size is too small for one to be confident about the findings. Also, the examination of academic performance needs to be expanded to a large number of students with Down syndrome across several subject areas.

REFERENCES

Brown, L., Jones, S., Troccolo, E., & Heiser, C. (1972). Teaching functional reading to young trainable students: Toward longitudinal objectives. *Journal of Special Education, 3,* 237–246.

Butterfield, E. C. (1961). Provocative case of over-achievement by a Mongoloid. *American Journal of Mental Deficiency, 66* (61), 444–448.

Dalton, A., Rubino, C., & Hislop, M. (1973). Some effects of token rewards on school achievement of children with Down's syndrome. *Journal of Applied Behavior Analysis, 6,* 251–259.

Englemann, S., & Carnine, D. (1969). *DISTAR: Arithmetic 1. An instructional system.* Chicago: Science Research Associates.

Freagon, S., Peters, C., & Brandt, D. (1984). [Report to the Illinois Developmental Disabilities Council]. Unpublished manuscript.

Fredericks, H., Baldwin, V., Grove, D., Moore, W., Riggs, C., & Lyons, B. (1978). Integrating the moderately and severely handicapped preschool child into a normal day care setting. In M. Guralnick (Ed.), *Early intervention and the integration of handicapped and nonhandicapped children.* Baltimore: University Park Press.

Gottlieb, J., & Leyser, Y. (1981). Facilitating the social mainstreaming of retarded children. *Exceptional Education Quarterly, 1* (4), 57–69.

Hamre-Nietupski, S., & Nietupski, J. (1981). Integral involvement of severely handicapped students within regular public schools. *The Journal of the Association for the Severely Handicapped, 6* (2), 30–39.

Knox, M. (1983). Changes in the frequency of language use by Down's syndrome children interacting with nonretarded peers. *Education and Training of the Mentally Retarded, 18* (3), 185–190.

MacMillan, D. L., & Borthwick, S. (1980). The new educable mentally retarded population: Can they be mainstreamed? *Mental Retardation, 18* (4), 155–158.

Peck, C. A., & Semmel, M. I. (1982). Identifying the least restrictive environment (LRE) for children with severe handicaps: Toward an empirical analysis. *The Journal of the Association for the Severely Handicapped, 7* (1), 56–63.

Rynders, J. (1982). Research on promoting learning in children with Down syndrome. In S. Pueschel & J. Rynders (Eds.), *Down syndrome: Advances in biomedicine and the behavioral sciences* (pp. 389–451). Cambridge, MA: Academic Guild.

Rynders, J., Johnson, R., Johnson, D., & Schmidt, B. (1980). Producing positive interaction among Down syndrome and nonhandicapped teenagers through cooperative goal structuring. *American Journal of Mental Deficiency, 85* (3), 268–273.

Rynders, J., Spiker, D., & Horrobin, M. (1978). Underestimating the educability of Down's syndrome children: Examination of methodological problems in recent literature. *American Journal of Mental Deficiency, 82* (5) 440–448.

Seagoe, M. V. (1965). Verbal development in a Mongoloid. *Exceptional Child, 31,* 269–275.

Stainback, S., Stainback, W., Strather, M., & Dedrick, C. (1983). Preparing regular classroom teachers for the integration of severely handicapped students: An experimental study. *Education and Training of the Mentally Retarded, 18* (3), 203–209.

Elementary Education
for Children
with Down Syndrome

Jean M. Zadig

✦✦✦

Chapter 7 has presented the "bad news." The literature with regard to the education of elementary school pupils with Down syndrome is not only inconclusive, it is virtually nonexistent. How are these children progressing? What is the range of their educational potential? What are their functional academic skills at a specific age or grade level? What will be their long-term retention of those skills? On a national basis, where are they being educated, and to what degree are they being mainstreamed? What are the effects of educational integration? None of the answers to these questions is known.

Fredericks, Mushlitz, and DeRoest have described the school placement of 74 Oregon children with Down syndrome, and the skill levels of a subset of these. They note that there seems to be no discernible relation between educational placement and academic performance. It even seems unlikely that IQ was a factor in determining whether a child was placed in a developmental disabilities class, a separate class for those who are mentally handicapped, or a resource room. The degree to which these pupils were mainstreamed and the academic progress that they made is very disappointing. Only *one* of the Oregon pupils had reached a grade equivalency of 3.8 in reading; only *one* had reached an equivalency of 2.4 in math. The author has concluded that many professionals and parents have an expectation that the child with Down syndrome will make substantial progress toward normalcy, given a supportive home and appropriate education. While academic achievement is obviously only one part of life success, it is surely not an inconsequential one.

Probably it is fair to note that the Oregon experience is, in several respects, quite different from that of many other states. In Oregon, there were no public elementary school programs for children with Down syndrome 15 years ago. In Massachusetts, 15 years ago, all public school districts were educating such children. The state schools had been closed to new child admissions for several years, due in part to the well-known efforts of the late Burton Blatt. There have never been many private schools for handicapped children; such programs have tended to be utilized by the wealthy or the very poor. From the latter have come children whose families have been unable to care for them, making out-of-home placement necessary; currently, foster placement and adoption are usually considered even in those cases. The author believes, unfortunately without hard evidence, that virtually all Massachusetts public school pupils with Down syndrome are integrated with normal elementary school pupils at least to the minimal extent described in Chapter 7.

There is, however, a tendency to integrate the younger child to a greater degree; not only are the years before age 10 viewed as the "golden" ones for children with Down syndrome, but these are also the years before the "academic gap," particularly in written language, becomes difficult to manage. There are more program options at the nursery, kindergarten, and primary levels. Early education is mandated from age 3, but many parents appear to use the public special needs program to obtain the needed special services and small group instruction, while enrolling their child in a second program for normalization. Children with Down syndrome are found in a variety of private nursery and kindergarten programs, as well as in Head Start and day care programs.

Ungraded primary classes and "transition classes," resource rooms, developmental classes, and "substantially separate classes" are all utilized; as in Oregon, the factors determining the choice are often quite arbitrary. The skills that are taught in a class are supposed to match the needs of each pupil, and that, of course, depends on the appropriateness of the individualized education program (IEP) and the ability of the staff to implement it. Given Massachusetts's apparently longer experience of educating children with Down syndrome, it is, according to the author, all the more scandalous that she and her colleagues have no data to show for it. A whole generation of children with Down syndrome have gone from preschool to vocational training and there is only a vague idea of what the children and the providers of the educational services have accomplished.

FUNCTIONAL LEARNING

In an unpublished doctoral dissertation, Weisenfeld (1983) looked at the IEPs of 41 elementary pupils with Down syndrome; most were Massachusetts public school pupils. He analyzed the content of the IEPs with a view to comparing the maturationally based or stage theory model with a functional model, in which skills taught would have some immediate or future usefulness to the student. Academics figured as an objective on 100% of those IEPs. But the reading materials that may have been employed and the uses to which reading may have been put are cause for concern. Also reason for concern is a math curriculum that may require students to practice add-combinations year after year, while neglecting to teach the use of a pocket calculator, a digital watch, or a coin sorter, for keeping quarters and nickels in their proper places. There is so much to learn and so little time to learn it, that teachers must make every minute count. And sometimes common sense does not figure prominently in the curriculum.

Common sense is, arguably, the most functional of all learned behavior. The author was so impressed one night at the supermarket by the resource-fulness of a young woman with Down syndrome. The author's attention was first drawn to the young woman's shakily printed shopping list, which she deciphered with some difficulty. Having caught the author's eye, the woman decided that she was the right height and degree of neighborliness to be approached. "Will you get me one of those pickle jars up there?" she asked, indicating the top shelf, far beyond her reach. Subsequently, she approached the author again. "Is this Lo-Cal dressing?" (It seemed that a housemate was on a diet.) Obviously, the young woman's home/school situation had had quite a success in training common sense.

By contrast, the picture of mentally retarded adolescents wasting their time on activities that have no relevance for them is all too familiar. The author remembers a "state school" class decades ago, where the teacher used five pictures reproduced from a coloring book as the cornerstone of her curriculum. When the members of her class could color the kite to this teacher's satisfaction, they moved on to the sailboat; after that, came the robin. Good work habits and careful attention to staying within the lines were thought to flow from this activity. This teacher reported with great indignation that the parents of one 17-year-old boy had removed him from the school and set him to digging ditches, so that they could collect his wages. (This, although he had only completed the sailboat!)

Much progress has been made in offering more appropriate education to secondary pupils. But is it possible that some of the same issues have not been addressed at the elementary level? Perhaps the question "Why does this child need to be learning *this* task at *this* time ?" should be asked. The answer may simply be, "Because he or she will enjoy it." or "Because it is what other children his or her age learn." But still, the question *should* be asked. If functional language competency, the ability to function appropriately in a variety of social contexts, and an attractive appearance are critical factors in secondary placements and success, these areas should be given considerable attention at earlier levels. (By attractive appearance, the author does not imply cosmetic surgery, but good grooming and personal hygiene, apparel that follows local norms, and, if possible, some degree of conformity to weight norms for height and age.) In examining the IEPs of her clients, the author does not see objectives in those areas. Perhaps this is one instance where noncompliance with the IEP is practiced with justification.

DECIDING WHAT TO TEACH

The point has been made (Weisenfeld, 1983) that the technology of *how to teach* appears to be more advanced than the knowledge of *what to teach* and in what sequence. There is often a distressing absence of setting priorities among IEP objectives. The most famous example at the clinic at The Children's Hospital in Boston was 7-year-old Martha's IEP, on which the first objective was, "Martha will learn to keep her thumb out of her mouth at all times." (One suspects that if little Martha were to get her hands on some interesting educational materials, she might find her thumb unavailable for sucking, anyway.) The problem of not seeing the forest for the trees is not a new one for educators. And the current requirement of spelling out a whole year's objectives is fraught with perils. (It is clearly better than not having any projections, but the author often looks at the paltry list of what the child will learn and thinks, "that's ALL?") Frequently the staff who will implement this IEP in the coming year have not yet arrived on the scene when it is being formulated, and, predictably, the student's progress is somewhat different from what was anticipated. There is also considerable "soft" evidence that special and regular educators seldom refer to those IEP objectives as the months go by.

Regardless of the program prototype in which the elementary school–age child with Down syndrome finds him- or herself, the curriculum has certain commonalities. Until the child is ready for a formal academic curriculum, "readiness activities" figure prominently. These are appropriate for the younger child but become less so as the years pass and the child has clearly not made the hoped-for progress. (For the 12-year-old child, readiness activities demand the question, "Readiness for what?") Other objectives on the IEP are in the areas of language, motor function, "academics," and social/adaptive function. It is certainly possible that all of these areas can be addressed in the education program to the profit of the student; unfortunately, this is not always the case. The author agrees with Fredericks et al. that social learning has not received enough attention in the schools, or in many homes, for that matter. For all children, it is obviously a critical factor in school and life success and happiness. It is not clear to the author that teachers and parents of children with Down syndrome have seriously considered what social/adaptive skills are going to be needed in the environments toward which the children are moving (e.g., secondary, vocational, community living). It is also not clear when they think the children should learn those life skills and how they should learn them. In fact, the suspicion is inescapable that teachers and parents structure the environment to suit the functional level of the client, rather than looking ahead to preparing the client for a particular environment. "Responsive environments" are desirable, but surely there is a responsibility to see that the children are challenged to reach their potential. Isn't that why parents and teachers spread the good news about the triumphs of children with Down syndrome who live and work in near-normal environments? This doesn't just happen; it is years in the making.

TRANSITION TO ADOLESCENCE

Just before the onset of the dreaded transition to post-elementary education, parents often panic. They think of a dozen reasons why their child should not move up to the middle school or the junior high school; this, in spite of the fact that special needs pupils are usually not advanced to these schools until they are a year or so older than their normal peers. Of course youngsters with Down syndrome are short of stature and often exhibit less mature behavior. Of course junior high schools are "jungles" where all manners of vice abound. But the dangers of alcohol abuse, smoking, and worse are surely less of an issue for children with Down syndrome than for normal children! And there is no evidence that keeping a mentally retarded young person with much younger pupils has a maturing effect on him or her; common sense suggests that the opposite effect can be expected. Where are the social role models, the recognition of the adolescent thrust toward independence? How will the child know which sneakers are "in" and which jeans are "out?" Of course the elementary school is safe and comfortable. But that's part of the problem. The author knows a mother who complains that her daughter with Down syndrome is left by the school bus at a school entrance that is far from her own classroom. "Anything could happen as she traverses that enormous building," the mother says. But the teacher remarks, "How marvelous that Marian travels all that way alone, nodding a greeting to familiar people, stopping off at her locker, and demonstrating to herself and all the world, 'I can handle this by myself.' " The early proponents of normalization warned that normalization entails risk. Growing up in the United States entails enormous risk in itself. But the risk is lower for individuals with special needs if the problems that they will encounter are anticipated and they are taught strategies for handling various situations. Clearly, parents and teachers cannot wait until the "child with Down syndrome" becomes "the adult with Down syndrome" before training for adulthood is begun. Like sex education, training for mature social interaction cannot be delivered in a single "innoculation" at age 16, 18, or 21. They must be prepared all along the way.

TEACHING READING

Since space is limited, this part of the response focuses briefly on one curricular area that is particularly important: reading. Literacy, often defined generally as reading at the fifth/sixth grade level, is considered an essential tool in our culture; albeit one that approximately 10% of the adult population in the

United States lacks. The author is not familiar with any study documenting the percentage of individuals with Down syndrome who are literate, but her suspicion is that only a tiny minority are. She also does not know if one should make one's peace with that, berate the teachers, or demand new and better instructional methods and materials. Given the probability that reading at the fifth or sixth grade level is not "in the cards" for most with Down syndrome, how should reading as a focus of curriculum for the child with Down syndrome be approached? Are primary level reading skills useful? Is it valuable to be able to decode words, if comprehension lags far behind?

The author feels that any reading skills at all are of potentially enormous value to the person with Down syndrome. She also believes that students who continue to demonstrate progress in and motivation for reading should continue with daily reading instruction at least until age 16. Reading is not an all-or-none proposition; it may be viewed along a continuum of representational or symbolic communication. Experience with nonverbal clients with cerebral palsy, many of whom have the intelligence and the motivation to learn an alternative mode of communication, shows that even persons with severe mental retardation can learn simple communication using 3-dimensional objects or photographs. For others, rebuses or Blissymbols may be employed when alphabetic symbols are too complex. The usefulness of sight words should not be underestimated either, since words such as STOP and EXIT, two universally familiar sight words, can literally save a life. Probably parents and teachers do not stress the expansion of a sight vocabulary enough because they tend to see this as a laborious and inefficient way of acquiring reading skills. However, much of the world's population routinely does it this way. The author once asked a special educator from Japan how he taught all of those characters to mentally retarded pupils and he responded quickly, "Oh, we don't. We teach them to read Japanese words in your alphabet!"

Many teachers are comfortable with using basal reading approaches with young mentally retarded pupils, even though the materials lack practical application at the early stages. However, if a child of 10 has spent half of his or her life trying to master sound/symbol associations without success, a better use should be found for that child's time. The age of 10 is not the time, in the author's opinion, when different developmental reading approaches should be tried, while the child grows increasingly frustrated and discouraged. It is the time to move to a reading program where a functional sight vocabulary is derived from the child's own needs and experiences, and is practiced in ways that provide the child with intrinsic rewards for mastering his or her assignment.

There is, of course, for many individuals, an intrinsic delight in reading. For the child with Down syndrome, this extends even to the carrying of books to and from school or the library. The personal satisfaction of decoding squiggles on a paper is akin to the exhiliration of deciphering symbols on the

Rosetta stone. Reading the TV guide, the menu at a fast-food emporium, or the rules at the swimming pool are normalizing experiences. The use of books and magazines for leisure should also be fully developed in persons whose leisure opportunities will be more circumscribed than those of most individuals. A walk through any children's library reveals that books available at any level, even the preprimer, have much to offer to adults, as well as children: singing poetry, gorgeous illustrations, and nonfiction titles abound. But more than all of this, the tasks of daily living constantly provide opportunities to apply simple reading skills: making or using a shopping list, selecting products from the store shelves, banking, using public transportation, following simple maps, choosing a greeting card for a loved one, using the telephone directory, sorting mail in a residence or place of work, reading a note from Mom, or following a recipe. The list could go on and on.

CONCLUSION

There is even a place for teaching strategies to handle the situations where skills fall short of the need. A wise teacher of severely retarded young adults was once asked, "How can you let your students go to Boston alone when they can't read to find their way back?" "No problem," he replied. "As soon as they come into the program we start practicing how to take a position on the platform where the end car will be. After the cars have come in they look around for a friendly face and say, 'Was that the Arborway car? It came in so fast I didn't see the front.' "

The lack of research on the education of elementary school–age children with Down syndrome is shocking and must be remedied if parents and teachers are to serve them well. Let it be resolved to move quickly in this area, so that curricula, teaching methods, materials, and settings may be planned for maximizing their potential.

REFERENCES

Weisenfeld, R. B. (1983). An empirical basis for the content analysis of individual education programs (IEPs) for Down's syndrome children (Doctoral dissertation, Kent State University). *Dissertation Abstracts International, 4410A*.

Chapter 8

Secondary Education
for Students
with Down Syndrome
Implementing Quality Services

Barbara Wilcox and G. Thomas Bellamy

Until quite recently, special education programs for high school students suffered from pervasive, though benign, professional neglect. Rarely were teachers or related service professionals trained to meet the specific needs of older students with handicaps; there were few curricula or instructional materials relevant to their age level; and there were virtually no program models demonstrated to be both effective and appropriate for the high school environment. That this has now changed is evident both in legislation and in federal initiatives. For example, PL 98-199 amended the language of PL 94-142 to refer to handicapped children and *youth* (rather than simply children), and also established a discretionary grant program to improve special education at the secondary level. The highly visible federal initiative on transition from school to work and adult life (Will, 1984) has also directed considerable professional attention to the quality and effectiveness of special education preparation in the nation's high schools.

Concern for the quality of secondary special education comes at a critical time. The first generation of students to grow up enjoying a free appropriate public education has now reached high school. Unlike their cohorts of earlier generations, these students have been able to attend local public school programs rather than be transferred to institutional settings. As a consequence,

The Oregon High School (OHS) Project was supported by contract 300-81-0408 from the Special Needs Section, Office of Special Education Programs, U.S. Department of Education, to the University of Oregon. The authors wish to acknowledge the contributions of Shawn Boles, John McDonnell, and Heidi Rose, which were important to the success of the project. Thanks go as well to the teachers, students, parents, and administrators of the OHS classrooms who helped the authors learn what they needed to know.

there has been rapid expansion in the number of students with moderate and severe handicaps in community high schools. Such expansion provides both the pressure and the opportunity to examine services, and to define excellence for high school programs serving students with more intense educational needs.

The literature addressing high school for students with severe handicaps has generally taken one of two forms. A growing number of studies have reported the acquisition, generalization, and maintenance of skills functional for adolescents and young adults. There are, for example, demonstrations of teaching grocery shopping (McDonnell, Horner, & Williams, 1984; Nietupski, Welch, & Wacker, 1983; Wheeler, Ford, Nietupski, Loomis, & Brown, 1980) and other purchasing skills (Storey, Bates, & Hanson, 1984), telephone use (Horner, Williams, & Steveley, 1984), simple meal preparation, and use of mass transit, as well as a variety of community jobs (e.g., Certo, Mezzullo, & Hunter, 1985). The second strand of the high school literature comprises those papers that advance a particular value framework for the organization of secondary programs (Bellamy & Wilcox, 1980; Brown et al., 1979; Sailor & Guess, 1983; Williams, Vogelsberg, & Schutz, 1985). While such position papers are important, few data are available to indicate whether the program features advocated are either achievable or useful in local educational programs.

Though students with Down syndrome are an identifiable group, the literature specifically focused on high school students with Down syndrome is virtually nonexistent. However, many studies report the participation of adolescents with Down syndrome (e.g., McDonnell et al., 1984; Nietupski et al., 1983; Wheeler et al., 1980). Authors of position papers focus more broadly on the educational concerns of all youth with handicaps, including those with Down syndrome. The fact that students with Down syndrome function across a range of ability levels may serve to make them less visible in the literature than in the classroom.

The purpose of this chapter is to review the status of high school programs for students with Down syndrome. In essence, this requires attention to three basic questions: What are the goals of high school for students with Down syndrome? How can the educational system be changed to achieve those goals? What are the actual effects of such changes? The authors' response to these questions derives from an effort begun at the University of Oregon in 1980, to develop, install, and evaluate exemplary high school services for students with moderate to severe handicaps.

GOALS OF HIGH SCHOOL PROGRAMS

Ongoing debate about the purposes of regular education notwithstanding, there exists a well-established ideological foundation for defining the goals of secondary schooling for students with moderate to severe handicaps. In earlier writings, the authors proposed the preparation for and transition to successful adult living as the mission of secondary special education. Successful adult living, they have argued, could be usefully indexed by an individual's productivity, independence, and integration into the community (Wilcox & Bellamy, 1982). The adoption of these same features as the explicit goals of programs funded under the Developmental Disabilities Act Amendments of 1984 demonstrates the breadth of current support for this view of quality in adult life.

Though measures of the adult status of special education students are useful in clarifying the mission of secondary special education and in providing a long-term view of program effectiveness, they are less useful in evaluating the impact of program improvements. Follow-up measures are both delayed and unavailable to most decision-makers. In addition, an individual's status on follow-up measures is affected by many variables other than the quality of schooling. For example, the gains of an excellent vocational program in the high school can be quickly lost if post-school services do not match the competence and skills of the student. The availability of supported employment programs which emphasize wages and integration (rather than traditional day activity and workshop programs which emphasize "readiness"), can dramatically affect the employment status of a school-leaver. Likewise, if a community has no small, family-scale residential services for persons with severe handicaps, it is unlikely that students will graduate to the least restrictive residential option, no matter how good their skills or preparation.

The definition of desired adult life-styles provides a framework for articulating more immediate program features that are logically or empirically related to distant outcomes. The definition of successful graduates as productive, independent, and integrated citizens helps generate program features, or qualities, that could serve as indices of the success of high school programs: a logical analysis suggests that quality high school programs should be integrated, age appropriate, community referenced, future oriented, comprehensive, effective, and involve parents (Bellamy & Wilcox, 1980).

THE SYSTEMS CHANGE EFFORT

The context for the discussion of the educational system's ability to implement these qualities in high school programs is the Oregon High School (OHS) model. The OHS model is a replicable guide for planning and operating a secondary program for students with moderate and severe handicaps. The authors adopted a program replication strategy for systems change (Paine, Bellamy, & Wilcox, 1984) because of the continuing discrepancy between "best practice" and "normal practice." Simply continuing to demonstrate that extraordinary quality could be achieved with extraordinary resources in special grant projects seemed to miss the critical need to implement quality services under normal conditions and constraints.

The process of using replicable models in program improvement efforts involves two components: 1) a program *model*, which delineates how education should be designed and delivered; and 2) an implementation *process*, which outlines systematic procedures for installing the program model in natural service settings. The program model is a collection of best practice procedures that are standardized and defined in operations manuals for teachers and their supervisors (Wilcox, McDonnell, Bellamy, & Friedman, 1984; Wilcox, Rose et al., 1984). The implementation process is described in staff training and start-up guides, and includes methods for installing the procedures in a new setting and assessing the degree of model implementation. To be useful in program improvement efforts, such models should be usable in a variety of normal service settings by persons other than model developers, and achieve valued outcomes for service consumers (Paine et al., 1984).

Program Model

The OHS model was designed for use in high school classrooms for students with moderate and severe handicaps, which are located on a regular high school campus. The model can be adopted and fully installed with the personnel and resources that are normally available to a single secondary classroom. In a strict sense, however, OHS is not a classroom model, since it emphasizes instruction in the larger high school environment, in the community, and in the home. The OHS model comprises the following elements:

1. A *curriculum* that is organized as a catalog of activities reflecting important opportunities and demands of integrated community environments, rather than goals from academic sequences or developmental pinpoints. The catalog is used to plan individualized education programs (IEPs). The domains in the curriculum are referenced to major aspects of adult life (work, leisure, and personal management), and academic skills are taught only in the context of actual activities. There is an emphasis on performing complete activities (with prostheses or adaptations as necessary) rather than on the mastery of isolated skills.
2. *IEP procedures* that follow a negotiation format and result in activity goals in work, leisure, and personal management domains. IEPs are completed in the spring so that teachers can do necessary development of community-based instructional programs prior to the start of school in the fall. The selection of goals does not follow a predetermined sequence; instead, goals are selected based on what is important for individual

students to learn. Choosing IEP goals from an activities catalog is very similar to the situation a person faces when selecting gifts or personal items from any mail order catalog: there are many interesting items, but limited resources available! The choice of objectives takes into account family values and life-style, and the IEPs that result from such a process are, understandably, individualized.

3. *Instruction* that emphasizes procedures for general case programming (e.g., Horner, Sprague, & Wilcox, 1982) and techniques for community-based training. The model presumes that teachers know how to teach in the classroom (to analyze activities, present cues, reinforce or correct student responses, take data, and modify programs); and that the challenge is to build student performance in settings in the community where no training occurred. For many students, training includes a heavy reliance on the use of alternate performance strategies or partial participation (Brown, Branston-McLean et al., 1979) to support community involvement.

4. *Classroom organizational procedures* that build a classroom schedule based on student IEPs, utilize peers as tutors and advocates, schedule regular contact with parents, and provide measures of overall classroom effectiveness. Probably the unique—and most important—contribution of the model is its organizational structure for teachers. The model applies current management technology to the operation of an exemplary classroom. The organizational system allows data-based decision making to occur at the level of classroom operation, not just at the level of individual student programs.

5. *Administrative policies and procedures* that support community-based training. This includes changes in both administrative procedures and personnel roles, especially for related service staff. In a community-based program, related service personnel consult and/or train skills in community settings rather than provide therapy in isolation.

6. *Procedures for planning the transition* from school to adult services, so that services are comprehensive, reflect parent/family priorities, and continue uninterrupted.

Implementation Procedures

Support for model implementation included 5 days of training for the classroom teacher and his or her supervisor in Eugene, Oregon, at an established OHS classroom; approximately 5 days of technical assistance on location at the field test sites; weekly telephone contact; and quarterly reviews of model implementation. Quarterly implementation reviews served as the basis for identifying and scheduling any additional technical assistance or training events.

RESULTS OF MODEL IMPLEMENTATION

The first set of questions to ask about the OHS model concerns the extent to which it could be used under normal circumstances in high school programs for students with moderate to severe handicaps. The OHS model was implemented in eight high schools between fall, 1981, and fall, 1984, and now operates in nine classrooms in Oregon (with additional sites recently established in Utah and Washington). The implementation data presented here refer only to the original eight sites. (For a more complete discussion of data collection methods and results, the reader is referred to Wilcox & Bellamy, 1984).

Site Demographics The classrooms that implemented the OHS model differed with regard to district size, administrative and community characteristics, distance from model developers, teacher skill and experience, and classroom staffing. Table 1 summarizes the characteristics of each implementation site.

Student Characteristics In Oregon, services to students with moderate and severe handicaps are delivered noncategorically through programs for persons classified as trainably mentally retarded. This program designation includes all students with measured IQs less than 50 who also have significant problems in adaptive behavior. These programs serve students who otherwise might be labeled moderately, severely, or profoundly retarded; autistic; deaf-blind; or multiply handicapped. As a consequence, classroom groupings tend to be heterogeneous rather than focused on one particular disability category or level of functioning. Practically, most students with Down syndrome are served in programs with this designation, although some may attend special education services for students with mild learning problems. At the close of the 1983–1984 school year, 80 students were served in the OHS classrooms, with a range of 6–14 students per site. Students ranged in age from 16 to 21 years. Of this number, 25 (or 30%) were identified as having Down syndrome.

Level of Implementation Figure 1 presents the level of implementation in each of the original eight OHS replication sites as measured through external review using a checklist of critical program features. During the 1982–1983 school year, the level of implementation for sites 1–5 (as listed in Figure 1) ranged from 83% to 96%. An examination of the level of implementation in the fall of 1982, and 1983, indicates a drop in the number of model elements in place attributable to the planning and start-up activities expected each new year. However, in the fall of 1983, this drop is considerably less dramatic, indicating that the model became easier to implement with practice.

Data on the level of implementation for classrooms that adopted the model more recently (sites 6–8, as listed in Figure 1, received training in March, 1983, with technical assistance in June and September) indicate sys-

Table 1. Descriptive information on implementation sites as of fall 1981

	Characteristics of local education agency					Characteristics of teachers					Characteristics of site	
	Distance from Eugene (miles)	Demographic status	Average per pupil expenditure 1981–1982	TMR classrooms	Secondary TMR classrooms	Sex	Age	Years teaching	Years at site	Total staff	Total students	Target class size
North Eugene High School	—	urban	$6,950	15	8	M	–30	1	1	1 T[a] 2 A[b]	1,000	14
South Eugene High School	—	urban	$6,950	15	8	M	–30	1	1	1 T 2 A	1,150	11
McMinnville High School	86	small town	NA[c]	4	1	F	50+	11	3	1 T 1½ A	625	10
Ashland Senior High School	181	small town	NA		4	M	30+	4	2	1 T ½ VocT[d] ½ A	720	7
Crater High School	166	rural	NA	1	3	F	30	1	1	1 T 1 A ½ VocT	1,029	7

(continued)

209

Table 1. (continued)

	Characteristics of local education agency					Characteristics of teachers					Characteristics of site	
	Distance from Eugene (miles)	Demographic status	Average per pupil expenditure 1981–1982	TMR classrooms	Secondary TMR classrooms	Sex	Age	Years teaching	Years at site	Total staff	Total students	Target class size
Central High School	70	rural	NA	4	2	F	30	5	3	1 T 1 A	750	8
Jefferson High School	120	inner city	$12,000	26	11	F	30+	3	3	1 T 2 A S/L[e] OT/PT[f] VocT Beh Sp[g]	2,000	13
Columbia High School	150	small town	$12,000	26	11	F	30+		3	1 T 2 A S/L OT/PT VocT Beh Sp	1,000	11

[a] Teacher.
[b] Aide.
[c] Information not available from district.
[d] Vocational teacher.
[e] Speech-language pathologist.
[f] Occupational therapist or physical therapist.
[g] Behavior specialist.

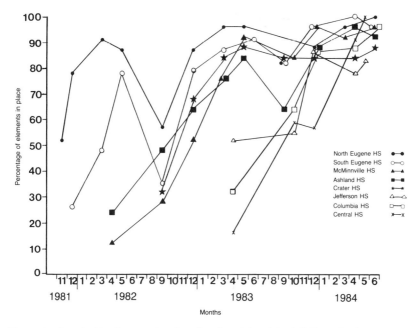

Figure 1. Level of implementation found at the eight original OHS replication sites, as measured at each review.

tematic improvement in the number of model elements in place (range = 83%–100%; mean = 95%). These data suggest that significant changes in curriculum, IEP development, classroom organization, and instructional procedures can be accomplished within a relatively short period by teachers of varying skills in classrooms and communities with differing resources.

Utility and Feasibility of the OHS Model Data indicate that classroom teachers rate the overall utility of OHS systems and procedures quite highly (a mean of 5.4 on a 6-point scale where 6 indicates "maximum utility"). They also indicate the overall effort required to adopt and implement the OHS model to be within reason (3.6 on a 6-point scale where 6 equals "maximum effort"). Descriptive data on the distribution of teacher time shows that teachers in classrooms implementing the OHS model report working an average of 8.3 hours per day or 41.5 hours per week. Compared with Sykes's (1984) data that regular education teachers work an average of 46 hours per week, the time required to implement the OHS model seems reasonable. Data suggest that the adoption and implementation of the OHS model is both possible and feasible within typical resource constraints.

Satisfaction with the OHS Model The satisfaction of persons affected by the OHS model is high. Figure 2 presents results of surveys done with parents, support personnel, special education administrators, and building

A Summary of the OHS Consumer Satisfaction Rating
1981–1982   1982–1983

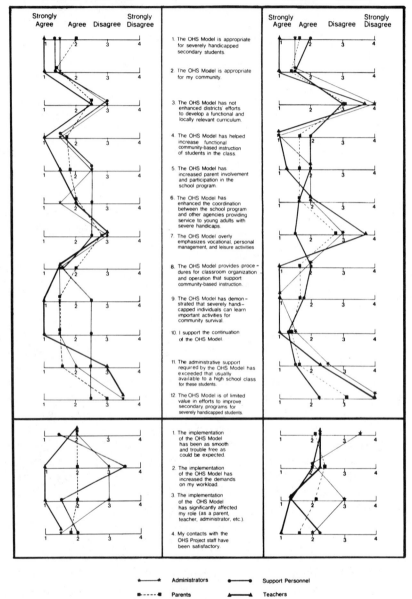

Figure 2.   A summary of the OHS consumer satisfaction rating for 1981–1982 and 1982–1983.

principals. Results indicate that these groups were pleased with the student outcomes and classroom-level changes that the model had produced, and that they supported continued use in their respective settings.

PROGRAMMATIC IMPACT

A second and more basic set of questions to ask about the OHS model relates to effects on the quality of services provided to students in participating classrooms. As noted earlier, the authors began work on the OHS model by formulating a set of program features, or qualities, that reflected the literature on normalization, professional opinion papers, court decisions, and best practices in existing educational services. Though these qualities seemed to be supported broadly by service providers and advocates, they have not always been highly visible in the actual operation of high school programs for students with moderate and severe handicaps.

In an attempt to reduce the discrepancy between belief and practice, the authors found the need to be as explicit with classrooms as they have taught teachers to be explicit with students; that is, to formulate goals as behavioral objectives. Before they could expect to see the identified program qualities translated into practice, they had to define those qualities in a way that could be measured, and then set standards or criterion levels for acceptable performance. That process, in turn, was followed by regular measurement, comparison of performance to the established standard, and a decision to continue or adjust classroom procedures and resources. These procedures constituted the OHS Implementation Checklist (available from the authors) and the process for quarterly site reviews. The remainder of this chapter reviews each of the qualities identified by Bellamy and Wilcox (1980) as important, and reports on the degree to which those qualities have been realized by programs using the OHS model.

High School Should be Integrated

The integration of students with moderate and severe handicaps typically involves locating a special class on a regular high school campus where there is opportunity to share resources and nonacademic experiences with same-age peers who have no identified handicaps. Integration is not equivalent to the mainstreaming of students with moderate to severe handicaps into regular classes, but rather emphasizes the importance of learning opportunities provided by interactions with nonhandicapped peers.

The value of integration with normal peers is reflected in litigation (*Halderman v. Pennhurst State School and Hospital,* 1977), legislation (the least restrictive educational environment provisions of PL 94-142), and professional opinion (e.g., Brown, Branston et al., 1979; Certo, Haring, &

York, 1984; Gilhool & Stutman, 1978). One of the most salient characteristics of the environments in which students must ultimately function is frequent interactions with persons without disabilities. It is only logical to duplicate this feature in settings charged with preparation for adult living. Further support for the importance of integration is provided by Hasazi, Gordon, and Roe (1985), who found that most special education graduates who were employed had found their jobs through a "self-family-friend" network. Such a network would appear much less likely to develop if high school afforded no opportunities for friendships with persons without disabilities.

Status Report All classrooms that implemented the OHS model (and, indeed, virtually all classrooms for high school students with moderate to severe handicaps in the state of Oregon) are located on regular high school campuses. This allows students labeled moderately or severely handicapped to participate in the offerings of the regular high school curriculum, such as slimnastics, weight training, wood shop, horticulture, and home economics. Such participation is selected through the IEP process. Students are typically accompanied by a classroom aide or peer tutor who provides the assistance needed to follow a modified curriculum (e.g., using picture recipe cards to prepare a simple one-dish meal rather than reading a recipe).

A standard of the OHS model is that each student should have at least five scheduled daily contacts with nonhandicapped peers. Across all students in all eight OHS classroom sites, scheduled contacts ranged from 4 to 11 per day. Those contacts occurred in integrated classes, in-school jobs, regular school events (such as lunch, travel on the regular school bus), and work with peer tutors. All eight classrooms had formal programs of peer tutoring as a way of facilitating interaction between special education students and students in the regular curriculum. The number of tutors participating in a classroom ranged from 6 to 43 per term.

Concern for students' integration out of school and after school is addressed by encouraging participation in extracurricular and community events as IEP goals. Students had objectives, particularly in the leisure domain, that targeted performance of learned skills after school hours. Several of the schools using the OHS model established integrated social service clubs whose mission was to increase the out-of-school integration of students with severe handicaps. Clubs have been sponsored by schools themselves (for example, the North Eugene Highlander Advocates; Sprague & Wilcox, 1984) or through affiliation with other organizations (for example, the Sky Club at Central Point, supported through the Kiwanis Club). These extracurricular clubs foster integrated group and individual events outside school hours. Youth with severe handicaps and their nonhandicapped peers "hang out" at shopping malls, attend school games and events, enroll in community center programs, and visit each other's homes. Data from the Highlander Advocates illustrate the potential of such extracurricular clubs. During a 6-month period, the 14 students with moderate and severe handicaps attending the ''Basic Skills Class'' at North Eugene High School averaged nearly nine after school activities (range=1–24). A recent evaluation of the group (Shapiro, 1985) showed that parents of students with and without handicaps strongly support the club's integration objectives.

The success of the integration of students with severe handicaps into Oregon's high schools is perhaps most apparent in a statewide survey of parent attitudes toward integration (Winsley, 1983). Winsley asked parents of students with moderate to severe handicaps about their feelings toward integrated school programs. All respondents reported that they would select an integrated school over a segregated school placement. Parents whose children had earlier attended an institution or segregated school program were even stronger in their support for school integration. When asked about the benefits of integration, parents identified not only direct benefits to their son or daughter, but also the opportunity to educate nonhandicapped peers.

High School Should Be Age Appropriate

The quality of age appropriateness highlights the relevance of a student's chronological age in selecting instructional tasks and activities. The requirement that tasks be appropriate to students' ages is not meant to ignore the fact that students with severe handicaps have basic skill deficits. Rather, it accentuates the similarities with age-peers, and avoids the stigmatizing effects of using tasks and activities that are associated with young children (large piece puzzles, blocks, color- and coin-naming exercises, and so on).

A commitment to providing age-appropriate programming requires that the school day and extracurricular activities of nonhandicapped students be referenced in program design. Useful indices of age appropriateness might include the location of the classroom, its materials and decor, and the nature of the instructional goals established for students.

Status Report   As of spring, 1984, all schools using the OHS model located the classroom for students aged 16–21 on a regular high school campus. (Since then, one district has created a class of students 19–21 years of age and located it on a college campus.) Rather than creating specialized environments that duplicate resources within the high school, OHS classrooms typically contain the same furniture and materials as other classrooms. Students labeled as having moderate to severe handicaps have lockers, student identification cards, and other perks associated with being a high school student. The classrooms follow the regular bell schedule of the high school and students participate in assemblies and other all-school events. Goals selected on students' IEPs represent activities typical of age-peers (e.g., eating at fast food restaurants, traveling on mass transit, shopping for clothes and other personal items).

216 / WILCOX AND BELLAMY

High School Should Be Community Referenced

Just as many regular education teachers may "teach to the test," so might teachers of adolescents with severe handicaps "teach to the community," since community competence is the ultimate test of school effectiveness. Attending to community demands and opportunities has dramatic implications for the structure of curriculum, the selection of objectives, and the location of instruction. A community-referenced curriculum replaces traditional academic or developmental domains (e.g., reading or math; gross motor, social, or cognitive) with categories that derive from the basic demands of adult functioning: work, leisure, and independent living. Goals are selected for individual students, not because they come next in a developmental or logical sequence, but rather because they are valued activities in the student's home and community. There is an emphasis on skills that are functional (i.e., whose performance is frequently required in the actual community environment) and on criteria that relate to the demands and expectations of the community. Teaching *to* the community, if done effectively, also requires teaching *in* the community.

Status Report All classrooms using the OHS model use the "activities catalog" (Wilcox & Bellamy, 1982; Wilcox & Bellamy, 1987) as their curriculum. The catalog provides a generic organizing structure within which locally available activities can be listed to facilitate both assessment and choice among possible objectives. In addition to requiring the activities catalog, the OHS model establishes standards for training in the community. The standards specify that students aged 16–17 spend at least 25% of their instructional week in community training, and that students aged 18–21 spend at least 35% of their time in the community learning activities targeted on the IEP. The actual range of community training time was 20%–45% for the younger student group and 30%–100% for the older students. Though direct training in the community is critical, studies also show that combining community-based training with carefully designed classroom simulations maximizes the effectiveness of instruction (McDonnell, 1984; McDonnell et al., 1984).

High School Should be Comprehensive

High school programs should provide students with whatever training and support they need to become as productive, integrated, and independent as possible. All students, regardless of the nature or extent of their handicaps, need training to develop competence in work, leisure, and personal management domains. Despite the fact that individual teachers may lack the skills to provide certain program components (e.g., they may not know how to develop work training sites or how to run a janitorial crew), schools should make a concerted effort to develop the resources necessary to support students in all needed training activities. Indices of a program's comprehensiveness include the balance of goals on student IEPs and the extent of work training provided.

Status Report   The curriculum and IEP structure of the OHS model emphasizes the need to select work, leisure, and personal management goals for all students. The leisure and personal management goals target activities such as shopping for groceries or clothing items, using fast food restaurants, swimming at the YMCA, and completing a high school weight training class. Work training varies along two dimensions: the type of job performed (e.g., food service worker, janitor, day care aide, library aide, greenhouse assistant) and the training format (e.g., work crew, individual job, or enclave). All students have job training in the community; some also hold additional work training responsibilities in the school, but these are not prerequisites to community-based training.

High School Should Be Future Oriented

A future orientation is a natural and necessary complement to community referencing. While a strict community-referenced approach would presumably result in programming in and for existing work, leisure, and residential opportunities, the environments currently available are, in many cases, less than satisfactory. Innovations in both employment and residential programs suggest that current services do not constitute a representative sample of what will be available in the future. It is not unreasonable to expect adult service programs to be smaller, afford greater access to the community, provide regular opportunities for integration, and enable persons with severe disabilities to earn nontrivial wages. Schools should prepare students for this future, not for the perpetuation of current day and residential services, where wages and opportunities for integration are low.

Status Report   Two aspects of OHS implementation sites illustrate future orientation: the emphasis on vocational training and the procedures for transition planning. Vocational training in the OHS model sites emphasizes student training in actual community job sites, and avoids preparation for traditional sheltered settings. Training for each student samples several job clusters and occurs across several formats (Sowers, Lundervold, Swanson, & Budd, 1980; Sprague, Paeth, & Wilcox, 1983). These training formats correspond to exemplary strategies for providing remunerative and integrated supported employment for adults with severe disabilities (see, for example, Mank, Rhodes, & Bellamy, 1986). Students are trained for state-of-the-art programs, even though such programs may not yet be available in their communities.

Because of the complexity of the transition from school to work and adult life, the OHS model includes several requirements that relate to transition. The first is that each program develop a "transition manual" (e.g., McDonnell, Sheehan, & Wilcox, 1982) for use by parents and teachers. The manual describes the operation of post-school services in general, delineates criteria that parents might use to evaluate post-school services for their sons and daughters, and presents data on the outcomes available to participants in local work and residential programs. Transition plans are developed as an extension of the IEP process. A formal plan developed for each student aged 19 years or older directs parent and professional attention to major decisions (work, residence, income and medical support, estate planning, and so on), and results in the definition of tasks and timelines that will maximize the probability of a smooth transition to the least restrictive post-school services.

High School Should Involve Parents

Parent involvement in the special education program serving their son or daughter is a major intent of PL 94-142. That involvement can take a variety of forms, including participation in the development of IEPs, home-based instruction, community training, data collection, participation in program design, and advocacy both for improved educational services and for increased post-school options. The values parents hold are more important and more apparent in educational programming for secondary students because there are no defensible skill sequences to guide the selection of goals for the IEP. There is, for example, no logical or necessary relation between learning to shop for groceries, learning a food service job, and attending an aerobics class at the community center. Decisions about which task is taught first, the amount of time invested, and the expected approximation to normal (rather than adapted) performance depend, not on logic, but on the value judgments of parents and professionals. Consequently, parents should play a much more powerful role in the selection of instructional objectives than is normally the case. The logical basis for supporting increased parent involvement is complemented by recent studies indicating that parent involvement in the school and post-school services may be directly related to employment outcomes achieved by school-leavers with disabilities (Hasazi et al., 1985; Schalock, Wolzen, Feis, Werbel, & Peterson, 1984).

Status Report   The OHS structure for curriculum and IEP development significantly increases the potential for parent influence in the secondary program. IEPs developed using an activities catalog represent a radical departure from IEPs in which a curriculum sequence defines instructional goals for the ensuing year. With the catalog, parents review and select from the array of work, leisure, and personal management activities that are available in the community and could be taught to their son or daughter. The IEP meeting is structured so that parents take the lead in nominating activity goals. After parents, and then school staff, have suggested goals in each domain, the meeting follows a negotiation format to agree on 10–15 goals for the following year. The meeting format encourages identification of goals for the home environment where the parents assume primary responsibility. However, such home goals typically focus on providing opportunities for the student to practice learned skills at home rather than expecting active training by a parent.

A standard of the OHS model is that classroom staff have contact with each family at least once every 2 weeks to follow up on IEP goals targeted for the home and to share information about student status on other activities. These contacts take the form of scheduled phone calls, notes, or visits. There is a system for teachers to record contacts so that no family is intentionally (or unintentionally) overlooked.

High School Should Be Effective

Effectiveness is a key criterion in any service. Regardless of other features, a program that is not effective can be viewed as unduly restrictive (Laski, 1979). Effectiveness can be addressed on several levels: 1) the extent to which a program achieves specified goals for individual students, 2) the extent to which teachers and classroom staff use procedures that support student progress, and 3) the extent to which the program effects life-style change for the students served.

Status Report For the 80 students served during the 1983–1984 school year, 85% of the 1,024 established IEP goals were addressed. Of the goals addressed, 62% were still in progress at the end of the year, 34% were completed or on maintenance, and 4% had been dropped. Although meeting IEP objectives is only one measure of effectiveness, its importance is increased when one considers the nature of the objectives. Student IEPs targeted activities such as working as a dishwasher in a local restaurant, completing transactions at a bank, bowling, using the school store, using vending machines, and riding public mass transit. Objectives were only considered "met" when students could perform in the environments in which these activities normally occur.

Several measures of staff performance were gathered to determine the extent to which high school programs using the OHS model were effective. The model includes a standard that students receive instruction for at least 80% of the time allocated on the schedule; measures of instructional time were gathered regularly with training data. A direct observation instrument (Adler, 1982) was used to assess whether teachers and other instructional staff used appropriate instructional delivery. A final aspect of program effectiveness was the standard that classroom staff would complete at least 80% of their scheduled noninstructional tasks each week. Such tasks included calls to parents, materials development, contacts with work training sites in the community, and monitoring of peer tutors and students participating in regular curriculum offerings. Although not all sites met established standards at each quarterly review, rarely were discrepancies substantial or persistent across successive evaluations.

The weekly activities interview (WAI) was developed in an attempt to assess the impact of the OHS model on the life-style of the students served. The WAI asked parents/caregivers of a student attending an OHS classroom to report whether the student had participated in any of 56 activities once or more than once during the previous week. Four weekly telephone calls were conducted and combined to yield a score representative of student life-style. The WAI was administered each spring and fall on a voluntary basis. Data show that participation in an OHS classroom significantly affected community integration. The mean community integration score indicated that the typical OHS student engaged in 58 community integration events per 4-week period during the times when the WAI was administered. This figure compares favorably with a mean community integration score of 46 obtained with an earlier version of the WAI (prior to OHS implementation), and with a score of 52 for students in traditional high school classrooms not using the OHS model (Sowers, 1982). Further, WAI data from the subset of students who participated in OHS classrooms for at least 2.5 years averaged 77 community activities per 4-week period. This is about 20 more activities on average than the aggregate score for all OHS students and approximately 1.5 times that found by Sowers (1982) for comparable students. Students who were long-term participants in model classrooms show a steady progression across time in their average community integration score, from 63 in spring, 1982, to 89 in spring, 1984, with a slight and unexplained reversal in fall, 1983.

SUMMARY AND RECOMMENDATIONS

The major issue confronting parents and professionals concerned with quality secondary education for individuals with Down syndrome is not procedural development, but rather the implementation of available procedures. In recent years, there have been dramatic developments in methods and procedures specifically focused on high school programs. There are now curriculum models that support integration and community competence. Such curricula, in turn, have generated IEP procedures that promote genuine parent involvement and program individualization. With the emphasis on a functional, community-referenced curriculum, procedures for community-based training and a technology of instructional programming that increases the generalization of behavior change (e.g., Horner, McDonnell, & Bellamy, 1986) have emerged. Organizational management systems are available to help the teacher manage classroom staff and meet the demands of a community-based program. Though undoubtedly there will be further improvements in these areas, the pressing problem today is how to use what is known. The clear message of the Oregon High School Project is that any interested high school can provide exemplary services to its students with moderate to severe handicaps.

There are several variables that may influence the ease or speed of the needed translation from best practice to common practice. The quality of personnel preparation programs is one obvious factor. By ensuring that future teachers learn contemporary best practice technologies, teacher training programs will facilitate the installation of the best available procedures in the common classroom. Special education training programs that promote a specialization at the secondary level, and those that offer internships in integrated educational settings, will do much to foster the development of the particular skills required to deliver best practice services to adolescents with moderate to severe handicaps.

If recent developments in curricula, instructional procedures, and other areas are to produce broad changes in the system, then developers must take care to ensure that the materials and procedures they propose are, indeed, usable. It is not sufficient that a group of hand-picked teachers can use new procedures under the direct tutelage of their inventor; rather, there should be the expectation that procedures be field tested with teachers in circumstances that sample the range of intended use, and that procedures be revised to fit the resources typically available.

Informed parents will, themselves, influence the speed with which what professionals know becomes what teachers practice: The placement of adolescents with moderate to severe handicaps in special schools or in elementary schools can continue only if parents tolerate segregated and age-inappropriate programs. Parent advocacy can bring about the integrated and age-appropriate placements that are basic to quality services. To the extent that parents hold a vision of what is possible in high school programs for students with severe handicaps, they will be able to advocate local school improvements.

The use of standardized program models is a key variable in installing best practice procedures in ongoing service settings. Results from the implementation of the OHS model lend support to the model replication strategy as one important way of gaining the use of exemplary practices in integrated service programs.

REFERENCES

Adler, E. (1982). *The effect of public posting of comparative classroom performance data on staff instructional related time.* Unpublished doctoral dissertation, University of Oregon, Eugene.

Bellamy, G. T., & Wilcox, B. (1980). Secondary education for severely handicapped students. Guidelines for quality services. In B. Wilcox & A. Thompson (Eds.), *Critical issues in the education of autistic children and youth.* Washington, DC: Office of Special Education.

Brodsky, M. M. (1983). *A statewide follow-up study of the graduates of school programs for trainable mentally retarded students in Oregon: 1977–1981.* Unpublished doctoral dissertation, University of Oregon, Division of Special Education and Rehabilitation, Eugene.

Brown, L., Branston, M. B., Hamre-Nietupski, A., Johnson, F., Wilcox, B., & Gruenewald, L. (1979). A rationale for comprehensive longitudinal interactions between severely handicapped students and nonhandicapped students and other citizens. *AAESPH Review, 4,* 3–14.

Brown, L., Branston-McLean, M. B., Baumgart, D., Vincent, L., Falvey, M., & Schroder, J. (1979). Using the characteristics of current and subsequent least restrictive environments in the development of curricular content for severely handicapped students. *AAESPH Review, 4,* 407–424.

Certo, N., Haring, N., & York, R. (Eds.), (1984). *Public school integration of severely handicapped students: Rational issues and progressive alternatives.* Baltimore: Paul H. Brookes Publishing Co.

Certo, N., Mezzullo, K., & Hunter, D. (1985). The effect of total task chain training on the acquisition of busperson job skills at a full service community restaurant. *Education and Training of the Mentally Retarded, 20,* 148–156.

Gilhool, T., & Stutman, E. (1978). Integration of severely handicapped students: Toward criteria for implementing and enforcing the integration imperative of PL 94-142 and Section 504. In *LRE: Developing criteria for the evaluation of the least restrictive environment provision* (pp. 191–227). Philadelphia: Research for Better Schools.

Halderman v. Pennhurst State School and Hospital, 466 F. Supp. (E. D. Pa. 1977).

Hasazi, S. B., Gordon, L. R., & Roe, C. A. (1985). Factors associated with the employment status of handicapped youth exiting high school from 1979–1983. *Exceptional Children, 51,* 455–469.

Horner, R. H., McDonnell, J. J., & Bellamy, G. T. (1986). Teaching generalized behaviors: General case instruction in simulation and community settings. In R. H. Horner, L. H. Meyer, & H. D. Fredericks (Eds.), *Education of learners with severe handicaps: Exemplary service strategies* (pp. 289–314). Baltimore: Paul H. Brookes Publishing Co.

Horner, R. H., Sprague, J., & Wilcox, B. (1982). General case programming for community activities. In B. Wilcox & G. T. Bellamy (Eds.), *Design of high school programs for severely handicapped students* (pp. 61–98). Baltimore: Paul H. Brookes Publishing Co.

Horner, R. H., Williams, J. A., & Steveley, J. D. (1984). Acquisition of generalized telephone use by students with severe mental retardation. Manuscript submitted for publication.

Laski, F. J. (1979). Legal strategies to secure entitlement to services for severely handicapped persons. In T. Bellamy, G. O'Connor, & O. Karan (Eds.), *Vocational rehabilitation of severely handicapped persons: Contemporary service strategies.* Baltimore: University Park Press.

Mank, D., Rhodes, L., & Bellamy, G. T. (1986). Four supported employment alternatives. In W. E. Kiernan & J. A. Stark (Eds.), *Pathways to employment for adults with developmental disabilities* (pp. 139–153). Baltimore: Paul H. Brookes Publishing Co.

McDonnell, J. (1984). *Effects of in vivo and simulation-plus-in vivo training on the acquisition and generalization of a grocery item search strategy by high school students with severe handicaps.* Unpublished doctoral dissertation, University of Oregon, Eugene.

McDonnell, J., Horner, R., & Williams, J. (1984). A comparison of three strategies for teaching generalized grocery purchasing to high school students with severe handicaps. *Journal of the Association for Persons with Severe Handicaps, 9,* 123–133.

McDonnell, J. J., Sheehan, M., & Wilcox, B. (1982). *Effective transition from school to work and adult services: A procedural handbook for parents and teachers.* Unpublished manuscript, University of Oregon, Eugene.

Nietupski, J., Welch, J., & Wacker, D. (1983). Acquisition, maintenance, and transfer of grocery item purchasing skills by moderately and severely handicapped students. *Education and Training of the Mentally Retarded, 18,* 279–286.

Paine, S., Bellamy, G. T., & Wilcox, B. (Eds.). (1984). *Human services that work: From innovation to standard practice.* Baltimore: Paul H. Brookes Publishing Co.

Rose, H. (1984). *Non-instructional interventions: Affecting the way adolescents with severe handicaps spend their time outside school.* Unpublished doctoral dissertation, University of Oregon, Eugene.

Sailor, W., & Guess, D. (1983). *Severely handicapped students: An instructional design.* Boston: Houghton Mifflin.

Schalock, R. L., Wolzen, B., Feis, P., Werbel, G., & Peterson, K. (1984, May). *Post-secondary community placement of mentally retarded individuals: A five year follow-up analysis.* Paper presented at the annual convention of the American Association on Mental Deficiency, Minneapolis.

Shapiro, I. (1985). *An evaluation of an integrated extracurricular social service club.* Unpublished master's thesis, University of Oregon, Eugene.

Sowers, J. (1982). *Validation of the weekly activity interview (WAI): An instrument to measure the lifestyle of severely handicapped secondary students.* Unpublished doctoral dissertation, University of Oregon, Eugene.

Sowers, J., Lundervold, D., Swanson, M., & Budd, C. (1980). *Competitive employment training for mentally retarded adults: A systematic approach.* Unpublished manuscript, University of Oregon, Specialized Training Program, Eugene.

Sprague, J. (1981). *Vending machine use: An analysis of a general case programming strategy to induce generalization to a full range of examples.* Unpublished master's thesis, University of Oregon, Eugene.

Sprague, J., Paeth, M. A., & Wilcox, B. (1983). *Community work crews for severely handicapped high school students.* Unpublished manuscript, University of Oregon, Specialized Training Program, Eugene.

Sprague, J., & Wilcox, B. (1984). *Organizing a social service club for handicapped and nonhandicapped students.* Unpublished manuscript, University of Oregon, Eugene.

Storey, K., Bates, P., & Hanson, H. B. (1984). Acquisition and generalization of coffee purchase skills by adults with severe disabilities. *The Journal of the Association for Persons with Severe Handicaps, 9*(3), 178–195.

Sykes, G. (1984). The deal. *The Wilson Quarterly, 8,* 59–77.

Wheeler, J., Ford, A., Nietupski, J., Loomis, R., & Brown, L. (1980). Teaching moderately and severely handicapped adolescents to shop in supermarkets using pocket calculators. *Education and Training of the Mentally Retarded, 15,* 105–111.

Wilcox, B., & Bellamy, G. T. (1982). *Design of high school programs for severely handicapped students.* Baltimore: Paul H. Brookes Publishing Co.

Wilcox, B., & Bellamy, G. T. (1984). *The Oregon High School Project: Final report* (U.S. Department of Education Contract #300-81-0408). Eugene: University of Oregon.

Wilcox, B., & Bellamy, G. T., (1987). *A comprehensive guide to The Activities Catalog: An alternative curriculum for youth and adults with severe disabilities.* Baltimore: Paul H. Brookes Publishing Co.

Wilcox, B., McDonnell, J., Bellamy, G. T., & Friedman, D. (1984). *The Oregon High School Model: Classroom operations manual.* Eugene: University of Oregon, Specialized Training Program.

Wilcox, B., Rose, H., Adler, E., Baird, P., Falco, R., Proulx, B., Rickerson, P., & Sprague, J. (1984). *The Oregon High School Model: Administrators' and supervisors' manual.* Eugene: University of Oregon, Specialized Training Program.

Will, M. (1984). *Bridges from school to working life: Programs for the handicapped.* Washington, DC: Clearinghouse on the Handicapped.

Williams, W., Vogelsberg, R. T., & Schutz, R. (1985). Programs for secondary-age severely handicapped youth. In D. Bricker & J. Filler (Eds.), *Severe mental retardation: From theory to practice.* Reston, VA: The Council for Exceptional Children.

Winsley, G. (1983). *A survey of parents' attitudes toward school integration.* Unpublished master's thesis, University of Oregon, Eugene.

The Oregon High School Secondary Education Model for Students with Down Syndrome

Denis W. Stoddard

The quality of secondary education for students with Down syndrome represents a major issue facing the human services field. Fortunately, this is an issue that appears to be set for change.

The benefits of PL 94-142 have not only resulted in a larger number of students with Down syndrome and other significant disabling conditions entering secondary education programs; the act has also "taught" large numbers of parents and other advocates, now politically seasoned, to expect and obtain reasonable educational services in less restrictive, more integrative environments. Along with the larger numbers of students to serve, and a greater number of more effective parents/advocates with higher expectations, have come the programmatic development and government support for change referred to by Wilcox and Bellamy in Chapter 8. (See also U.S. Department of Health and Human Services, 1984, for additional guidelines for change.) In the author's opinion, the critical need, growing political pressure, documented performance capability of persons with handicaps, and current public policy support have irreversibly targeted secondary education and adult services for major changes, changes that will be of great benefit to persons with Down syndrome. The major change agent is, and will continue

Preparation of this chapter was made possible by Project 84-28a, which is a collaborative effort of the Cincinnati Center for Developmental Disorders and Comprehensive Training and Development Institute, Inc., funded under PL 98-527 in accordance with the goals established by the Ohio Developmental Disabilities Planning Council and administered by the Ohio Department of Mental Retardation and Developmental Disabilities. The work presented and/or expressed herein does not necessarily reflect the position or policy of the Ohio Department of Mental Retardation and Developmental Disabilities or the Ohio Developmental Disabilities Planning Council, and no official endorsement by the above agencies should be inferred.

to be, astute, persistent parents who simply will not put up with a less-than-best effort on the part of service delivery and support systems.

Wilcox and Bellamy's chapter sets the direction needed for this wave of change. Their Oregon High School (OHS) secondary education program model provides the means for bringing about the changes needed. This response discusses a few key aspects of their chapter, and the OHS model, so as to sharpen the prospects for change.

VALUE-BASED PROGRAM DESIGN

Too often it seems that disproportionate fiscal, administrative, and political concerns overshadow quality-of-life concerns in the design, development, and operation of human services. In the author's opinion, the two crucial strengths of the Oregon High School (OHS) secondary education model are its solid ideological foundation and its demonstrated practical replicability. The OHS model ties its indicators of success to important quality-of-life values similar to those proposed by other leaders in the field. For example, Wehman and Moon (1985, p. 3) listed the following nine critical employment services values for persons with developmental disabilities:

1. Employment in integrated settings
2. Decent pay
3. The need for vocational choices
4. Avoiding "charity" work
5. Vocational training to reflect local labor needs
6. Parent involvement in planning
7. Parent education relative to social security laws
8. Community based vocational training
9. Systematically planned transition

From the author's own experience in using a simple values clarification tool (Stoddard, 1985), there seems to be a near consensus among parents, administrators, teachers, and related professionals on the basic values that should direct secondary education and other programs for individuals with Down syndrome. This apparent consensus is not, however, reflected in the secondary education programs generally experienced by individuals with Down syndrome. There are probably many reasons for this, some of which have been alluded to in the introductory remarks to this section and described in the Wilcox and Bellamy chapter.

What is needed? One answer is the adoption of the OHS or similar model. Another partial answer (one that could be used while getting ready to implement the OHS or similar model) is to employ sound, value-based guidelines as a type of program review checklist when making decisions within existing systems. Both the OHS model's successful high school program qualities list and the Wehman and Moon list could serve this function. Another more general list developed in a project of the Ohio Developmental Disabilities Planning Council (Deinstitutionalization Task Force, 1983a) is one that the author has generally found useful to recommend to parents, teachers, and others who participate in general and/or individual educational and vocational planning sessions.

A major dilemma is not disagreement over values, but rather is the lack of practical means for using agreed upon values in day-to-day as well as long-range program decision making. For just such practical use, the Ohio Developmental Disabilities Council values statement has also been produced in the form of a rubber stamp which can be imprinted in an IEP notebook, a conference attendee's packet, or any other material that would be handy in future program decision-making meetings. Often what is needed is not more sophisticated knowledge, but rather a practical means for using simple truths already known. The rubber stamp's imprint reads as follows:

Developmental Disabilities Quality Assurance Checklist

The purpose of providing services to people with developmental disabilities is to assist them in maximizing their:
- INDEPENDENCE AND HUMAN DIGNITY
- PRESENCE AND PARTICIPATION IN COMMUNITY LIFE
- STATUS AS VALUED COMMUNITY MEMBERS
- POTENTIAL FOR GROWTH AND DEVELOPMENT

Another checklist, offered by the Rehabilitation Research and Training Center (1984) in Virginia, is intended specifically for parents of high school students with mental retardation. The seven recommendations are given under the heading "Getting Your Child Ready for Employment."

1. Continue to reinforce the importance of work with your son or daughter
2. Be sure your child's current IEP addresses employment training
3. Actively support the teacher's effort to teach vocational skills
4. Encourage the school to arrange vocational training in actual worksites
5. Arrange part-time or volunteer work for your daughter or son
6. Emphasize physical fitness, stamina, and personal appearance
7. Be in touch with your local rehabilitation agency prior to graduation to arrange a smooth transition from school to work

Again, as with the OHS model, these recommendations give practical ideas consistent with sound, value-based principles.

OHS MODEL REPLICABILITY: A CONSUMER PERSPECTIVE

What might educational administrators, teachers, parents, and support personnel expect as they assume the task of adopting and replicating the OHS model? Wilcox and Bellamy reported that the satisfaction of persons affected by the OHS model is high.

The OHS model, while requiring significant systemic change, a bit more work for nearly everyone, and some additional challenges for administrators, is appropriate, effective, and well worth the effort. The curriculum might possibly benefit from being expanded, but there is no argument about the value and usefulness of what it presently contains. Considering that worthwhile change rarely occurs easily, the Wilcox and Bellamy summary of OHS results amount to a remarkably positive endorsement by consumers.

OHS SECONDARY EDUCATION PROGRAM DESIGN AND INSTRUCTIONAL TECHNOLOGY: NEED ONE EXCLUDE THE OTHER?

Early in their chapter, Wilcox and Bellamy indicate that the literature describing high school programs for students with moderate to severe handicaps has generally taken two forms. The first might be called *instructional technology studies* reporting "the acquisition, generalization, and maintenance of skills functional for adolescents and young adults." The second might be called secondary *program design papers* "that advance a particular value framework for the organization of secondary programs." The important point is then made by them that "few data are available to indicate whether the program features advocated are either achievable or useful in local educational programs." Fortunately for state-of-the-art purposes, they do an admirable job of providing data demonstrating how the OHS model, basically a value-based program design approach, is both achievable and useful in local educational programs in Oregon. The comments that follow are not intended to detract from their highly successful effort, but rather are intended to suggest possible enhancements of a system already demonstrated to be of significant worth.

Recently, in doing some reading in a classic work on strategic planning (Steiner, 1979), the author came across the following consideration. If an organization had to choose, which of the following would most assure organizational success: 1) an excellent overall strategic plan with a somewhat inadequate internal management system; or 2) an excellent internal mechanics or management system, but with a nonexistent or poorly defined strategic planning system?

Steiner (1979) suggested that chances for success would be far greater with an excellent strategic plan and a less effective internal operation. (The best option, of course, is not to have to choose, but to have the best of both worlds—an excellent overall plan aimed in the appropriate direction, with the best possible internal operations.) In this author's opinion, the OHS model provides an excellent strategic plan or general system design, and could incorporate instructional technology components that, together with its current design, would represent the best possible internal operations as well.

REFOCUS ON PERSONS WITH DOWN SYNDROME

A typical characteristic of individuals with Down syndrome is that they have a difficult time learning things. Often this is the major distinction between them and individuals with other types of disabilities. This would seem to indicate that a "best practice" approach should encourage and incorporate at least some of the best instructional technologies available for use by teachers working with individuals with Down syndrome. Ideally, these should be value-based technologies consistent with the OHS model. The work of the late Marc Gold provides an excellent example of a highly developed and effective instructional technology that shares the ideological foundation inherent in the OHS model. Gold's training system has also proven itself to be effective in working with individuals with Down syndrome in such varied vocational areas as operation and maintenance of lawn care equipment (Marc Gold and Associates, 1978), assembling electronic printed circuit board assemblies for NASA (National Children's Center, 1978), and performing a variety of food preparation tasks (cutting, weighing, portioning, and cooking) for Red Lobster restaurants (Marc Gold and Associates, 1982). (Also see Gold, 1980a, 1980b.)

Wilcox and Bellamy, however, indicate that "the model presumes that teachers know how to teach in the classroom (to analyze activities, present cues, reinforce or correct student responses, take data and modify programs)." This implies that nothing was done to enhance the specific instructional skills of the teachers, support staff, or parents; yet, at least based on the author's experience, less than adequate instructional competencies on the part of persons filling instructional roles continues to be a significant problem influencing both expectations of and effectiveness with students with Down syndrome.

Materials and expertise in this area, at least as far as readily identifiable skills are concerned, have been developed and available for over 14 years (Hall, 1971). Examples of easily implemented life skill and complex vocational skill instructional materials have been distributed for over 8 years (see for example, Gibson & Stoddard, 1977; Reynolds, Johns, & Stoddard, 1977). There is no question that Wilcox and Bellamy have the expertise necessary to instruct staff members in how to teach persons who have a difficult time learning. It is also clear that they are experienced in applying this expertise in the area of job training. In discussing a summer job training and placement program, Clarke, Greenwood, Abramowitz, and Bellamy (1980) described the successful training of CETA-eligible nonhandicapped 16- to 21-year-olds who, in turn, served as co-workers and on-site job trainers for secondary level students labeled moderately or severely retarded (2 of the 10 students discussed had Down syndrome). The following were included in the instructional skills taught to the co-worker/trainers: positive reinforcement, use of assistance in training, task analysis, and data collection.

The choice of not to include a component on instructional competencies may be a matter of a perceived necessary trade-off with a concern that additional demands on instructors might result in rejection of the OHS model. The consumer satisfaction data reported by Wilcox and Bellamy, however, seem to indicate a willingness to take on extra work because it is both appropriate and worth the effort.

Given that the intent of the OHS model is to provide best practice secondary education programming, how might instructional technology training, at least for teachers, be incorporated into the model? Even more important, what impact might this have for students with Down syndrome?

Briefly, the OHS Model is designed currently to be suitable for normal conditions and constraints. Under these conditions, staff are trained in the OHS model during a 5-day training period. This is followed by 5 days of technical assistance, telephone contacts, and quarterly reviews. It is suggested that their same proven format could be used with 3–5 days being added at the beginning of training and with 1–2 days of observation, feedback, and related technical assistance being added as a part of the regularly scheduled contact and review sessions.

Another suggestion is to add higher paying job training options to the OHS jobs catalog. Adding these more complicated jobs seems feasible with the addition of recommended enhanced job analysis and training skills of the staff. Additional employment outcomes might then be possible (see Rehabilitation Research and Training Center, 1985). The question of whether jobs have been, or should be, passed over because of training requirements must be asked.

CHALLENGES FOR THE FUTURE

The result of adding consumer training in instructional technology to the OHS model could be assurance that optimally prepared instructors would be ready to pursue all relevant secondary education training needs of individuals with Down syndrome. Meeting the future secondary education needs of students with Down syndrome will be a question of implementation and refinement of known and agreed upon philosophies, programs, and techniques. The major future challenge to mainstreaming, at least in this author's opinion, will be that of providing a structure that develops and maintains successful interactions between persons with Down syndrome and nonhandicapped individuals. Part of the structure needs to take form in providing sound support networks.

Informal supports are support networks such as families, friends, neighbors, and peer groups, or organizations such as churches, schools, work groups, and clubs that offer friendship and assistance in problem solving and obtaining needed assistance. Often, interactions in these support networks reflect a reciprocal relationship. Persons with disabilities receive support and, in turn, offer friendship and help. (Deinstitutionalization Task Force, 1983b, p. 1)

As Perske (1983) so aptly stated:

People were meant to complement each other. Where I am strong, you may be weak. At points where you excel, I may be all thumbs. And the ultimate tragedy takes place when I reject you because of your handicaps and you reject me because of mine. Then we live apart . . . and we die apart. We die without ever really knowing each other or experiencing the rich contributions each could have made to the other's life. (p. ii)

A difficulty lies in the fact that personal relationships or informal supports are largely just that, personal and informal and difficult to define and program in an organized, systematic way. And yet, secondary education programs for students with Down syndrome must accept the challenge of preparing students for a productive and satisfying adult life. Personal relationships form an essential part of successful adult living. The OHS model provides a direction and, as reported, a foundation for further research and development in this area.

REFERENCES

Clarke, J. Y., Greenwood, L. M., Abramowitz, O. B., & Bellamy, G. T. (1980). Summer jobs for vocational preparation of moderately and severely retarded adolescents. *Journal of the Association for Persons with Severe Handicaps, 5* (1), 24–37.

Deinstitutionalization Task Force. (1983a). *Future directions in adult services* (p. 1–4). Columbus: Ohio Developmental Disabilities Planning Council.

Deinstitutionalization Task Force. (1983b). *Promoting quality community living through formal support services and informal supports* (p. 1). Columbus: Ohio Developmental Disabilities Planning Council.

Deinstitutionalization Task Force Project. (1985). Personal relationships for persons with developmental disabilities. *Proceedings of a conference on informal supports* (pp. 14–37). Columbus: Ohio Developmental Disabilities Planning Council.

Gibson, D., & Stoddard, D. W. (1977). *Electronics assembly manual—A "try another way" task analysis system for training moderately and severely handicapped individuals in electronics assembly skills.* Washington, DC: The National Children's Center.

Gold, M. W. (1980a). *Marc Gold: "Did I say that?".* Champaign, IL: Research Press.

Gold, M. W. (1980b). *Try another way. Training manual.* Champaign, IL: Research Press.

Gold, M., & Associates. (1978). *The California project: Final report of a state wide training project.* Sacramento: California Department of Rehabilitation and Health.

Gold, M., & Associates. (1982). *The Ohio Employee Development Project: Final report.* Columbus, OH: U.S. Department of Labor, Ohio Bureau of Employment Offices for the Comprehensive Employment and Training Act.

Hall, R. V. (1971). *Managing behavior: Part 3. Applications in school and home; Part 4. New ways to teach new skills; part 5. A teachers guide to writing instructional objectives.* Lawrence, KS: H and H Enterprises.

National Children's Center. (1978). *Project Skills: Final report of an electronics assembly training and employment program.* Washington, DC: Department of Health, Education, and Welfare, Region III, Office of Human Development, Developmental Disabilities Office.

Perske, R. (1983). In Deinstitutionalization Task Force, *Promoting quality community living through formal support services and informal supports* (p. ii). Columbus: Ohio Developmental Disabilities Planning Council.

Rehabilitation Research and Training Center. (1984). Improving the employability of mentally retarded citizens. *RRTC Newsletter, 1* (2).

Rehabilitation Research and Training Center. (1985). Improving the employability of citizens who are mentally retarded. *RRTC Newsletter, 2* (1).

Reynolds, A. T., Johns, M., & Stoddard, D. W. (1977). *Travel training manual: A task analysis approach for training moderately and severely developmentally disabled individuals in the use of public transportation.* Washington, DC: The National Children's Center.

Steiner, G. A. (1979). *Strategic planning: What every manager must know* (p. 5). New York: The Free Press.

Stoddard, D. W. (1985). *Some value orientations* [Values clarification training materials]. Columbus, OH: Comprehensive Training and Development Institute.

U.S. Department of Health and Human Services. (1984). *A program inspection on transition of developmentally disabled young adults from school to adult services* (754-021/4548). Washington, DC: U.S. Government Printing Office.

Wehman, P., & Moon, M. S. (1985). *Critical values in employment programs for persons with developmental disabilities* (p. 3). Richmond: Virginia Commonwealth University, School of Education, Rehabilitation Research and Training Center.

Chapter 9

Language and Communication Characteristics of Children with Down Syndrome

Jon F. Miller

✝✝✝

Children with Down syndrome are particularly at risk for language learning problems for reasons beyond the associated cognitive deficits. First, there is an increased frequency of middle ear infection, which is frequently associated with delayed language acquisition in normal children (Brandes & Elsinger, 1981; Downs, 1980). Frequent middle ear infection can result in hearing loss, which is always associated with language learning problems. Second, the deficits in motor coordination associated with Down syndrome may adversely affect the synchrony of motor movements required of the speech production system, including respiration, phonation, and articulation of the palate, tongue, lips, and jaw (Bless, Swift, & Rosen, 1985). Third, cognitive deficits specific to Down syndrome may result in language learning problems beyond those commonly associated with mental retardation (Miller, Chapman, & MacKenzie, 1981). And fourth, there can be decreased expectations for performance of mentally retarded individuals, which frequently result in learned incompetence or lack of appropriate experience (Coggins & Stoel-Gammon, 1982). Any one of these factors can result in deficits in language acquisition; taken together, they represent a formidable puzzle to unravel in order to understand the forces affecting language growth in this population.

The writing of this chapter was supported in part by Core Research Support to the Waisman Center on Mental Retardation and Human Development from NICHD, Grant #2 P30 HDO3352, 1985. The author would like to express his thanks to Gloria Streit, Pam Laikko, John Rynders, and Robin Chapman for their critical comments.

The focus of this chapter is language learning in individuals with Down syndrome, with a consideration of all of the factors affecting the acquisition and use of language as a symbolic system. Prior to the discussion of the studies of children with Down syndrome, the general themes in the research on the language characteristics associated with mental retardation are reviewed. These themes include investigations of cognitive characteristics and the extent to which they are necessary for language learning, and investigations of the nature of the language acquired by individuals with mental retardation (i.e., is it delayed or deviant relative to normal acquisition?). Investigations of the speech and language performance of children with mental retardation have focused, in general, on the major determinant factors for acquiring a language system, including cognitive constructs, environmental facilitation, and physiological limitations, both perceptual and motor.

LANGUAGE ACQUISITION AND MENTAL RETARDATION

There can be little doubt that children with mental retardation do not demonstrate the same language behaviors as normal children of the same chronological age. However, despite a variety of methods used to study the various etiologies resulting in mental retardation, the results of most studies indicate that children with mental retardation use normal linguistic forms and do not produce bizarre language patterns, such as unique word combinations, invented word meanings, or novel discourse characteristics (Duchan & Erickson, 1976; Graham & Graham, 1971; Kamhi & Johnston, 1982; Lackner, 1968; Miller et al., 1981; Naremore & Dever, 1975; Newfield & Schlanger, 1968; Ryan, 1975; Semmel, Barritt, Bennett, & Perfetti, 1967; Yoder & Miller, 1972). Mental retardation is a behavioral classification resulting from a variety of etiologies, including: metabolic and genetic syndromes; disease processes; trauma, both pre- and postnatally; and cultural and familial influences (Miller et al., 1981). It is impressive that despite a variety of brain syndromes, children with mental retardation learn the standard form of their native language.

Attempts to characterize the language performance of persons with mental retardation have evolved over time, resulting in several competing points of view over the past 25 years. Initially, a major issue was whether the language of these persons was quantitatively or qualitatively different (i.e., delayed or deviant relative to nonverbal cognitive skills). This controversy was derived in large part from different ideas about the relation between language and cognitive skills. The view of quantitative differences is consistent with the idea that developments in language are directly contingent on developments in cognition. Such a view predicts that language skills are always consistent with cognitive development or mental age, and never advanced or delayed relative to nonverbal mental age development (Graham &

Graham, 1971; Lackner, 1968; Lenneberg, Nichols, & Rosenberger, 1964). Further, quantitative differences argue for similar cognitive structures, with learning rate the primary problem, which results in language learning being characterized as "slow motion" normal development. The qualitative or deviant development view of the language of children with mental retardation argues that language learning is delayed relative to the performance level predicted by mental age (Newfield & Schlanger, 1968; Semmel et al., 1967). Delays in language development relative to mental age are interpreted as deviant language performance, compared to the synchrony of development of chronological age, mental age, and language in normal children. Several studies have supported the deviant view. However, the majority of research has supported the position that language development in children with mental retardation follows the same course and sequence as that of normal children but progresses at a slower rate (i.e., it is quantitatively different) (Miller & Yoder, 1974; Ryan, 1975; Yoder & Miller, 1972). In general, the language performance of children with mental retardation has been found to be similar in form and content to that of normal children matched for mental age or linguistic stage of development.

Both the delay and deficit views recognize that cognitive development is essential for language development. The delay position implies that development in cognition is sufficient for language to develop, and the deficit view recognizes that additional child characteristics are necessary for language growth. Both of these views, however, oversimplify the complexities of the language itself and the acquisition process, viewing it as unidimensional and static over time. Neither considers the role of social factors, the impact of language on cognition, or the influence of specific linguistic capabilities on language development, which are prominent ideas in current theories of language development (Bates & MacWhinney, 1979; Slobin, 1985; Wells, 1980). Recent surveys of the relation between language and cognition (Cromer, 1981; Finch-Williams, 1984; Leonard, 1978; Miller, Chapman, Branston, & Reichle, 1980) have suggested a correlational relation, in which language development proceeds generally at the rate of cognitive development, but depending on environmental events, may be slightly behind or ahead of cognitive skills. Such a view recognizes the central role the child's environment must play in language acquisition, which includes providing both quality and frequency of language and nonverbal experiences leading directly to increasing knowledge of the world.

Studies of children with mental retardation have supported this correlational view of the language-cognition relationship, documenting differences in language performance not accounted for by cognitive status. Two studies have investigated the profiles of language comprehension and production in relation to nonverbal cognitive development in children with moderate and severe mental retardation (Miller, Chapman, & Bedrosian, 1978; Miller et al., 1981). Significant asynchronies were found in the profiles of these children, who were functioning developmentally between 7 months and 7 years. The studies found three profiles of language skills: 25% of the subjects had delays in productive language relative to comprehension and cognitive skills, 25% of the subjects had delays in both comprehension and production of language relative to cognitive skills, and 50% had comprehension and production skills commensurate with cognitive skills. One-half of the subjects studied (i.e., the first two groups) did not match the generalization of retarded performance (i.e., "slow motion" normal performance). The delays could not be attributed to hearing or speech-motor deficits. They were evident at several levels of cognitive skill, from Piaget's sensorimotor stage V through late preoperational development (Piaget & Inhelder, 1969). The subjects at each cognitive stage were of various chronological ages. Perhaps language skills fail to develop at the same pace as other cognitive skills in some children as they get older either due to etiology or other intervening factors. The variation in development found in individual children across specific linguistic features (vocabulary, syntax, and semantics in both comprehension and production) may be due to social or environmental differences.

In another study, Kamhi and Johnston (1982) found frequency differences among linguistic characteristics they attributed to social and motivational behaviors rather than deficits in cognitive or linguistic abilities. This study is important in that it proposes different underlying processes for different language characteristics. Frequency of use of specific linguistic forms is attributed to social aspects of the conversational context or to motivation. Differences in frequency of use would not be interpreted as reflecting differences in linguistic or cognitive knowledge. Taken together, these studies suggest that the social interaction, including language input and maternal responsiveness, may explain the individual variation in language learning in children with mental retardation.

To summarize, previous research on children with mental retardation has resulted in several very general conclusions about their communication. The language performance of such children has been described as following the same developmental pattern as normal children when matched for mental age or linguistic stage. Despite differences in etiology, the majority of research has documented similar performance across linguistic domains. While language and communication skills are clearly delayed relative to chronological age, many of the differences disappear when children with mental retardation are compared to children of similar mental abilities. Other studies (Kahmi & Johnston, 1982; Miller et al., 1981) have documented differences in language not attributable to cognitive deficits. In investigating language and communication skills in children with Down syndrome, one must evaluate language skills relative to their underlying processes, cognitive as well as social, recognizing the complexity of the language system as it is used in speaking and listening.

LANGUAGE AND DOWN SYNDROME

The research literature dealing with the language behavior of children with Down syndrome has reviewed many of the same issues associated with mental retardation in general, including the components of language behavior and the internal and external (cognitive and environmental) forces associated with language development. The goal of this chapter is to document what is known about language acquisition in Down syndrome so that improved methods for facilitating language growth and change can be developed.

What specific areas of expertise must be developed in order to learn a language? Consider that the child must acquire the sound system, vocabulary, and grammar to convey an unlimited set of meanings derived from his or her knowledge of the world. Learning and using a language system requires the development of both comprehension and production skills to allow its use in socially appropriate ways—to give and get information in conversation, tell stories, argue, persuade, and accomplish all of the other functions for which language is used. Normal children acquire their language over the course of childhood, with more advanced communicative skills added in the early teenage years (deVilliers & deVilliers, 1985). Children demonstrate linguistic performance at the onset of the 2nd year, comprehending and producing single word utterances. Development proceeds rapidly through age 5, when the basics of syntax for simple sentences have been mastered. The ability to convey a range of information—including marking past and definite future events, simple spatial relationships, and primitive causal constructs—has also developed. The essential elements of conversation skills have also been mastered. Vocabulary size is estimated to be 23,700 different words at age 7 (Smith, 1941), indicating an accelerating vocabulary acquisition rate of 7–10 new words a day. Any characterization of retarded language development must view the individual features of the language system (i.e., phonology, syntax, semantics, and pragmatics) as they develop independently and in synchrony with each other in speaking and listening.

As mentioned previously, there are several characteristics associated with Down syndrome that put these children at particular risk for language deficits beyond their cognitive deficits. They have increased incidence of otitis media resulting in hearing loss. They may have speech-motor control problems resulting in deficits in speech intelligibility. There may be specific cognitive deficits associated with language learning, and differences may exist in expectation for performance. All of these characteristics will affect language interaction patterns, stimulation, and responsivity. The requirements for language development include intact perceptual, cognitive, and speech-motor systems, and a stimulating and responsive linguistic environment (Miller, 1981). Children with Down syndrome are at risk for language problems resulting from potential deficits in any one of these essential areas.

The majority of work viewed in this chapter compares the performance of children with Down syndrome to normal children in order to address the following question: Are children with Down syndrome acquiring language at the same rate and in the same sequence as normal children? In the majority of studies, normal children and children with Down syndrome have been matched on chronological age, mental age, and, recently, language level in an effort to uncover any differences in language performance between the two groups. Baumeister (1967, 1984) pointed out the dangers inherent in matching studies, particularly in inferring underlying processes from similar to different performance characteristics between normal children and children with mental retardation. While the comparative studies are, necessarily, reviewed in detail, the parallel theme of this chapter is the emerging language competence of children with Down syndrome.

DO CHILDREN WITH DOWN SYNDROME HAVE A DISTINCTIVE PATTERN OF LANGUAGE DEVELOPMENT?

The literature on productive language development of children with Down syndrome reveals a pattern of increasing linguistic deficit with advancing chronological age (CA). A summary of the results of 16 studies can be found in Table 1. As chronological age advances, deficits in language development below mental age (MA) expectations are more likely to be found. Table 1 also includes the developmental age or linguistic stage of the persons studied, when available. Together, these studies investigated 226 individuals with Down syndrome, ranging in chronological age from 6 months to 49 years.

Syntax and Semantics

Several studies have reported that the language skills of children with Down syndrome fail to keep pace with their increasing cognitive abilities (Harris, 1983; Rogers, 1975; Wiegel-Crump, 1981). Wiegel-Crump (1981) studied the growth of syntax in 80 children with Down syndrome, with CAs of 6–12 years, and nonverbal MAs of 2–6 years. While she found no difference between home-reared and institutionalized subjects, she found significant MA effects at each level (2, 3, 4, 5, and 6 years). Compared to the norms on the Developmental Sentence Scoring task (Lee, 1974), children with Down syndrome with MAs of 2 years performed at the 50th–60th percentile and subjects with MAs of 3–6 years performed at the 10th–15th percentile. Little change was noted in the language skills of the 3–6 year MA group. Their language was characterized as stereotypic, repetitive, and inflexible. Rogers

Table 1. Summary of studies on the productive language development of persons with Down syndrome

Source	N	Chronological age	Developmental level	Outcome
Wiegel-Crump, 1981	80	6–12 yrs.	2–7 yrs.	As DS[a] subjects got older, deficits in syntax got larger. Productions were stereotypic, repetitive, and inflexible.
Rogers, 1975	17	4.5[b]–16.1 yrs.	3.11 yrs.	All DS subjects below MA[c] comparison for syntax, 70% below in vocabulary, and 60% below in semantics. Language deficits more pronounced in older (CA[d]) DS subjects.
Leuder, Fraser, & Jeeves, 1981	8	17–37 yrs.	3–7 yrs.	Significant linguistic deficits and discourse abilities.
Price-Williams & Sabsay, 1979	9	29–49 yrs.		Deficits in syntax and intelligibility over discourse skills.
Rondal, 1978a	14	5–12 yrs.	2–2.5 yrs.	No overall difference in syntax development between DS and language-matched normals. Differences noted at more advanced language level.
Harris, 1983	10	2.6–6.9 yrs.	MLU[e] 1.18–1.32	Younger DS children are like matched normals, but older DS children use different means to expand utterances; may use different acquisition strategies.
Layton & Sharifi, 1978	9	7.4–12.2 yrs.	3.2–5.8 yrs.	Similar range of semantic structures expressed, MA- and language-matching results in similar semantic functioning.
Coggins & Stoel-Gammon, 1982	4	5.1–6.9 yrs.	Ling. stage I	No differences in DS performance, and requests for clarification responded to.
Coggins, Carpenter, & Owings, 1983	4	5.1–6.9 yrs.	18–24 mos.	DS and normals equivalent in use of gestures and vocalization. Range of communicative infants similar,

(continued)

Table 1. (continued)

Source	N	Chronological age	Developmental level	Outcome
				commensurate with cognitive and linguistic development.
Owens & MacDonald, 1982	6	20–89 mos.	36–48 mos.	No differences in communicative interactions expressed by DS and normals at linguistic stages I and II.
Coggins, 1979	4	3.1–6.3 yrs.	Ling. stage I	Same diversity of meanings expressed by DS and normal children.
Rondal, 1978b	21	3–12 yrs.	MLU 1.0–1.5 1.75–2.25 2.5–3.0	DS and normal children's language increases in complexity as MLU increases. No differences were found between groups except TTRs[f] were higher in DS, indicating advanced lexical development.
Scherer & Owings, 1984	4	5.1–6.9 yrs.	MLU 1.6–2.0	Responses to maternal questions same in frequency and type as normal children at same MLU.
Greenwald & Leonard, 1979	20	10–54 mos.	8–18 mos.	Communication abilities consistent with cognitive development, advances in older CA DS children, some using words.
Leifer & Lewis, 1984	10	18–23 mos. 3.5–4.5 yrs.	MLU 1.0–1.5	Responses to maternal questions delayed in DS children compared to normal subjects matched on MLU.
Jones, 1980	6	6–24 mos.	8–19 mos.	No difference in DS vocalization compared to normals matched on developmental age. Differences in quality of interaction, DS mothers were directive, less responsive to child, and initiated more speech.

[a]DS is used in place of Down syndrome in order save space in this summary material.
[b]4.5 yrs. = 4 yrs., 5 mos.
[c]Mental age.
[d]Chronological age.
[e]Mean length of utterance.
[f]Type-token ratio.

(1975) reported that of 17 subjects tested on the Raynell Test of Language Performance, all 17 had scores below those of MA comparisons for language structure, 13 of 17 subjects had lower scores on vocabulary, and 11 of 17 subjects had lower scores on language content. Six of 17 subjects had good speech intelligibility, and a significant relation was found between speech intelligibility and language structure scores. Surprisingly, Rogers found the comprehension scores of the older children with Down syndrome (10–16 years) to be significantly worse than their production scores. All of the children with Down syndrome showed significant language deficits relative to their nonverbal mental abilities. These two studies, which investigated almost 100 subjects with Down syndrome, using cross-sectional research designs, document a pattern of increasing linguistic deficit with age.

The strategy of matching normal children and children with Down syndrome on general language ability is used when relations among language characteristics are being investigated and when differences in language development would confound the results. Usually investigators use mean length of utterance (MLU), which is a calculation of the child's average spoken utterance length in words or morphemes. This measure is interpreted as an index of general syntactic development (Brown, 1973; Miller, 1981), and therefore allows comparisons of specific syntactic devices or semantic and discourse features. Several studies of younger children with Down syndrome have documented similarities in language and communication abilities when directly compared to normal subjects matched on their stage of language development by MLU. (Note the developmental level of these children in Table 1.)

Harris (1983) studied 10 children with Down syndrome and 10 normal children to determine the validity of MLU as a linguistic matching technique. His subjects with Down syndrome ranged in CA from 2.6 to 6.9. No MA data were reported. He found that the language of his younger subjects with Down syndrome closely resembled the language of normal children of the same MLU stage. However, the older subjects used different means to expand their utterances, suggesting different language learning strategies that are evident only as both children with Down syndrome and normal children become older and acquire more advanced language skills.

Coggins (1979) found that children with Down syndrome and normal children expressed the same range of meanings, as coded by semantic relation categories in extensive free speech samples. The four subjects with Down syndrome were in linguistic stage one, MLU = 1.0–2.0, the earliest stage of language development. Normal children pass through this stage between 12 and 24 months of age. Rondal (1978b) found no differences between the language performance of his 21 subjects with Down syndrome as compared to the language of normal children matched for MLU. As MLU increased, language complexity increased, expressing the same range of meanings. The children with Down syndrome showed more advanced vocabulary development than the normal children at the same MLU stage. Owens and Mac-

Donald (1982) studied the expressive communication ability of six subjects with Down syndrome and six normal subjects at linguistic stages I and III, MLU = 1.0–2.0 and 2.5–3.0, respectively. No differences in the range or frequency of communicative behaviors expressed verbally were found. The children with Down syndrome and the normal children used language equally well across a range of communicative situations (e.g., requesting, commenting, answering, naming). Coggins, Carpenter, and Owings (1983) found similar results investigating four subjects with Down syndrome and four normal subjects all at linguistic stage I, in sensorimotor stage VI, and having MAs of 18–24 months. They coded communicative behavior which was expressed either gesturally or verbally. They found that both the range and proportional use of communication behaviors were the same for the subjects with Down syndrome and the normal subjects.

The often reported preference for gestural expression over verbal expression among children with Down syndrome by educators, parents, and speech-language pathologists has been examined by several investigators. Using a well-documented coding scheme, Coggins and Carpenter (1981) reported similar use of vocal and gestural means of expression. Greenwald and Leonard (1979), however, found that children with Down syndrome, as compared to normal children of similar language and cognitive stages, used more gestures than verbal means in expressing imperatives and declaratives. Coggins et al. (1983) studied the free speech of their subjects while playing with their mothers. Greenwald and Leonard (1979) used an elicitation technique developed by Snyder (1978). Differences in performance may be due to differences in the communicative demands of the two situations, one coding naturally occurring events, the other setting up contingencies to evoke a communicative response. One could speculate that when communication is demanded, the children with Down syndrome use gestures over words, but that they can express the same range of communicative events verbally as their normal counterparts when they are not under communicative pressure.

Phonology

In an investigation of 10 children with Down syndrome, premeaningful vocalizations for the first 15 months of life were reported by Smith and Oller (1981). They found substantial similarities between children with Down syndrome and normal children. Both groups began to produce canonical, reduplicated babbling at 8–8 1/2 months of age. The development of vowels and consonants showed similar patterns for the first 15 months of life. Stoel-Gammon (1980) reported on the articulation problems of four children with Down syndrome in Brown's (1973) early and late stage I of linguistic development. The articulatory patterns were reported in relation to their overall language performance, as well as their articulation errors in terms of phonological processes. The results indicate that while subjects are able to produce nearly all of the consonant phonemes, correct production in conversational speech was usually limited to a particular position in the word; the position varied across subjects. The phonological processes that account for the speech sound errors are similar to those reported for young normal children. The phonological abilities of the four children with Down syndrome are comparable to or better than their general language ability, as measured by their mean length of utterance.

The findings of Smith and Oller (1981) and Stoel-Gammon (1980) confirmed that children with Down syndrome exhibit knowledge of the phonological rules for speech-sound combination commensurate with their general language ability. Phonological rule knowledge may be appropriate for those children with Down syndrome who have fairly intelligible speech. Speech intelligibility remains, however, a consistent problem among individuals with Down syndrome. Intelligibility problems can be directly attributed to the oral and facial anomalies associated with the condition, affecting the jaws, tongue, teeth, and gingival and mucosal structures (Sanger, 1975) and the speech-motor control of these structures (Bless et al., 1985). The tongue is frequently reported to be too large for an undersized oral cavity and protruding from the mouth. Motor control of all oral structures is negatively affected by the general hypotonia associated with Down syndrome. In addition, there is evidence for a general motor deficit in Down syndrome that particularly affects coordination and timing of motor movements. The range of speech intelligibility in the syndrome is, therefore, attributable to both structural and motor control deficits.

Intelligibility of speech intrudes on all of the other aspects of productive language development discussed. Given the range of intelligible speech, one wonders how subjects were selected for a study of productive language. Informal surveys of researchers frequently result in comments about the high frequency of unintelligible speech. Paul Berry (personal communication, 1984), for example, who is conducting a longitudinal study of 60 children with Down syndrome and their families in Queensland, Australia, reported that the majority of his 5- and 6-year-olds were unintelligible. Elicitation tasks were required to study productive language because, without knowing in advance what was being said, their speech was not interpretable. Better reporting of subject-selecting criteria must be made if the results are to generalize to the full population of children with Down syndrome, rather than only to those who have mostly intelligible speech.

Discourse

Discourse is defined in this chapter as any analysis of language units larger than an utterance, particularly the contingent relations between utterances in conversation, narration, or other pragmatic speaking conditions. In an investigation of children's strategies to clarify utterances when they are not under-stood by a speaking partner, Coggins and Stoel-Gammon (1982) found that all four of their subjects with Down syndrome were sensitive to their speaking partner's request for clarification. This was evidenced by either a repetition or a revision of the utterance. The results document that by linguistic stage I, children with Down syndrome have mastered this major aspect of human communication, as would be expected of normal subjects at the same level of linguistic development.

Leuder, Fraser, and Jeeves (1981) and Price-Williams and Sabsay (1979) have documented the advance of communicative competence over linguistic skills in adult subjects with Down syndrome. These studies investigated con-versational skills, discovering that subjects used a variety of strategies for gaining attention and clarifying utterances when they were not understood. The subjects tended to use discourse strategies to establish topic, and relied on posture and gestures to indicate appropriate social distance with strangers. In general, subjects with Down syndrome used nonverbal interaction strategies over verbal means of communication. Both Price-Williams and Sabsay (1979) and Leuder et al. (1981) concluded that adults with Down syndrome lack the linguistic means for expression of their experience and knowledge of the world, but that their communicative competence is intact to the extent that their severe linguistic deficits permit.

Another study of the discourse skills of three subjects with Down syn-drome documented advanced communicative skills when language skills more closely correspond to mental abilities (Nisbet, Zanella, & Miller, 1984). The three subjects in this study were 12 and 15 years of age and, educa-tionally, were mainstreamed into a normal high school. Free speech samples were recorded in conversation with peers and with a normal student of the same chronological age. All of the subjects were rank-ordered according to their social and communicative competence. Analysis revealed that all of them demonstrated more advanced linguistic competence as they assumed more competent speaking roles, by adjusting their language ability to take charge of the conversation, asking more questions, introducing more topics, and using longer utterances. This study complicates the view of increasing linguistic deficit with age, clearly contradicting the trend noted in the majority of studies reviewed. Where language skills have developed in children with Down syndrome, overall communicative competence appears to be finely tuned.

Studies of chronologically younger children with Down syndrome have documented similar development of language structure, semantic expression, and discourse features compared to normal children matched for MA and general language level (Coggins, 1979; Coggins et al, 1983; Coggins & Stoel-Gammon, 1982; Greenwald & Leonard, 1979; Harris, 1983; Jones, 1980; Owens & MacDonald, 1982). As chronological age increases, to 3–4 years, differences in language performance are reported, not simply an increased slowing down of the acquisition process (Rogers, 1975; Rondal, 1978a; Wiegel-Crump, 1981). It is not clear at this point whether: 1) the deficits associated with advancing age are the result of differences in environmental support for language learning that may decrease with increasing age, 2) there is difficulty in learning the more complex linguistic means to express conceptually complex ideas, or 3) these conceptually complex ideas have not been acquired. Examples of these complex ideas are past, present, and future time concepts; concepts of space and the relation between individuals and objects in space; and concepts of causality (i.e., agent-action-object relations). It is also possible that the outcome of the premature appearance of Alzheimer disease in persons with Down syndrome is being seen (Miniszek, 1983). Only through longitudinal investigation of the language development of children with Down syndrome, including their comprehension and expression of linguistically and cognitively complex notions such as time, will one begin to understand the relation between chronological age, environmental influences, and the cognitive characteristics of Down syndrome.

Vocabulary

The development of vocabulary appears to be independent of other linguistic features in children with Down syndrome. Rondal (1978b) reported that children with Down syndrome have advanced vocabulary diversity over normal children of the same MA and linguistic stage. They use a larger vocabulary when conversing with their mothers in free play than younger normal children in the control sample. Rondal concluded that this lexical advance is present in his subjects because their advanced age reflects more experience, both linguistic and nonlinguistic. He argued that vocabulary, as opposed to other aspects of language, is a direct outcome of environmental experience. Is this advanced development or elaborated development within the same developmental stage? Miller et al. (1978) and Miller et al. (1981) found similar advances in vocabulary in their population of multiply handicapped, and moderately to severely retarded children, who had developmental ages of 7 months–7 years. Apparently, increased vocabulary diversity is not a particular characteristic of children with Down syndrome. It may be a function of experience, as Rondal (1978b) suggested or of language intervention or special education, as postulated by Miller et al. (1981).

Paradoxically, several studies have shown that children with Down syndrome exhibit significant deficits in referential looking behavior, the ability to establish joint reference to objects. Jones (1979, 1980) documented that subjects with Down syndrome, aged 8–22 months developmentally, engaged in less than one-half of the referential looking than their matched normal developmentally subjects. Gunn, Berry, & Andrews (1982) found that the looking behavior of children with Down syndrome had an interpersonal rather than referential quality. Sinson and Wetherick (1982) found differential social interaction patterns which lead to isolation in children with Down syndrome. This was attributable to the subjects' failure to observe the conventions of mutual gaze. These studies together suggest a difference in visual behavior essential to establishing prelinguistic interaction patterns (Schaffer, Collis, & Parsons, 1977); referential communication (Gray, 1978); and language development (Ryan, 1974). Referential looking is a major method of initiating interaction (Jones, 1980) and the establishment of joint reference is essential for vocabulary learning. If these skills are deficient, then why do children with Down syndrome appear to show advanced vocabulary development?

First, vocabulary may be advanced in the number of different words produced relative to total words in a conversation, but may not mark or code more complex conceptual meaning. Second, the data to date are production data only, without corroboration of this population's ability to comprehend advanced meaning or more diverse vocabulary at the same level of conceptual complexity. Third, there is evidence to suggest that lexical and relational meaning may be deficient in subjects with Down syndrome in later periods of development and in subjects who are chronologically older. Several studies have documented that the meanings conveyed by individuals with Down syndrome in conversations are restricted to the here and now (Layton & Sharifi, 1978; Leuder et al., 1981; Rondal, 1978a). Apparently, individuals with Down syndrome fail to transcend time and space in their productive language, talking instead about objects and events immediately present in both time and space.

Comprehension

There are few studies of the language comprehension skills of individuals with Down syndrome, or of the relation between comprehension and production. Several studies have reported on related aspects of comprehension performance.

In two experimental intervention studies, Holdgrafer (1981, 1982) reported variable training rates between comprehension and production for subjects learning plural ''s.'' He interpreted this result as supporting the independence of the two modes in development. Language can develop independently in comprehension and production in children with Down syndrome. This view contrasts sharply with the widely held assumption that comprehension precedes production in language learning (Bloom, 1974; Ingram, 1974). How far comprehension precedes production through the developmental period is not well understood in normal development. In one of the best studies of this relation, Benedict (1979) reported a 5-month gap with comprehension preceding production for the second year of life in a longitudinal study of normal children. Hartley (1982) reported specific comprehension deficits for sequential or syntactic tasks, suggesting right hemisphere dominance for language processing in individuals with Down syndrome. This is in contrast to left hemisphere dominance in normal speakers. The Miller et al. (1981) study documented that comprehension always precedes production, but that production does not always follow the development of comprehension in children with mental retardation. Significant deficits in production relative to comprehension frequently occur.

In two studies of the responses of children with Down syndrome to maternal questions (Leifer & Lewis, 1984; Scherer & Owings, 1984), conflicting results are reported. Scherer & Owings (1984) found that all four of their children with Down syndrome produced appropriate contingent responses to maternal requests for information, clarification, acknowledgment, and action. Correct response rates were 70%–80% for all categories except requests for information, for which two subjects supplied the correct form but not the correct information. They concluded that their subjects perform like normal children of the same linguistic stage. Leifer & Lewis (1984), however, found that the overall response rate of their six children with Down syndrome, four language-matched normal children, and four children matched in age to the language-matched normal group was very low. Appropriate responses to maternal questions were almost nonexistent for the age-matched normal children at 3%, 15% for the language-matched normal children, and 31% for the children with Down syndrome. As well as more frequent appropriate responses, the children with Down syndrome demonstrated advanced responding to directive questions, using more vocalized responses than action responses. Developmentally, action responses precede vocalized responses. Leifer and Lewis (1984) argued that children with Down syndrome show general delays in development compared to chronological age–matched normal children, as well as differences when language level matches are compared. The children with Down syndrome show superior response performance to maternal questions. Leifer and Lewis contended that children with Down syndrome follow a different sequence in the development of syntax and conversational skills than normal children.

Differences in the outcome of these two studies can be attributed to two factors. First, Scherer and Owings (1984) studied children in late stage I (MLU 1.6–2.0) and Leifer and Lewis (1984) studied children at early stage I (MLU 1.0–1.5). Second, the language matches of the Leifer and Lewis study were based on MLU, a production measure, ignoring the fact that children's comprehension abilities show substantial change while they are at the one-word stage of language production (Benedict, 1979; Miller et al., 1980). Leifer and Lewis assumed similar comprehension development based on production ability, an assumption that is not warranted in persons with mental retardation. While production levels were matched, the nature of the response differences reported suggest that the group with Down syndrome had more advanced comprehension skills. Rather than following a different sequence of development, they are simply displaying developmentally advanced responses to maternal questions. This study exemplifies the problem of attempting to match subjects at the one-word level of production on the basis of MLU measures. The one-word period of development extends through most of the second year of life. Matching at this level violates the logic proposed by Brown (1973) for using MLU, that is, as an index of structural development.

A recent study by Bless et al. (1985) found that all of their nine subjects with Down syndrome showed delays in both comprehension and production, as compared to their nonverbal cognitive status. These children were functioning between 5 and 8 years developmentally and were tested on measures of vocabulary and syntax. This is the only study of the relations among linguistic variables in both comprehension and production. It confirmed increasing deficits at advanced developmental levels in both comprehension and production. Further, this study documented significant speech-motor problems contributing to the expressive language difficulty of individuals with Down syndrome.

Summary of the Language
Characteristics of Children with Down Syndrome

Earlier in this chapter, it was asked if individuals with Down syndrome exhibited specific profiles of language behavior that might be interpreted as evidence for the unique language learning abilities associated with Down syndrome. The answer must be "no" at this time, due primarily to the lack of research on language comprehension for any linguistic characteristic, and the failure of production studies to examine the more advanced aspects of syntax and semantics in favor of more general investigations of pragmatics. Primarily, the review in this chapter has documented the limitations of what can be learned from cross-sectional research. Developmental relations involving changing synchronous interactions require longitudinal study.

Children with Down syndrome show an increasing linguistic deficit in relation to their nonverbal cognitive status with increasing chronological age. This pattern may be the result of specific cognitive deficits associated with the syndrome (including limited capacity for complex representation through language), physiological limitations of perception or motor performance, or a failure of the environment to support language learning through a protracted developmental period. There are few data to support the cognitive deficit view (Cicchetti & Pogge-Hesse, 1982), although three recent investigations have pointed out the increased interest in cognitive, information-processing explanations of the language deficits in persons with Down syndrome. Kahn (1985) found similar cognitive structures in organic (Down syndrome) and nonorganic retarded children. Lincoln, Courchesne, Kilman, and Galambos (1985) found, using electrophysiological measures, that children with Down syndrome process some types of information slower than MA- and CA-matched normal children. Ellis, Deacon, and Wooldridge (1985) found evidence for structural memory deficits (in short-term memory) in persons with mental retardation, one-third of whom had Down syndrome. The complexities of tracing specific correlates to language learning becomes more apparent with advancing research.

Physiological links to deficits in language acquisition and use have not been established beyond assumed co-occurrence where deficits in perception or motor performance were found. Studies must be undertaken to uncover profiles of performance, noting change over time.

The last factor, the environment, can be investigated through two sources: studies of maternal language input, and the outcome of language intervention studies. An examination of the literature dealing with the language environment of individuals with Down syndrome follows. It first identifies the factors associated with language facilitation in natural environments and then reports the outcomes of environmental manipulation on language development.

WHAT ARE THE CHARACTERISTICS OF THE LINGUISTIC ENVIRONMENT OF CHILDREN WITH DOWN SYNDROME?

Chapman (1981) reviewed in detail the role of mother-child interaction on language development in the second year of life. She concluded that input plays a demonstrable role in language development when it is specifically contingent upon the child's initiated actions and utterances. She went on to say that it is the linguistically responsive environment, rather than the linguistically stimulating one, that should accelerate language acquisition in the 1- to 2-year-old child. The most important operating principle for the mother seems to be: "Pay attention to what the child is doing and saying" (Chapman, 1981, p. 224).

A number of studies have investigated the assertion that parental expectations due to early knowledge of the condition of Down syndrome affects parent-child interactions. The general pattern that emerges from these studies is as follows. First, both mothers and infants with Down syndrome are less responsive to each other (Stevenson & Leavitt, 1983). Second, mothers of infants with Down syndrome talk to their children more and tend to talk at the same time that their infants are vocalizing (Berger & Cunningham, 1983). Third, mothers of children with Down syndrome speak at a faster rate, producing more utterances per unit time than mothers of normal children (Buckhalt, Rutherford, & Goldberg, 1978). Fourth, mothers of children with Down syndrome are more directive, intrusive, and controlling (Eheart, 1982; Jones, 1979, 1980). Fifth, not all mothers of these children are alike; that is, individual differences in patterns of interaction exist. Thus, maternal sensitivity and directiveness are independent features of maternal behavior (Crawley & Spiker, 1983).

Studies of mothers' speech directed toward their children with Down syndrome have assumed that linguistic complexity is an index of maternal sensitivity to the child's linguistic development. This assumption predicts that maternal language that is judged as too complex or too simple would inhibit language development, while maternal language just above the child's level of linguistic mastery would facilitate language development. The majority of studies have found that maternal language addressed to children with Down syndrome is similar in complexity to that addressed to normal children (Mitchell, 1980; O'Kelley-Collard, 1978; Rondal, 1978a). Two studies, however, produced contradictory results. Mahoney (1983) found that mothers' speech input to young children with Down syndrome did not change over the course of 10 months and was unrelated to the child's behavior. Glaser, Schwethelm, Haffner, and Mahoney (1984) found that mothers of children with Down syndrome produced 79% of their directives toward mother-initiated activities and only 21% of their directives in relation to child-initiated activities. Significantly more directives were successful in changing or facilitating child activities if the activities were child initiated rather than mother initiated. Mothers continued to be successful when they followed the child's lead.

In contrast to the language production literature, the mother-child interaction and maternal language input literature paint a picture of an early lack of maternal responsiveness, followed by a period of adjustment to the child's growing language competence. This view is supported by a study of general responsiveness of mothers to their handicapped children, including children with Down syndrome (Brooks-Gunn & Lewis, 1984). Prior to the onset of intelligible speech, mothers and children with Down syndrome appear mismatched in their communicative interactions. Obviously, these competing pictures (i.e., one of responsiveness and one of lack of responsiveness) should not coexist, if views of normal development are correct. Some insight in the conflicting mother-child literature is provided by Crawley and Spiker (1983), who showed that mothers of children with Down syndrome vary widely in the dimensions of directiveness, sensitivity, and elaborativeness. Mothers who combine sensitivity and directiveness in ways that provide stimulative value may have more competent infants. The maternal characteristic of directiveness has emerged as the most descriptive of mothers of handicapped children. Consider that most intervention programs involve maternal stimulation, some recommending increasing stimulation of all types. It is probable that researchers are recording the results of some of their own advice, correctly or incorrectly interpreted by the mothers of children with Down syndrome.

An increasing awareness of individual variation in the behavior of children with Down syndrome is seen as a function of variation in the child's cognitive and linguistic abilities, hearing level, speech intelligibility and environmental support for language. This chapter now turns to the experimental literature on language intervention with these children as a final window into their language performance.

CAN LANGUAGE INTERVENTION FACILITATE THE LANGUAGE DEVELOPMENT OF CHILDREN WITH DOWN SYNDROME?

Language Intervention

Bricker and Carlson (1981) discussed the convergence of research in cognitive, affective, and linguistic processes in producing new views of language intervention. Intervention programs not accounting for the relation between and among these major domains will be deficient in promoting language as a useful communicative tool. Further, Bricker and Carlson called for an increased emphasis on intervention in the first year of life, prior to the expectation of intelligible speech. Finally, they called on interventionists to exploit the rich interactive feedback networks and reciprocal environmental contexts that exist in the child's environment. In other words, they urged interventionists to do what normal mothers and their children do but to do it more frequently, being particularly responsive to the child's activities and topics, and to the child's communicative needs within his or her environment.

The language intervention literature reviewed in this chapter demonstrates the effectiveness of various teaching techniques. For example, operant conditioning techniques are effective in establishing verbal imitation responses and improving speech intelligibility (Farb & Thorne, 1978; Mac-Cubrey, 1971; Nelson, Peoples, Hay, Johnson, & Hay, 1976). Parent training will not generalize from the laboratory to new contexts (e.g., the home) without instruction (Salzberg & Villani, 1983). Children with Down syndrome show more difficulty in attaining verbal solutions to learning tasks versus nonverbal solutions, which argues the presence of a verbal learning deficit (Rynders, Behlen, & Horrobin, 1979). Training mothers of children with Down syndrome in the use of behavior modification techniques will lead to improved language, self-help skills, and motor and social behavior (Bidder, Bryant, & Gray, 1975). The control of verbal input, lexically and structurally, will improve these children's identification of the target stimuli and improve learning. Also, teacher responsiveness by itself is not sufficient for learning, but must be paired with specification of what is to be learned (Filler, 1976). Together, these studies show that a variety of training techniques can change the language behavior of children with Down syndrome.

Most impressive, however, are the documented effects on children's language development associated with changing maternal interaction style. The approaches to intervention that have had the most productive results are those that have employed developmental interaction models to improve the mother's interaction style, and primarily to improve maternal responsiveness. Seitz (1975) reported on the use of such a model with three mothers of children with Down syndrome. All three children showed gains in language, as documented by an increase in MLU and by an increase in the number of utterances per session, from an average of 42 to 126. The mothers' behavior also significantly changed the children's compliance to the mothers' commands. Compliance increased from 43% to 98% over the 8 weeks of the study. MacDonald, Blott, Gordon, Spiegel, and Hartmann (1974) reported an increase in MLU, and in structural complexity associated with generalization of parent training to new settings. Parents were trained to imitate and expand child utterances. During the last 3 months of the 5-month study, there were gains equivalent to 3 months of development at the same linguistic stage as Brown's (1973) normal subjects. In a large scale follow-up study, Baker, Heifetz, and Murphy (1980) evaluated 95 children 14 months after parent training. The mothers continued to show growth in the trained skills in three of four areas. Forty-four per cent of the families judged the training to continue to be very useful, and most had incorporated the teaching activities into daily routines.

Ludlow and Allen (1979) conducted a 10-year follow-up of English children who were enrolled in an early intervention program. This program had been introduced to reduce the progressive decline in developmental quotients of children with Down syndrome. All of the 143 children with Down syndrome enrolled in the study were followed. Three groups were investigated. Group A received parent counseling regarding behavior management and techniques to facilitate cognitive, motor, and language development. Group A's program appears to have resembled those of Seitz (1975) and MacDonald et al. (1974), and included periodic visits to a developmental clinic to monitor performance and provide feedback to parents. In group B, the children with Down syndrome were living at home, but the families did not participate in the counseling or developmental clinic programs. In group C, the children with Down syndrome were institutionalized by the second year of life. The group A children showed significantly higher scores than the children in the other two groups on IQ and developmental scales, particularly in personal-social and speech-language development. Mahoney and Snow (1983) investigated cognitive level as a possible predictor of the outcome of language training. Their subjects were 14 children with Down syndrome, ranging in age from 24 to 36 months, and all performed at or below the one-word stage of language production. The experimenters used the MacDonald and Horstmeier (1978) Environmental Language Intervention Program to train parents to facilitate language development. Outcomes of the intervention program were significantly correlated with performance on sensorimotor scales of cognitive development. Children at later sensorimotor stages gained the most and those at earlier stages gained the least from language training.

An Australian study of 36 children with Down syndrome enrolled in an early intervention study that trained mothers to facilitate the language growth of their children reported that all children showed increases in developmental quotients (Clunies-Ross, 1979). Gains were particularly noticeable in social and language areas, with examples cited of children's DQs (developmental quotients) exceeding CA. Younger children made bigger gains than chronologically older children. Finally, Cheseldine and McConkey (1979) analyzed the spontaneous language training strategies of parents. They found that after the mothers were told to teach language, but not how to go about it, three mothers improved their language facilitation strategies and four mothers did not change. Given further opportunity to improve, including direct instruction, two more mothers improved over the control mothers, as evidenced by reduced directiveness and increased responsiveness.

Sign Language Training

The practice of sign language instruction has emerged over the past 10 years in response to children with Down syndrome's failure to learn oral language to the level expected by parents or the educational system. The logic for such instruction is based on two assumptions. First, the child has the cognitive capacity to acquire a representational system. Second, the child has specific deficits that prohibit the acquisition or use of oral language (e.g., a severe speech motor deficit or significant hearing loss). Frequently, however, assumptions are made about the ease of learning a visual language system over spoken language. Such assumptions tend to ignore the fact that both sign language and speech require the same degree of cognitive representational skills, and that both are complete language systems. The issue is complicated by the existence of several sign systems, each of which is fairly independent. Central to the issue, however, is the question of whether teaching sign language facilitates language learning. That is, will children with Down syndrome be able to express themselves more completely using sign language than they could using oral language? Two studies have addressed this question.

Romski and Ruder (1984) investigated the acquisition of agent-object combinations in two conditions: speech alone and speech combined with sign (total communication). The subjects were 10 children with Down syndrome, 3–7 years of age. There were no significant differences found for the two conditions. However, the children exhibited a wide range of individual patterns of development. Romski and Ruder cautioned against automatic adoption or rejection of manual sign systems as a part of oral language training. The second study (Weller, 1981) found that both oral and Signed English training for parents were effective in facilitating language and cognitive growth in 15 children with Down syndrome, 18–36 months of age. Further, they found that the use of signs did not inhibit oral language development.

While the oral language versus sign language controversy is far from settled, preliminary data suggest a wide range of individual variation in the skills necessary for language learning. These skills must be carefully evaluated relative to prognosis for language development with either an oral or manual system. The child learning sign is limited to communicating with other signers. The child with no language does not communicate. Signing may enhance oral language development for some children. Signing programs should be considered transitional and augmentative to the development of oral language skills.

Summary

The language intervention studies with children with Down syndrome show that their language behavior can be facilitated with early intervention. Intervention programs emphasizing mothers' language interaction style are particularly effective in increasing language performance. These programs emphasize decreasing the directiveness and complexity of maternal language spoken to the child, increasing responsiveness to the child's initiated behavior (both verbal and nonverbal), and increasing responsiveness to child-initiated topics and the child's communicative needs. Early intervention with families of children with Down syndrome can significantly improve the rate of language development in children with Down syndrome. It appears that a paraphrase of Chapman's (1981) operating principles for mothers of normal children, "Follow the child's lead and respond to their speech and actions," should be adopted by language interventionists as well.

Although early intervention using a directed stimulation model is effective in promoting language learning, there is neither a clear understanding of the specific contingent behaviors leading to language growth nor of how they may change over time. It is the latter of these two points that is particularly troublesome to those concerned with the language development of children with Down syndrome, given the expectation of decreasing language skills over time relative to the development of other skills areas. It is clear that the factors that govern language growth and change in both normal and disordered populations are only beginning to be understood. Clearly there is a great need for further research into the language skills of children with Down syndrome.

QUESTIONS FOR FUTURE RESEARCH

1. Is there developmental continuity in development among linguistic elements, vocabulary, syntax, semantics, and pragmatics, within and between both comprehension and production?

2. Are there individual differences in the patterns of language acquisition that can be explained by characteristics of language input, speech intelligibility, hearing status, or cognitive skills?
3. Can environmental intervention significantly improve language performance? When should intervention begin? Over what period of time is it effective? Can one teach a language system to the child with Down syndrome or can one only provide a supportive environment conducive to language learning?
4. Do early patterns of development predict later performance?

In considering the first question, future research must invoke multidimensional models of speech and language performance. At minimum, these models should include consideration of language comprehension and production; phonology, syntax, semantics, and discourse features; nonverbal cognitive abilities; speech motor performance; and hearing status. The linguistic environment of the child with Down syndrome must also be included. These models must account for developmental change as well as provide for the description of deviant performance at the lexical, utterance, and discourse levels. Such models would provide the bases for hypothesis generation as well as for the evaluation of experimental language interventions.

In order to answer the second, third, and fourth questions, a way to conduct longitudinal research on language change in this population needs to be found. Two major problems must be overcome. First, current funding cycles of 3–5 years preclude studying anything more than 1 year of development. Second, many children with Down syndrome in the United States are in some type of early intervention/special education program. Mechanisms must be developed to bring the researcher into the intervention/special education circle so they can learn which practices work and which ones do not. An example of a productive strategy can be found in Gibson and Ingram (1983). In this study, a parent and a researcher combined efforts to conduct a longitudinal study of a child with delayed language. The result is an impressive study with a very rich data base. Parents, ''bring a researcher home to dinner.'' Researchers, listen to what parents have to say, and take heed of their concerns. The goal is the same: improved communication for children with Down syndrome.

Longitudinal research demands long-term commitment on the part of researchers, requiring at least 10 years to study 5 years of longitudinal development. Most researchers consider this very high risk research, given that one-third to one-fourth of a career may be at stake. Funding mechanisms and support networks must be developed to form communities of scholars who will work jointly with families of children with Down syndrome.

New tools will have to be designed and implemented to overcome the data analysis problems inherent in language research. The development of computer analysis techniques may provide the significant advances necessary to make longitudinal research possible. Computers can be used to analyze free speech samples, as well as to gather data on language comprehension (Miller & Chapman, 1984). Computer formats for free speech sample analysis provide a standard for transcription that can be read by clinicians and researchers alike. Data exchanges for language data of various populations must be encouraged (MacWhinney & Snow, 1985). Longitudinal research will require a great deal of data and data analysis. The use of computers for exchange and analysis of the data will finally bring true longitudinal study of communication development in children with Down syndrome into the realm of reality.

REFERENCES

Baker, B. L., Heifetz, L. J., & Murphy, D. M. (1980). Behavioral training for parents of mentally retarded children: One-year follow-up. *American Journal of Mental Deficiency, 85,* 31–38.

Bates, E., & MacWhinney, B. (1979). A functionalist approach to the acquisition of grammar. In E. Ochs & B. Schieffelin (Eds.), *Developmental pragmatics* (pp. 167–214). New York: Academic Press.

Baumeister, A. (1967). Problems in comparative studies of mental retardates and normals. *American Journal of Mental Deficiency, 71,* 869–875.

Baumeister, A. (1984). Some methodological and conceptual issues in study of cognitive processes with retarded people. In P. Brooks, R. Sperber, & C. McCauley (Eds.), *Learning and cognition in the mentally retarded* (pp. 6–38). Hillsdale, NJ: Lawrence Erlbaum Associates.

Benedict, H. (1979). Early lexical development: Comprehension and production. *Journal of Child Language, 6,* 183–200.

Berger, J., & Cunningham, C. C. (1983). Development of early vocal behaviors and interactions in Down's syndrome and nonhandicapped infant-mother pairs. *Developmental Psychology, 19,* 322–331.

Bidder, R. T., Bryant, G., & Gray, O. P. (1975). Benefits to Down's syndrome children through training their mothers. *Archives of Disease in Childhood, 50,* 383–386.

Bless, D., Swift, E., & Rosen, M. (1985). Communication profiles of children with Down syndrome. Unpublished manuscript, University of Wisconsin, Waisman Center on Mental Retardation and Human Development, Madison.

Bloom, L. (1974). Talking, understanding, and thinking. In L. Lloyd (Ed.), *Language perspectives: Acquisition, retardation, and intervention* (pp. 285–312). Baltimore: University Park Press.

Brandes, P., & Elsinger, D. (1981). The effects of early middle ear pathology on auditory perception and academic achevement. *Journal of Speech and Hearing Disorders, 46,* 301–307.

Bricker, D., & Carlson, L. (1981). Issues in early language intervention. In R. Schiefelbusch & D. Bricker (Eds.), *Early language: Acquisition and intervention* (pp. 477–516). Baltimore: University Park Press.

Brooks-Gunn, J., & Lewis, M. (1984). Maternal responsivity in interactions with handicapped infants. *Child Development, 55,* 782–793.

Brown, R. (1973). *A first language.* Cambridge, MA: Harvard University Press.

Buckhalt, J. A., Rutherford, R. B., & Goldberg, K. E. (1978). Verbal and nonverbal interaction of mothers with their Down's syndrome and nonretarded infants. *American Journal of Mental Deficiency, 82*, 337–343.

Chapman, R. (1981). Mother-child interaction in the second year of life: Its role in language development. In R. Schiefelbusch & D. Bricker (Eds.), *Early language: Acquisition and intervention* (pp. 201–250). Baltimore: University Park Press.

Chapman, R., Miller, J., MacKenzie, H., & Bedrosian, J. (1981, August). *The development of discourse skills in the second year of life.* Paper presented at the 2nd International Congress for the Study of Child Language, University of British Columbia, Vancouver, British Columbia, Canada.

Cheseldine, S., & McConkey, R. (1979). Parental speech to young Down's syndrome children: An interview study. *American Journal of Mental Deficiency, 83*, 612–620.

Cicchetti, D., & Pogge-Hesse, P. (1982). Possible contributions of the study of organically retarded persons to developmental theory. In E. Zigler & D. Balla (Eds.), *Mental retardation: The developmental-difference controversy* (pp. 277–318). Hillsdale, NJ: Lawrence Erlbaum Associates.

Clunies-Ross, G. G. (1979). Accelerating the development of Down's syndrome infants and young children. *The Journal of Special Education, 13*, 169–177.

Coggins, T. E. (1979). Relational meaning encoded in the two-word utterances of stage 1 Down's syndrome children. *Journal of Speech and Hearing Research, 22*, 166–178.

Coggins, T. E., & Carpenter, R. L. (1981). The communicative intention inventory: A system for observing and coding children's early intentional communication. *Applied Psycholinguistics, 2*, 235–251.

Coggins, T. E., Carpenter, R. L., & Owings, N. O. (1983). Examining early intentional communication in Down's syndrome and nonretarded children. *British Journal of Disorders of Communication, 18*, 98–106.

Coggins, T. E., & Stoel-Gammon, C. (1982). Clarification strategies used by four Down's syndrome children for maintaining normal conversational interaction. *Education and Training of the Mentally Retarded, 17*, 65–67.

Crawley, S. B., & Spiker, D. (1983). Mother-child interactions involving two-year-olds with Down syndrome: A look at individual differences. *Child Development, 54*, 1312–1323.

Cromer, R. (1981). Reconceptualizing language acquisition and cognitive development. In R. Schiefelbusch & D. Bricker (Eds.), *Early language: Acquisition and intervention* (pp. 51–138). Baltimore: University Park Press.

deVilliers, P., & deVilliers, J. (1985). The acquisition of English. In D. Slobin (Ed.), *The cross-linguistic study of language acquisition.* Hillsdale, NJ: Lawrence Erlbaum Associates.

Downs, M. (1980). The identification of children at risk for middle ear effusion problems. *Annals of Otology, Rhinology and Laryngology, 89* (3, Part 2), 168–171.

Duchan, J., & Erickson, J. (1976). Normal and retarded children's understanding of semantic relations in different verbal contexts. *Journal of Speech and Hearing Research, 19*, 767–776.

Eheart, B. K. (1982). Mother-child interactions with nonretarded and mentally retarded preschoolers. *American Journal of Mental Deficiency, 87*, 20–25.

Ellis, N. R., Deacon, J. R., & Wooldridge, P. W. (1985). Structural memory deficits of mentally retarded persons. *American Journal of Mental Deficiency, 89*, 393–402.

Evans, D. (1977). The development of language abilities in mongols: A correlational study. *Journal of Mental Deficiency Research, 21*, 103–117.

Farb, J., & Thorne, J. (1978). Improving the generalized mnemonic performance of a Down's syndrome child. *Journal of Applied Behavior Analysis, 11*, 413–419.

Filler, J. W., Jr. (1976). Modifying maternal teaching style: Effects of task arrangement on the match-to-sample performance of retarded preschool-age children. *American Journal of Mental Deficiency, 80*, 602–612.

Finch-Williams, A. (1984). The developmental relationship between cognition and communication: Implications for assessment. *Topics in Language Disorders, 5*, 1–13.

Gibson, D., & Ingram, D. (1983). The onset of comprehension and production in a language delayed child. *Applied Psycholinguistics, 4*, 359–376.

Glaser, K., Schwethelm, B., Haffner, P., & Mahoney, G. (1984, May). *The effects of maternal directives on the performance of Down syndrome infants.* Paper presented at the Annual Conference of the American Association on Mental Deficiency, Minneapolis.

Graham, J., & Graham, L. (1971). Language behavior of the mentally retarded: Syntactic characteristics. *American Journal of Mental Deficiency, 75*, 623–629.

Gray, H. (1978). Learning to take an object from the mother. In A. Lock (Ed.), *Action, gesture, and symbol: The emergence of language.* New York: Academic Press.

Greenwald, C. A., & Leonard, L. B. (1979). Communicative and sensorimotor development of Down's syndrome children. *American Journal of Mental Deficiency, 84*, 296–303.

Gunn, P., Berry, P., & Andrews, R. J. (1982). Looking behavior of Down syndrome infants. *American Journal of Mental Deficiency, 87*, 344–347.

Harris, J. (1983). What does mean length of utterance mean? Evidence from a comparative study of normal and Down's syndrome children. *British Journal of Disorders of Communication, 18*, 153–169.

Hartley, X. (1982). Receptive language processing by Down's syndrome children. *Journal of Mental Deficiency Research, 26*, 263–269.

Holdgrafer, G. (1981). Mode-relations in language learning by language-deficient retarded subjects. *Perceptual and Motor Skills, 53*, 520–522.

Holdgrafer, G. (1982). Teaching comprehension and production. *Perceptual and Motor Skills, 55*, 306.

Ingram, D. (1974). Comprehension and production. In R. Schiefelbusch & L. Lloyd (Eds.), *Language perspectives: Acquisition, retardation, and intervention.* Baltimore: University Park Press.

Jones, O. (1979). A comparative study of mother-child communication with Down syndrome and normal infants. In D. Schaffer & J. Dunn (Eds.), *The first year of life* (pp. 175–195). New York: John Wiley & Sons.

Jones, O. H. M. (1980). Prelinguistic communication skills in Down's syndrome and normal infants. In T. F. Field (Ed.), *High-risk infants and children: Adult and peer interactions* (pp. 205–225). New York: Academic Press.

Kahn, J. (1985). Evidence of the similar-structure hypothesis controlling for organicity. *American Journal of Mental Deficiency, 89*, 372–378.

Kamhi, A., & Johnston, J. (1982). Towards an understanding of retarded children's linguistic deficiencies. *Journal of Speech and Hearing Research, 25*, 435–445.

Lackner, J. R. (1968). A developmental study of language behavior in retarded children. *Neuropsychologia, 6*, 301–320.

Layton, T. L., & Sharifi, H. (1978). Meaning and structure of Down's syndrome and nonretarded children's spontaneous speech. *American Journal of Mental Deficiency, 83*, 439–445.

Lee, L. (1974). *Developmental sentence analyis.* Evanston, IL: Northwestern University Press.

Leifer, J., & Lewis, M. (1984). Acquisition of conversational response skills by young Down Syndrome and nonretarded children. *American Journal of Mental Deficiency, 88,* 610–618.

Lenneberg, E., Nichols, I., & Rosenberger, E. (1964). Primitive stages of language development in mongolism. *Research Publications: Association for Research in Nervous and Mental Disease, 42.*

Leonard, L. (1978). Cognitive factors in early linguistic development. In R. Schiefelbusch (Ed.), *Bases of language intervention.* Baltimore: University Park Press.

Leuder, I., Fraser, W. I., & Jeeves, M. A. (1981). Social familiarity and communication in Down syndrome. *Journal of Mental Deficiency Research, 25,* 133–142.

Lincoln, A. J., Courchesne, E., Kilman, B. A., & Galambos, R. (1985). Neurophysiological correlates of information-processing by children with Down syndrome. *American Journal of Mental Deficiency, 89,* 403–414.

Ludlow, J. R., & Allen, L. M. (1979). The effect of early intervention and preschool stimulus on the development of the Down's syndrome child. *Journal of Mental Deficiency Research, 23,* 29–44.

MacCubrey, J. (1971). Verbal operant conditioning with young institutionalized Down's syndrome children. *American Journal of Mental Deficiency, 75,* 696–701.

MacDonald, J. D., Blott, J. P., Gordon, K., Spiegel, B., & Hartmann, M. (1974). An experimental parent-assisted treatment program for preschool language-delayed children. *Journal of Speech and Hearing Disorders, 39,* 395–415.

MacDonald, J., & Horstmeier, D. (1978). *Environmental Language Intervention Program.* Columbus, OH: Charles E. Merrill.

MacWhinney, B. (1984). *Child Language Data Exchange System (CHILDES), MacArthur Foundation Project.* Pittsburgh: Carnegie-Mellon University.

MacWhinney, B., & Snow, C. (1985). The child language data exchange. *Journal of Child Language, 12,* 271–296.

Mahoney, G. (1983). A developmental analysis of communication between mothers and infants with Down's syndrome. *Topics in Early Childhood Special Education, 3,* 63–76.

Mahoney, G., & Snow, K. (1983). The relationship of sensorimotor functioning to children's response to early language training. *Mental Retardation, 21,* 248–254.

McCarthy, D. (1954). Language development in children. In L. Carmichael (Ed.), *Manual of child psychology* (pp. 492–630). New York: John Wiley & Sons.

Miller, J. (1981). *Analyzing language production in children: Experimental procedures.* Baltimore: University Park Press.

Miller, J., & Chapman, R. (1984). Disorders of communication: Investigating the development of language of mentally retarded children. *American Journal of Mental Deficiency, 88,* 536–545.

Miller, J., Chapman, R., & Bedrosian, J. (1978). The relationship between etiology, cognitive development, and language and communicative performance. *The New Zealand Speech Therapists' Journal, 33,* 2–17.

Miller, J., Chapman, R. S., Branston, M. B., & Reichle, J. (1980). Language comprehension in sensorimotor stages V and VI. *Journal of Speech and Hearing Research, 23,* 284–311.

Miller, J., Chapman, R., & MacKenzie, H. (1981). *Individual differences in the language acquisition of mentally retarded children.* Paper presented at the 2nd

International Congress for the Study of Child Language, Vancouver, British Columbia, Canada.

Miller, J., & Yoder, D. (1974). An ontogenetic language teaching strategy for retarded children. In R. Schiefelbusch & L. Lloyd (Eds.), *Language perspectives: Acquisition, retardation, and intervention* (pp. 505–528). Baltimore: University Park Press.

Miniszek, N. A. (1983). Development of Alzheimer disease in Down syndrome individuals. *American Journal of Mental Deficiency, 87*, 377–385.

Mitchell, D. R. (1980). Down's syndrome children in structured dyadic communication situations with their parents. In J. Hogg & P. J. Mittler (Eds.), *Advances in mental handicap research* (Vol. 2, pp. 161–194). New York: John Wiley & Sons.

Naremore, R., & Dever, R. (1975). Language performance of educable mentally retarded and normal children at five age levels. *Journal of Speech and Hearing Research, 18*, 82–96.

Nelson, R. O., Peoples, A., Hay, L. R., Johnson, T., & Hay, W. (1976). The effectiveness of speech training techniques based on operant conditioning: A comparison of two methods. *Mental Retardation, June*, 34–38.

Newfield, M., & Schlanger, B. (1968). The acquisition of English morphology by normals and educable mentally retarded children. *Journal of Speech and Hearing Research, 11*, 693–706.

Nisbet, J., Zanella, K., & Miller, J. (1984). An analysis of conversations among handicapped students and a nonhandicapped peer. *Exceptional Children, 51*, 156–162.

O'Kelley-Collard, M. (1978). Maternal linguistic environment of Down's syndrome children. *The Australian Journal of Mental Retardation, 5*, 121–126.

Owens, R. E., Jr., & MacDonald, J. D. (1982). Communicative uses of the early speech of nondelayed and Down syndrome children. *American Journal of Mental Deficiency, 86*, 503–510.

Piaget, J., & Inhelder, B. (1969). *The psychology of the child*. New York: Basic Books.

Price-Williams, D., & Sabsay, S. (1979). Communicative competence among severely retarded persons. *Simiotica, 26*, 35–63.

Rogers, M. G. H. (1975). A study of language skills in severely subnormal children. *Child: Care, Health and Development, 1*, 113–126.

Romski, M. A., & Ruder, K. F. (1984). Effects of speech and speech and sign instruction on oral language learning and generalization of action + object combinations by Down's syndrome children. *Journal of Speech and Hearing Disorders, 49*, 293–302.

Rondal, J. A. (1978a). Developmental sentence scoring procedure and the delay-difference question in language development of Down's syndrome children. *Mental Retardation, April*, 169–171.

Rondal, J. (1978b). Maternal speech to normal and Down's syndrome children matched for mean length of utterance. In C. E. Meyers (Ed.), *Quality of life in severely and profoundly mentally retarded people: Research foundations for improvement* (pp. 193–266). Washington, DC: American Association on Mental Deficiency.

Ryan, J. (1974). Early language development: Towards a communicational analysis. In M. Richards (Ed.), *The integration of the child into a social world*. London: Cambridge University Press.

Ryan, J. (1975). Mental subnormality and language development. In E. Lenneberg &

E. Lenneberg (Eds.), *Foundations of language development: A multidisciplinary approach* (Vol. 2, pp. 269–278). New York: Academic Press.

Rynders, J. E., Behlen, K. L., & Horrobin, J. M. (1979). Performance characteristics of preschool Down's syndrome children receiving augmented or repetitive verbal instruction. *American Journal of Mental Deficiency, 84,* 67–73.

Salzberg, C. L., & Villani, T. V. (1983). Speech training by parents of Down syndrome toddlers: Generalization across settings and instructional contexts. *American Journal of Mental Deficiency, 87,* 403–413.

Sanger, R. G. (1975). Facial and oral manifestations of Down's syndrome. In M. Koch & F. de la Cruz (Eds.), *Down's syndrome (Mongolism): Research, prevention and management* (pp. 32–46). New York: Brunner/Mazel.

Schaffer, H., Collis, G., & Parsons, G. (1977). Vocal interchange and visual regard in verbal and pre-verbal children. In H. R. Schaffer (Ed.), *Studies in mother-infant interaction.* New York: Academic Press.

Scherer, N. J., & Owings, N. O. (1984). Learning to be contingent: Retarded children's responses to their mothers' requests. *Language and Speech, 27,* 255–267.

Seitz, S. (1975). Language intervention—Changing the language environment of the retarded child. In M. Koch & F. de la Cruz (Eds.), *Down's syndrome (Mongolism): Research, prevention and management* (pp. 157–179). New York: Brunner/Mazel.

Semmel, M., Barritt, L., Bennett, S., & Perfetti, C. (1967). The performance of educable mentally retarded and normal children on a modified cloze task. *Studies in Language Learning and Language Behavior, 5,* 326–342.

Sinson, J. C., & Wetherick, N. E. (1982). Mutual gaze in pre-school Down's and normal children. *Journal of Mental Deficiency Research, 26,* 123–129.

Slobin, D. (1985). Cross-linguistic evidence for language-making capacity. In D. Slobin (Ed.), *The cross-linguistic study of language acquisition.* Hillsdale, NJ: Lawrence Erlbaum Associates.

Smith, B., & Oller, K. (1981). A comparative study of pre-meaningful vocalizations produced by normally developing and Down's syndrome infants. *Journal of Speech and Hearing Research, 46,* 46–51.

Smith, M. (1941). Measurement of the size of general English vocabulary through the elementary grades and high school. *Genetic Psychology Monographs, 24,* 311–345.

Snyder, L. (1978). Communication and cognitive abilities and disabilities in the sensorimotor period. *Merrill-Palmer Quarterly, 24,* 161–180.

Snyder, L. K., & McLean, J. E. (1976). Deficient acquisition strategies: A proposed conceptual framework for analyzing severe language deficiency. *American Journal of Mental Deficiency, 81,* 338–349.

Stevenson, M. B., & Leavitt, L. A. (1983). *Mother-infant interaction: A Down's syndrome case study.* Paper presented at the 2nd International Workshop on the "At Risk" Infant, Jerusalem.

Stoel-Gammon, L. (1980). Phonological analysis of four Down's syndrome children. *Applied Psycholinguistics, 1,* 31–48.

Weller, E. (1981). Comparison of oral and signed-English communication training with Down's syndrome children in a parent-assisted language intervention program. *Dissertation Abstracts International,* (University Microfilms).

Wells, G. (1980). Apprenticeship in meaning. In K. Nelson (Ed.), *Children's Language* (Vol. 2). New York: Gardner Press.

Wiegel-Crump, C. A. (1981). The development of grammar in Down's syndrome children between the mental ages of 2-0 and 6-11 years. *Education and Training of the Mentally Retarded, February,* 24–30.

Yoder, D., & Miller, J. (1972). What we may know and what we can do: Input toward a system. In J. McLean, D. Yoder, & R. Schiefelbusch (Eds.), *Language intervention with the retarded: Developing strategies* (pp. 89–110). Baltimore: University Park Press.

Response

Communication Intervention

DeAnna Horstmeier

Miller's review of the state-of-the-art research regarding the language and communication of individuals with Down syndrome was thorough, clear, and extremely well balanced with regard to the great variety of factors that make up a representational communication system. His own work has reflected a multidimensional approach to language that is revealed in the underlying issues that he developed in Chapter 9. The purpose of this response is to emphasize and augment two issues that Miller discussed.

INTELLIGIBILITY

Most investigators report substantial articulation disorders in individuals with Down syndrome, even exceeding those of non–Down syndrome delayed matches. In an older study, Schlanger and Gottsleben (1957) found that 95% of the institutionalized population of individuals with Down syndrome had substantial articulation deficits. A more recent study, by Dodd (1976), found that children with Down syndrome made over twice as many articulation errors as MA-matched children with other types of mental retardation and had 1½–2 times as many error inconsistencies, such as using different phonemes (sounds) to substitute for one incorrect phoneme. Silverstein, Ageno, Alleman, Derecho, & Gray (1985), investigating the adaptive behavior of adults with retardation, reported that subjects with Down syndrome showed greater social competence in every area except in the clarity of their speech. Little attention, however, has been paid to intelligibility in studies that have intervention implications for persons with Down syndrome.

The last 10 years have seen the reemergence of interest in child phonology (sound system), which emphasizes the child patterns of sound usage, as compared to adult phonology. Children seem to have orderly strategies to simplify the adult speech they are unable to reproduce exactly (Ingram, 1976). For example, children speaking in one- to two-word phrases often drop the final consonants in the words they use; hot cup becomes "hah kah." Would it be most effective to intervene on the sound /t/ and then the sound

/p/, or to help the child learn the strategy of using final consonants? Since phonological therapy looks at patterns of sound usage, it has been used successfully with multiple articulation errors.

Phonological rule analysis has been applied to the speech of children with Down syndrome. Investigators have found that individuals with Down syndrome use phonological processes similar to those used by normal language-learning children (Bleile, 1982; Bodine, 1974; Dodd, 1976; Stoel-Gammon, 1980). However, little use has been made of phonological process intervention for persons with Down syndrome, as reported in the literature. Moran, Money, and Leonard (1984), after a study of phonological processes in adults with retardation, concluded that when faced with multiple errors in a person with mental retardation, speech therapists should use phonological pattern therapy as is now being used with normal individuals (Ingram, 1976; Shreiberg & Kwialkowski, 1980; Weiner, 1979). Iglesias and Horstmeier (1978) reported on clinical phonological process intervention with clients with Down syndrome, ranging from preschool to adult age. Both the person with Down syndrome and his or her parents (or group home providers) were part of the therapy. Simple diagnostic and therapy procedures were designed. Many of the parents were able to conduct therapy under the direction of the therapists. All of the parents or group home providers were helped to use informal procedures to reinforce what was mastered in therapy.

The involvement of the individual's social environment for informal intelligibility training should be encouraged, no matter what type of therapy is used. The persons that interact with an individual with Down syndrome should insist on an appropriate level of clarity of speech or sign. The author's son Scott, a 15-year-old with Down syndrome, has had considerable language and articulation therapy. There are now very few sounds he cannot say correctly. He has been working at school on the /ch/ sound—with very little enthusiasm. The author has been so happy with his progression that she has not worked with him on that particular sound. One evening, their family went to Wendy's hamburger restaurant for dinner. They had challenged Scott to order something besides a hamburger. He told the girl at the counter that he wanted "Silly" (chili). "What?" she inquired, "Silly! Silly!" he continued in frustration. Finally, to his chagrin, he had to ask his mother to help. His request for a drink went smoothly. However, for dessert, he wanted chocolate chip cookies. One unintelligible plea for "soclate sip" made Scott point to the cookie display on the counter to clarify his order. At home, Scott started to work diligently on the /ch/ sound. If he temporarily lacked motivation, the author just had to remind him of "silly" at Wendy's to renew his zeal.

An additional possible problem can be that of the professional's perception of a person with Down syndrome. Bodine (1974) felt that the clinical picture held by some professionals of a person with Down syndrome, as having little language and talking in inarticulate grunts, along with the characteristic physical appearance of those with Down syndrome, may cause observers to underestimate their communication abilities and thus, have lower expectations of intervention efficacy.

Balkany, Downs, Jafek, & Krajicek (1979) had reservations about the expectations of professionals concerning the hearing of persons with Down syndrome. Over 78% of the individuals with Down syndrome tested had a significant hearing loss; 64% of those tested had a binaural loss (both ears). Over 80% of the losses were conductive in nature, with degree of loss ranging from mild to moderate (15–50 dB). Only 16% of the individuals had hearing aids. Balkany et al. attributed the low incidence of amplification to the widespread feeling that persons with mental retardation could not profit by normalized hearing through hearing aids. Amplification should be available to persons with Down syndrome when needed, especially during the early language learning periods. Further, much of the conductive loss was attributed to serous otitis media (fluid-filled middle ear), which is often present in children with Down syndrome. Tubes inserted in the middle ear for fluid drainage may improve hearing and should be available for individuals with Down syndrome.

Good clinical research should accompany a vigorous push toward effective intelligibility training. It is not clear, however, that the techniques of speech therapy and hearing intervention that are already in use for nondelayed persons are being vigorously pursued for persons with Down syndrome.

LINGUISTIC ENVIRONMENT:
MOTHER-CHILD INTERACTION STUDIES

A relatively recent development in the area of child language has been the investigation of mother-child interactions and the development of communicative competence. Characteristics of mother and child behaviors during social interaction acquired from studies of normally developing children and their mothers have been applied to observations of mothers and children with Down syndrome (see Chapter 9). Looking at the interactions of both partners in the discourse has shown that parent input affects child response and that, similarly, child behaviors affect parent input. Acknowledgment of the role of the parent in communication development has begun to change the way that intervention is designed (Cheseldine & McConkey, 1979; MacDonald, 1982; Seitz, 1975).

Now, however, it may be important to take a more critical look at how the mother-child studies are being translated into intervention. Rondal (1977) cited several studies (Buium, Rynders, & Turnure, 1974; Kogan, Wimberger, & Bobbitt, 1969; Marshall, Hegrenes, & Goldstein, 1973) in which the authors referred more or less implicitly to the familial linguistic environment of delayed children as deficit. Rondal's research, however, provided support for the similarity of maternal language when the children are matched for mean length of utterance (MLU) and not chronological age. Other studies, while confirming the basic similarity of maternal input, have shown differences (e.g., use of directives) that have been targeted for intervention by other practitioners (Eheart, 1982; Lombardino, 1978; MacDonald & Gillette, 1982). Intervention, however, may still operate from the deficit linguistic environment assumption. If a mother of a child with Down syndrome uses a strategy that is different from that of a mother of a normally developing child, does it necessarily mean that the different strategy is inappropriate?

Can global statements about parents of children with Down syndrome be made? Almost every study involving mothers and children with Down syndrome mentions the variability in both the children and in their mothers' strategies. For example, Alex, 20 months, has Down syndrome, and is just beginning to play with toys meaningfully. He does not explore much and does not occupy himself for long. Most annoying to his mother is his behavior of whining when he is bored. His mother intercedes, gets him toys, tells him to play with specific toys, and explains simply what to do with each toy. Observers count a higher percentage of directives than are typical with a mother having a normal child at Alex's developmental level.

If one looks only at the general research that has been done, one should teach the mother not to use as many directives with Alex. However, it is important to explore what happens in that individual situation.

1. Perhaps the mother's words gave the child just enough cues to manipulate the toys successfully. Then Alex will seek out these toys on his own. Perhaps he needs permission or a reminder that his mother is paying attention to him when he plays well. If the mother intervened with physical manipulation of the toys, the child might have let her take over. Under the above conditions, the mother's behavior would have been appropriate and adaptive to her specific child who is somewhat passive to the world about him.

2. Perhaps Alex reacts to his mother's directiveness by retreating farther away from her and hanging his head down. If continued, the withdrawing behavior will not facilitate Alex's learning, and his mother may feel somewhat rejected. Intervention can then be aimed toward making the interaction successful for both mother and child. Perhaps Alex would respond more if his mother modeled once how the toy worked, and then handed the toy to him. Perhaps the mother could play with the toy by herself or with another child so that Alex could observe until he shows interest. Intervention should be based on the parents' strengths, and they should not be made to feel guilty for the lags in their child's development.

3. Perhaps intervention should not be aimed at the mother or the child.

Perhaps the environment needs to be changed. The toys might not be placed at eye level or on a surface that is easy to play on (e.g., toy car on carpet). The toys themselves may be too simple or too complex for the child's developmental level. Alex could easily be bored with the toys because they are too familiar. Simple intervention with the situation may produce a much more alert child.

Intervention must, of course, stem from research findings. However, each situation must be treated individually, using a variety of alternatives. Both members of the dyad must be considered, along with the immediate environment, for communication intervention to be effective and efficient.

REFERENCES

Balkany, T., Downs, M. P., Jafek, B. W., & Krajicek, M. J. (1979). Hearing loss in Down's syndrome. *Clinical Pediatrics, 18* (2), 116–118.

Bleile, K. (1982). Consonant ordering in Down's syndrome phonology. *Journal of Communication Disorders, 15*, 275–285.

Bodine, A. (1974). A phonological analysis of the speech of two mongoloid (Down's syndrome) boys. *Anthropological Linguist, 16* (1), 1–24.

Buium, N., Rynders, J., & Turnure, J. (1974). Early maternal linguistic environment of normal and Down's syndrome language-learning children. *American Journal of Mental Deficiency, 79*, 52–58.

Chelseldine, S., & McConkey, R. (1979). Parental speech to young Down's syndrome children: An interview study. *American Journal of Mental Deficiency, 83*, 612–620.

Dodd, B. (1976). A comparison of the phonological systems of mental age matched normal, severely subnormal, and Down's syndrome children. *British Journal of Disorders of Communication, 11*, 27–42.

Eheart, B. K. (1982). Mother-child interactions with nonretarded and mentally retarded preschoolers. *American Journal of Mental Deficiency, 87*, 20–25.

Iglesias, A. (1978). *Assessment of phonological disabilities.* Unpublished manuscript, Temple University, Philadelphia.

Iglesias, A., & Horstmeier, D. (1978, May). *Speech intelligibility training.* Paper presented at the Down Syndrome Interest Group of the American Association of Mental Deficiency Convention, Miami.

Ingram, D. (1976). *Phonological disability in children.* New York: Elsevier.

Kogan, K., Wimberger, H., & Bobbitt, R. (1969). Analysis of mother-child interactions in young mental retardates. *Child Development, 40*, 799–812.

Lombardino, L. (1978). *Mothers' speech acts during play interaction with non-delayed and Down's syndrome children: A taxonomy and distribution.* Unpublished doctoral dissertation, Ohio State University, Columbus.

MacDonald, J. D. (1985). Language through conversation: A communicative model for language intervention. In S. Warren & A.K. Rogers-Warren (Eds.), *Teaching functional language* (pp. 89–122). Austin, TX: PRO-ED.

MacDonald, J. D., & Gillette, Y. (1982). *A conversational approach to language delay: Problems and solutions.* Columbus: Ohio State University.

Marshall, N., Hegrenes, J. R., & Goldstein, S. (1973). Verbal interactions: Mothers and their retarded children versus mothers and their nonretarded children. *American Journal of Mental Deficiency, 77* (4), 415–419.

Moran, M. J., Money, S. M., & Leonard, D. A. (1984). Phonological process analysis of the speech of mentally retarded adults. *American Journal of Mental Deficiency, 89,* 304–306.

Rondal, J. A. (1977). Maternal speech to normal and Down's syndrome children matched for mean length of utterance. In P. Mittler (Ed.), *Research to practice in mental retardation: Education and training* (Vol. 2, pp. 239–243). Baltimore: University Park Press.

Schlanger, B., & Gottsleben, R. H. (1957). Analysis of speech defects among the institutionalized mentally retarded. *Journal of Speech and Hearing Disorders, 22,* 98–103.

Seitz, S. (1975). Language intervention—Changing the language environment of the retarded child. In R. Koch and F. de la Cruz (Eds.), *Down's syndrome (Mongolism): Research, prevention and management* (pp. 157–170). New York: Brunner/Mazel.

Shreiberg, L., & Kwialkowski, J. (1980). *National process analysis: A procedure for phonological analysis of continuous speech samples.* New York: John Wiley & Sons.

Silverstein, A. B., Ageno, D., Alleman, A. C., Derecho, K. T., & Gray, S. B. (1985). Adaptive behavior of institutionalized individuals with Down syndrome. *American Journal of Mental Deficiency, 89* (5), 555–558.

Stoel-Gammon, C. (1980). Phonological analysis of four Down's syndrome children. *Applied Psycholinguistics, 1,* 31–48.

Weiner, F. (1979). *Phonological process analysis.* Baltimore: University Park Press.

SECTION III

PSYCHOSOCIAL ASPECTS

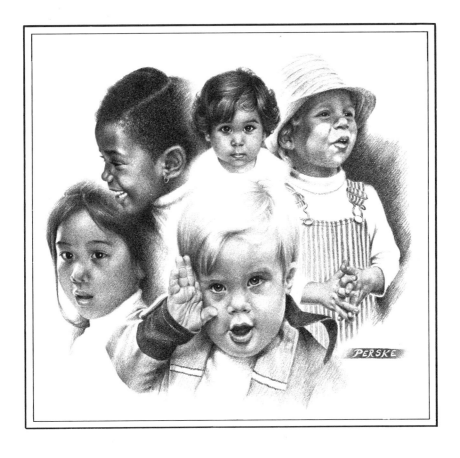

Introduction

Carol Tingey

✦✦✦

It is possible to look at the condition of Down syndrome from a variety of perspectives. Some perspectives contain a body of previously gathered information that can be adjusted and applied to the understanding of Down syndrome. For example, medicine and education are fields of study with facts, concepts, and findings gathered from ongoing professional experiences that can assist in the understanding of the general and specific concerns clustered around the condition of Down syndrome. It is possible to identify and describe how medical and educational practices need to be adjusted in order for service delivery systems to meet the physical and educational needs of individuals with Down syndrome. This identification and adaptation may not be possible in relation to psychosocial aspects. The psychological situation and the social situation are unique for each individual in that they relate to daily, informal, personal interactions rather than the organized delivery of services from a profession. Each individual has his or her own perceptions, and mental and behavioral characteristics. Each person has his or her own rank and status among the people with whom he or she interacts, and each person develops his or her own companions and interdependent relationships. Although there are times when people of the same family are similar, even children raised in similar situations respond to persons with Down syndrome with individual response patterns.

Each of us, as we grow and mature, is influenced by the services that we are provided through the medical and educational professions. We are, however, more intimately molded by our own individual psychological processes and those people with whom we live and those who regularly interact with us. Each of us is aware of things that we can do well, things that are difficult to do, and things that we see as almost impossible for us to do. Although one might remember a favorite physician and a favorite teacher, it is inconceivable to postulate that those individuals influenced our lives as much as our parents, grandparents, siblings, and even our neighbors.

There is, therefore, no single model or statistical analysis of psychosocial life for the general population that can be adapted to describe situations that are generally the same or different for individuals with Down syndrome. For this book, it was decided that psychosocial needs would be described by: 1) attitudes, acceptance, and awareness (How do people respond to the condition of Down syndrome?); 2) family considerations (What is the impact on the family?); and 3) socialization and maturation (What is the growth pattern of the individual with Down syndrome?).

Chapter 10

Attitudes, Acceptance, and Awareness
The Changing View
Toward Persons with Down Syndrome

Robert Perske

✛✛✛

Not long ago, the author's family nagged him for ignoring stop signs when he drove the car. Later, they warned him of approaching stop signs, and once or twice, with soft voices, they suggested a visit to the optometrist. Patriarchal power and pride was used to resist them—until the state driver's license examiner told him to get glasses or stop driving.

Of course, the ultimatum upset the author, until he put on his new prescription lenses. Then he saw stop signs three blocks away. The author peered into what used to be a distant blur and saw people—male and female people—and saw leaves on trees and flower petals and blades of grass in such vivid color and detail that his world view became happier and safer. Of course, it does not take an Einstein to know that the rest of the world was happier and safer, too.

Not long ago, most citizens thought that persons with Down syndrome should be out of sight and out of mind, away from the mainstream of society. Then came organizations like the Association for Retarded Citizens of the United States (ARC-US) and the National Down Syndrome Congress (NDSC), who began fashioning corrective lenses that help everyone see persons with Down syndrome more clearly than ever before. The following is a journalistic attempt to trace the progress of this effort toward attitudinal change.

A NEW VIEW IN THE MAKING

Consider some "headlines" taken from newsclips and the author's interview notes. (The real names of the persons in the stories have replaced the nouns and pronouns that usually appear in actual headlines.)

NATIONAL POSTER FEATURES MATT STARR BAR MITZVAH (National Organization on Disability, 1984)

JASON KINGSLEY STARS IN *FALL GUY* (UPI, 1984)

JOE CONNORS SERVES AS CONGRESSIONAL PAGE (Chafee, 1985)

RON SCHULTZ DROWNS TRYING TO SAVE FRIEND (Perske, 1980)

QUINCY EPISODE FEATURES DAVID MACFARLANE (National Broadcasting Corporation, 1982)

DAVID DAWSON CO-AUTHORS BOOK (Edwards & Dawson, 1983)

BLOOD BANK APPROVES JOE MAYER AS DONOR (Steward, 1979)

KEVIN LEE WRESTLES FOR GLENBARD HIGH (Perske, personal observation, 1982)

ROBERT MISSING DIES PULLING BROTHER FROM BURNING HOUSE (Perske, 1981, p. 49)

PAUL WILKE DRUMMER FOR WARREN HIGH (Association for Retarded Citizens—Minnesota, 1984)

DARSI HILTY GETS REGULAR DIPLOMA AT COLUMBIA HIGH (O'Callahan, 1982)

TINA DIRKSEN PLAYS "ANNIE" AT NEWTON SOUTH HIGH (Association for Retarded Citizens—Massachusetts, 1982)

TIM FREDERICKS MAKES LITTLE LEAGUE (Fredericks & Fredericks, 1980)

TOM HOULIHAN LONG-DISTANCE CALLS OLD FRIENDS AT CHRISTMAS (Perske, personal observation, 1984)

AL QUACKENBOSS EQUIPMENT MANAGER MILAN HIGH WRESTLING TEAM (Perske, 1985a)

MITCHELL LEVITZ CREATES OWN MIRACLE AT BAR MITZVAH (Walden, 1984)

BENGT OLSON OPERATES STAMPING PRESS FOR VOLVO (Perske, personal observation, 1969)

Like most headlines, these focus on celebrities and heroes in the movement, and fail to feature rank-and-file people who live in ordinary houses on ordinary streets and attend classes or work in the community. They fail to mention those persons with serious impairment who also have achieved higher rungs on their own developmental ladders, achievements that may be just as dramatic to them, their families, and friends. And, sadly, they fail to highlight heroic families who keep struggling to care for and train their children, even though their children suffer from degenerative conditions.

Even so, the headlines give a hint that a new view, a clearer, richer view, of persons with Down syndrome is now possible. Such stories would not have been considered authentic in 1968.

A SAMPLING OF AN OLDER VIEW

In April, 1968, *The Atlantic Monthly* published "The Right to Die," an article by *New York Post* journalist Bernard Bard and Joseph Fletcher, a professor at Episcopal Theological School in Cambridge, Massachusetts. Bard, upon learning that his newborn son, Philip, had Down syndrome, sent the child to a "sanitarium" in Westchester County to die, which the infant did on the eighth day of his life. Bard's article provided a step-by-step account of the birth and death of his son:

1. Bard stated that he himself had not seen anything wrong or repulsive about Philip, but that Dr. F., the physician, had provided numerous details about people with Down syndrome, all of them negative (p. 59).
2. Dr. F. described the sanitarium that was willing to accept Philip as one that "contains no oxygen, gives no inoculations, does no operations, and administers no 'miracle' drugs" (p. 61).
3. The sanitarium's administrator, Dr. K., was described as a "specialist in mental retardation for thirty years" who had examined every child with Down syndrome in Westchester County. He ran the sanitarium as a "hobby" (p. 61).
4. Dr. K.'s view of parents: "Some parents regularly visit their children here. They waste their lives trying to expunge a feeling of guilt that should not be there, instead of devoting themselves to their normal children" (pp. 61–62).
5. Dr. K. claimed support from the local clergy: "There are churches on all sides of me. Every one of these ministers agrees with me that it would not be moral, or serving God's will to prolong these lives" (p. 61).

On Philip's eighth day, he was placed in the sanitarium. A few hours later, the infant died of "heart failure and jaundice." Fletcher, who later became professor of Medical Ethics at the University of Virginia School of Medicine, supported the actions of Bard, Dr. F., and Dr. K.:

> Bernard Bard is a loving man. He is not a vitalist, which is the label philosophers attach to those who make an idol of life. . . . [He stated that physicians in obstetric situations often refrain from respirating newborn infants with Down syndrome.] Our statute and common law, that is our official morality, is thoroughly idolatrous and vitalistic. . . . People in the Bards' situation have no reason to feel guilty about putting a Down's syndrome baby away, whether it's "put away" in the sense of hidden in a sanitarium or in a more responsible lethal sense. It is sad, yes. Dreadful. But it carries no guilt. True guilt arises only from an offense against a person, and *a Down's is not a person* [italics added]. (Bard & Fletcher, 1968, pp. 62–64)

If this event had happened today, the NDSC, the ARC-US, The Association for Persons with Severe Handicaps (TASH), and other associations for persons with disabilities would have raised loud concerns. But that was 1968, and only a few isolated voices, like Gunnar Dybwad's (1970) spoke out against this clinically perfumed homicide. No organized movement made a formal protest.

And yet, veteran workers and volunteers cannot be too smug about this neglect. For example, the author worked in an institution for people with developmental disabilities at the time *The Atlantic Monthly* article appeared and many of his colleagues were on the fence regarding it. Many felt that John Langdon Down (1866) was correct when he described people with Down syndrome as "reversions to a primitive racial type."

In the author's opinion, professional libraries in 1968 contained bleak textbooks on "mongolism," pages filled with gloomy words, stomach-turning photographs, and a depressing "course of illness," predicting that most would die before age 10. Many professionals saw persons with Down syndrome as "no-program" people; the author recalls how an educator was laughed off an institution's grounds for trying to convince staff members that these persons could learn to read and write.

But that was 1968, and the views of that day differ from what many people now believe about persons with Down syndrome. This leads one to believe that a perceptual revolution has begun.

ISSUES INVOLVED IN PERCEPTUAL REVOLUTIONS

Changes in attitude happen slowly. It is much more comfortable to continue seeing familiar things. In a psychological experiment that deserves to be far better known outside the field, Jerome Bruner and Leo Postman (1949) placed average citizens before an apparatus that flashed playing cards before their eyes. The people were merely asked to identify the cards. Then, strange cards were introduced in the exposures (e.g., a red six of spades or a black four of hearts). Thomas Kuhn, in *The Structure of Scientific Revolutions* (1970, pp. 62–63) described the results:

1. People had a terrible time recognizing unfamiliar cards.
2. People usually failed to recognize unfamiliar cards even when the cards were exposed 4 times longer than the recognizable exposure rate of regular cards.
3. Even though people were told that the unfamiliar cards were in the sequence, they still became confused and uncomfortable. One person's recorded response: "I can't make the suit out, whatever it is. . . . I don't know what color it is now or whether it's a spade or a heart. . . . I'm not even sure now what a spade looks like. . . . My God!"

Kuhn used this and other experiments to show how even brilliant scientists have resisted new views that challenge old ones. He described in elaborate detail the agony people went through before they accepted the fact that the world is round, not flat; that the earth is not the center of the universe; that electricity is not a liquid; that X rays are real. His findings:

1. Perceptual revolutions take place after massive numbers of anomalous happenings and facts are discovered that cannot be explained by an old paradigm.
2. The anomalies are often discovered by accident. They are upsetting and painful, and they loosen stereotypes. Once they start appearing, they often keep multiplying until they force the discovery of a new paradigm.
3. New paradigms usually come through the work of two classes of people: the very young and people coming into a field fresh from another. (The point may be stretched, showing that veterans in the field can help with breakthroughs by staying close to the "youngsters" and the "transfers.")
4. As a new paradigm emerges, the textbooks on the issues must be rewritten.

Kuhn's ideas about perceptual revolutions may provide some basic principles for changing attitudes toward people with Down syndrome. (See Figure 1 for a visual representation of the model.)

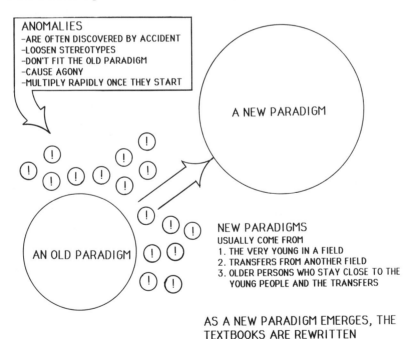

Figure 1. A visual representation of Kuhn's (1970) model.

KEY EVENTS IN THE PERCEPTUAL REVOLUTION
TOWARD PERSONS WITH DOWN SYNDROME

Although there are many other anomalous events, the following were key to the perceptual revolution toward persons with Down syndrome.

Parents organized Around 1950, mothers and fathers of persons with disabilities, confused by professional advice of the day that clashed with the dictates of their hearts, and feeling extremely alone with the problem, began searching for other families in the same situation. Some even advertised in newspapers. When they got together, they shared in one another's suffering for a time. Then, drawing strength from their togetherness, they rolled up their sleeves and developed the first community services. At first, professionals, observing these homespun little organizations in action, shook their heads in dismay. The author recalls how the clinical wisdom of that day tagged parents as traumatized, agitated, and helpless when it came to doing anything creative for their own child, and many professionals predicted that these parents' actions could only make things worse.

Local parent groups began to charter national organizations Lobbying and public attitude change efforts were initiated around 1953. Outstanding national organization newspapers described new perceptions and attracted new members to the organization. Many professionals joined the National Association for Retarded Children (now the ARC-US) for the remarkably informative *Children Limited,* a newspaper edited by veteran newspaperman Eric Sandahl. Now, many professionals join the NDSC to receive *Down Syndrome News.*

Jerome Lejeune and the 47th Chromosome In 1959, Lejeune discovered the 47th chromosome. By 1968, researchers in some institutions began recording systematic arrays of chromosomes in single cells (karyotypes) from residents with Down syndrome. At the time, it didn't seem like a very big deal to most professionals. But those attending the annual meeting of the NDSC in San Antonio in 1984, could not help but notice how parents surrounded keynote speaker Lejeune, thanked him, shook his hand, and hugged him.

The President's Panel In 1961, President Kennedy called for a national plan regarding mental retardation. His stirring message of October 11, coupled with his appointment of the President's Panel on Mental Retardation, led to the drafting of ''A National Action to Combat Mental Retardation'' in 1962 (PCMR, 1977).

Nigel Hunt In 1967, *The World of Nigel Hunt* was published. Although many leaders in the field saw persons with Down syndrome as being unable to read or write, this young man with Down syndrome nevertheless wrote a pithy, humorous story about high points in his life.

Who Shall Survive A film about infant death, entitled *Who Shall*

Survive, was shown in 1971, in the Eisenhower Theatre in the John F. Kennedy Center for the Performing Arts, in Washington, D.C. It was the first time the theatre was used. Sargent Shriver, representing the Kennedy Foundation, paused during his opening remarks while technicians pulled a small cannon onto the stage. They exploded a blank charge while other technicians, stationed throughout the theatre, took acoustical readings, since that was the first time that the new theatre had been filled with people (Menolascino & Perske, 1972).

The leaders in mental retardation from all over the world experienced a second cannon shot. They watched a 25-minute documentary showing how a newborn infant with Down syndrome and an intestinal blockage had been moved to a corner in the nursery of Johns Hopkins University Hospital, and was starved to death. Using the actual doctors and medical personnel involved, but with actors playing the real-life parents, the film traced the grisly, 15-day, step-by-step developments from birth until death. Unlike the 1968 Westchester County incident, a furor was raised. But even then, the reactions were not as intense as those surrounding later infant starvations.

Right to Education   In 1972, a Pennsylvania right to education case ruled that every child has the right to appropriate education. A panel of three judges made the decree in the case between the Pennsylvania ARC and the Commonwealth of Pennsylvania. One more precedent was set that slowly began to revise an older view toward all people with developmental disabilities (Perske & Smith, 1977).

National Down Syndrome Congress   In 1973, the NDSC was formed. This organization developed a sharper, more intense focus on issues surrounding the situation of Down syndrome. The organization further refined the advocacy begun by the National Association for Retarded Children in the 50s and 60s.

PL 94-142   In 1975, the Education for All Handicapped Children Act (PL 94-142) called for a "full service" public school education. This mandate may have increased the interaction between special and regular education, and it set the stage for face-to-face activities between students with disabilities and regular students.

Child's Rights versus Parent's Rights   When Phillip Becker's parents fought successfully in a California court, in 1980, to block lifesaving surgery for their 13-year-old son, dooming him to a slow and painful premature death, the rights of the child against the parents became an issue. And even though the Supreme Court refused to hear an appeal, letting the law stand, legal pressures continued until Phillip was awarded to the custody of foster parents. Recent reports have shown a young man, once destined to die, living a healthy, happy life. His current development has outstripped the earlier expectations of physicians who testified on behalf of his natural parents (Melberg, 1984).

Baby Doe   At first, it appeared to be just another quiet refusal to repair an easily corrected obstruction in the esophagus of a newborn infant with Down syndrome. It took place in 1982, in Bloomington, Indiana, with the Indiana Supreme Court saying that a starvation death was legal. But this time, people *moved*. Volunteer organizations began drafting petitions for the U.S. Supreme Court, and people willing to adopt the infant rushed to the scene. Unfortunately, the infant died before any further legal actions could be taken.

Even after the infant's death, the interest continued. Letter-writing campaigns and newspaper editorials abounded, and even President Reagan made what some view as one of his quickest, strongest, unilateral moves yet, when he threatened to withdraw federal funds from any hospital that ever did anything like that again. Baby Doe's death became something that was far from quiet.

SENSING THE DEPTH OF THE PERCEPTUAL REVOLUTION

How far has the movement come since *The Atlantic Monthly* article in 1968? Consider the following facts.

Within the movement's organizations and networks, the dignity, value, and rights of persons with Down syndrome have soared. A few workers and volunteers still hold to an older view, but they are usually removed from current hands-on technology and advocacy efforts.

With ordinary citizens, the perceptual revolution may not have come as far as those in the field think. Everyone does not understand yet. However, enough new information has been introduced to make the average citizen take a second look.

Many physicians have become kinder and more understanding toward persons with Down syndrome. But the "Dr. K.s" are still present in the world, ever ready to give bleak prognoses about persons with an extra chromosome. One can see a hopeful trend in the number of physicians who have become active members of organizations such as the ARC-US and the NDSC. But physicians who refuse to accept a higher valuing of these persons remain, in the author's view, the movement's largest problem. Without sympathetic, understanding physicians, the going, especially for "new" families, will always be tough.

Judging from the recent spate of news articles about persons with Down syndrome, many reporters have become healthy catalysts for this perceptual revolution. Some have become so caught up with what they observed in a family, a group home, a classroom, or a workshop, that they took copious notes and wrote long, spirited success stories. The only problem is that editors often cut the stories from, for instance, 50 column inches to 11, or they choose not to print them. (Editors know that successes do not sell newspapers as well as troubles do.) Even so, editors can be counted on to run hundreds of stories they would not have touched in 1968.

CURRENT EFFORTS THAT CAN HELP

Although it may not have been the primary goal, almost every effort on behalf of persons with Down syndrome also helps change public attitudes—legislative efforts, parent activities, technical breakthroughs, supported employment programs, generic recreation programs, and many others. Since 1968, ordinary citizens have observed the enthusiastic actions of many parents, professionals, and volunteers in community settings and many in the community now show an increased kindness and respect toward persons with Down syndrome. Even the gracious little things, like the way courageous parents take their children to public activities and send holiday greeting cards with pictures of their children with Down syndrome, have helped to make it more "in," more right, and somehow more godly to relate to people with disabilities than ever before.

Good Working Relations with the Media   Some organizations, even formal networks, now nurture individualized relationships with reporters who produce helpful pieces on behalf of persons with disabilities. Some organizations have been uncanny about making a reporter feel as if he or she had won a Pulitzer Prize for a story that helped the cause.

Leadership and Candor of Public Figures   Writer Emily Kingsley helps work people with disabilities into *Sesame Street. Quincy* and *Fall Guy* used actors with Down syndrome through the influence of writer-producer Lou Shaw. Syndicated columnist George Will produces penetrating commentaries when crucial situations like the Baby Doe and Phillip Becker cases hit the national press. The U.S. Office of Special Education and Rehabilitative Services moves forward as a no-nonsense, leading-edge organization under the leadership of Madeleine Will. Senator Lowell Weicker fights vigorously for legislation on behalf of persons with disabilities. Senator Hubert Humphrey openly discussed his grandchild with Down syndrome. Well-known people now seem more comfortable disclosing facts about their parentage of children with Down syndrome than they did at the time Dale Evans (1953) wrote about her daughter. And this situation doesn't apply only to Down syndrome. The disclosure by President John F. Kennedy of his sister's mental retardation helped change public attitude.

Creative Contact with Physicians   The problem with physicians looms so large that massive campaigns will need to be planned on many levels at the same time. Even so, one should never underestimate the power some parents have had in converting their own family physicians to more positive attitudes toward persons with Down syndrome. Of course, some parents failed and had to change doctors. But even so, something may have been gained in the trying. NDSC might consider a parent-training seminar in which successful parents describe the steps they took to change the attitudes of their physicians. Physicians can now earn continuing education credit for participation in conferences about Down syndrome (e.g., the first annual conference on research and practice in Down syndrome, NDSC & Utah State University, June, 1985).

Community and Family Living Amendments   The movement began as Senate Bill 2053 in 1984. In 1985, it became S.B. 873, with 9 co-sponsors; House Bill 2902 emerged as a companion bill—with 77 co-sponsors. If it fails, advocates will see that it reappears in another form until a federal law is voted that supports persons with disabilities in the community, and their families as well. When that happens, attitudes of the average citizen will be affected, just like they were when the Education for All Handicapped Children Act (Public Law 94-142) became a law.

State Zoning Laws   Few people would want to live next door to a fraternity house, a large rooming house, or a larger-than-family-size home for persons with disabilities, not even if it was a federally approved intermediate care facility. No matter how much they liked the people, their larger number could overwhelm neighbors and keep them at a distance. That is why many state zoning laws mandate that small group homes with six or less persons with disabilities be treated as single-family dwellings; in doing so, they have set the stage for healthy neighborhood relations.

Adoption Networks   Janet Marchese, the wife of a New York City policeman, who has been featured on network news programs and in magazine articles (see the May, 1983 issue of *McCalls*), runs a volunteer adoption program from the kitchen table of her White Plains home. She has successfully placed for adoption over 600 newborn infants with Down syndrome. The NDSC also maintains a list of people waiting to adopt infants with Down syndrome. Activities like this cannot help but influence many average citizens.

Children's Peer-Group Education   More and more students with disabilities are attending special education classes in their own neighborhood public schools. As that happens, more regular students will rub elbows with them in tutorial, advocacy, and guided-friendship programs being developed by forward-thinking educators. Brown (1979) pointed out that the future doctors, police officers, teachers, ministers—even the future parents of children with Down syndrome—are in the schools now. And the earlier people can understand and feel relaxed with persons with disabilities, the better. Someday, it may be proven that much of the jeering and derision that used to be hurled at children with disabilities really stemmed from a lack of involvement with such children at an early age.

Natural Reinforcement Programs for Good Neighborly Acts
Eight years ago, Gunnar Dybwad stated that more neighbors are for persons with disabilities than against them. These words were taken to heart during a series of national assignments conducted by the author. Over time, 158 neighbors were interviewed who lived near 87 well-run family-scale residences, each housing six or less persons with disabilities. The findings can hardly be considered scientific since a journalist's senses were used, rating each interview tape in one of three ways: friendly, indifferent, and hostile. Twenty-nine per cent were warmly involved with their neighbors with disabilities, 62% were indifferent, and only 9% were hostile (Perske, 1980, 1985b). Admittedly, most of these neighbors lived close to homes that leaders in the field claimed to be the best in their state. But the number of interviews with good neighbors moved the author to produce a novel, *Show Me No Mercy* (Perske, 1984), in an attempt to dramatize how valuable good neighbors could be to the Banks family and to Ben, their 16-year-old with Down syndrome.

This leads one to wonder if perhaps so much time and energy have gone to dealing with the loud neighborhood opposition, that the quieter, more caring neighbors have received little recognition and reinforcement. For example, staff writer Joseph Grace, in the March 19, 1985 issue of the *Bucks County Courier-Times,* reported that of 55 group homes in Bucks County, Pennsylvania, only 4 received neighborhood opposition (unfortunately, they received most of the press coverage, too).

Since educators are now quick to believe that unreinforced good behavior in students can fade, could that apply to neighbors, too? The day has come when new-breed professionals and volunteers will develop schemes for catching neighbors in the act of doing good to people with disabilities, then reinforcing them so naturally that the good neighbors will feel valued and their gracious acts will continue (Perske, 1985b).

Persons with Disabilities in Advertising "I am writing to you . . . about a matter of conscience . . . but, even more to the point, a matter of just plain good business sense" wrote Emily Kingsley of Chappaqua, New York, in one of her mailings to the nation's top advertisers (personal communication, 1985). "In America, where advertising has always been so responsive to demographic needs and to the pressures of various minority groups, it is surprising to me that the advertising industry continues to ignore the group which is acknowledged to be 'The *Largest* Minority'—that of the physically and mentally handicapped." Kingsley set the figure at 37 million, then added the spouses, the children, the extended families, and the concerned friends, to help corporate heads see a glaring chasm in their advertisement campaigns.

She cited another survey she carried out with parents of persons with disabilities: *"Every single letter tells me that people would buy the product whether they needed it or not.''* Her plea was so detailed and convincing, that executives have discussed the situation with her over the telephone. As efforts like these take place, the day will come when persons with Down syndrome will be seen doing ordinary things in the media, like appearing with other individuals in a Coca Cola ad, or sitting with other passengers in an Eastern Airlines Whisper jet.

Neighborhood Support Plans The Children's Clinic and Preschool, in Seattle, Washington, developed a 6-month project in which 16 families were given a budget of $200 per month, to be used for payments to relatives, friends, and neighbors for support services they rendered. With this money, the families managed to recruit 84 persons who helped with in-home training, respite care, babysitting, transportation, mending clothes, and the building of special equipment (Moore, Hamerlynck, Barsh, Spieker, & Jones, 1982). Six months later, when the payments ceased, 64% of the helpers continued their duties as volunteers. Although the program was designed to purchase added family support, the attitude change of some outsiders came as a happy surprise.

Efficient Media Monitoring Media persons now learn the hard way that demeaning statements about persons with disabilities can unleash a deluge of protests on an editor's or program director's desk. Those who organize on behalf of persons with disabilities are becoming keener and quicker about such monitoring. An article in the April 3, 1985 issue of *USA Today* serves as an example. In a featured interview, Jeff Lyon, the author of *Playing God in the Nursery,* approved of the death of Baby Doe in Bloomington, Indiana. He did not approve of the starvation method, but he upheld the parents' belief that the child was better off dead. His facts were pessimistic and he turned a blind side to the whole movement on behalf of persons with disabilities.

Before the sun had set, calls and telegrams reached the news room in Arlington, Virginia. NDSC, ARC-US, TASH, The Center on Human Policy, and others put organized protest efforts into motion and demanded a chance to present the other side of the story. Two days later, the editors had promised at least one such feature. One editor stated unofficially that no other article had evoked so many letters, telegrams, and telephone calls. A one-half page article by NDSC's executive director, Diane Crutcher, appeared in the April 25, 1985 issue of *USA Today.*

Parallel Attitude Change Campaigns In the case of the aforementioned *USA Today* issue, many organizations moved on the editorial offices, each in their own way. Power would have been lost if all efforts had been centralized into a single push. And yet, when ships in a convoy move in different directions, there can be disastrous effects. Not so in this case. Valuable interchanges of information took place between organizations, showing that the more public attitude change efforts there are, moving in the same direction, using their own resources and channels, the better it will be.

Fresh Perspectives from Self-Advocates In 1983, six Californians with developmental disabilities, one with Down syndrome, traveled throughout the state gathering the views of other persons with developmental disabilities on the services they received. With one advisor, a recorder/editor, and financing by the State Developmental Disabilities Council, they traveled 1,500 miles in California, talked to 150 people with disabilities, and recorded 70 hours of audio tapes. By oral training, not reading, they became expert on the Lanterman Developmental Disabilities Service Act, California's bill of rights and service delivery law. Anyone reading their report, *Surviving the System: Mental Retardation and the Retarding Environment (People First of California, 1984)*, will sense a fresh viewpoint emerging. Some points raised:

"The Lanterman Act pushes for development . . . but the system pushes back" (p. 9).

Some persons with disabilities talked about being treated as if they were only commodities, only things worth money to others (p. 8).

Questions were raised about being a Boy Scout at age 35 (pp. 14, 31).

Some persons with disabilities discussed how case managers told them they weren't ready to leave a residence when they knew they were being held back because of the money they brought into the service system (p. 56).

Some spoke about how they hated going bowling and to movies in large groups (p. 14).

Some felt successful services are rare because success is not rewarded (p. 58).

The task force members felt that every service provider should have a course in the Lanterman Act (p. 33).

Some talked about workshops that made them more retarded (p. 32).

Some hoped they would never have to work on another wind chime (p. 66).

Some made it plain that they should be seen as "primary consumers" (p. 7).

Others did indeed see themselves as "system survivors in retarding environments," as the title on the report implied (p. 7).

The report, with its pithy and candid statements, has, according to the California Council on Developmental Disabilities, become one of the most widely read documents they have produced. It has been in demand throughout the nation and has undergone multiple reprinting.

Now that self-advocates are being heard, they will be introducing perspectives that would have been totally ignored in 1968. For example: New Jersey, New York, Pennsylvania, and Connecticut held a combined self-advocate and professional retreat (InterServ, 1986) in which persons with disabilities were paired with high-ranking officials and professionals. They lived together (two people in each room) and attended sessions together. InterServ intended to show how face-to-face relationships can foster healthy attitude changes, more efficiently than mere didactic sessions could ever do.

A Concern for All Persons with Disabilities To deal only with public attitude change toward persons with Down syndrome tends to be awkward. For example, in the aforementioned *USA Today* article, Jeff Lyon (1985) opened his article by singling out persons with Down syndrome in alluding to persons with all kinds of disabilities. The public can be expected to generalize like this, too. Therefore, when it comes to changing attitudes, there is a strong need for groups advocating for persons with specific disabilities to pull for one another.

SUMMARY

The events highlighted in this chapter hint that there is a difference between the way persons with Down syndrome were viewed in 1968 and the way they are seen today. There has been an explosion of happenings leading to improved attitudes, acceptance, and awareness. A perceptual revolution has been taking place, but it is far from finished. Some individuals still cling to an older view based on misunderstanding, confusion, fear, and false assumptions about persons with Down syndrome. And such persons who fight to exclude individuals with disabilities from their circle of acceptance can cause disastrous setbacks.

And yet, the time may be right to apply Thomas Kuhn's ultimate question, testing whether this perceptual revolution is successful: Has this movement progressed to the point where *the textbooks are being rewritten?* The author of this chapter believes it has.

REFERENCES

Association for Retarded Citizens—Massachusetts. (1982, May). Tina Dirksen plays "Annie" at Newton South High School. *The ARC of Tomorrow* (annual convention program).
Association for Retarded Citizens—Minnesota. (1984, Summer). Paul Wilke drummer for Warren High. *Focus*.
Bard, B., & Fletcher, J. (1968). The right to die. *The Atlantic Monthly, 3,* 59–64.
Brown, L. (1979). Education for living. In R. Perske (Ed.), *The child with retardation today—The adult of tomorrow* (pp. 16–18). Arlington, TX: Association for Retarded Citizens of the United States.
Bruner, J., & Postman, L. (1945). On the perception of incongruity: A paradigm. *Journal of Personality, 17,* 206–223.
Chafee, J. (1985, June). *Joe Connors serves as page in Congress* [a press release]. Washington: Senate Office Building.
Crutcher, D. (1985, April 25). [Inquiry]. *USA Today*.
Down, J. (1866). Observations on an ethnic classification of idiots. *Report on Observations: London Hospital, 3,* 259–262.
Dybwad, G. (1970). Treatment of the mentally retarded—A cross-national view. In H. C. Haywood (Ed.), *Social-cultural aspects of mental retardation*. New York: Appleton-Century-Crofts.

Edwards, J., & Dawson, D. (1983). *My friend David*. Portland, OR: Ednick Communications.

Evans, D. (1953). *Angel unaware*. Los Angeles: Fleming H. Revell.

Fredericks, H. D., & Fredericks, D. (1980, June). Batter up: Baseball for children with disabilities. *Exceptional Parent*, p. 29.

Hunt, N. (1967). *The world of Nigel Hunt*. New York: Garrett Publications.

InterServ. (1986). *How we lived and grew together*. New York: Author.

Kuhn, T. (1970). *The structure of scientific revolutions* (2nd ed.). Chicago: University of Chicago Press.

Lyon, J. (1985, April 3). *USA Today*.

Lyon, J. (1985). *Playing God in the nursery*. New York: Norton.

Melberg, K. (1984, February). Whatever happened to Phillip Becker? *Dialect*.

Menolascino, F., & Perske, R. (1972, March). Afterthoughts on "Who Shall Survive." *Mental Retardation News*.

Moore, J., Hamerlynck, L., Barsh, E., Spieker, S., & Jones, R. (1982). *Extending family resources: Project of national significance*. Washington, DC: Administration on Developmental Disabilities.

National Broadcasting Corporation. (1982, February). *"Quincy" episode features David MacFarlane*. New York: Author.

National Organization on Disability. (1984, September). [The press release on Matt Starr]. Washington: Author.

O'Callahan, P. (1982, June 3). Darsi Hilty gets regular diploma at Columbia High. *Tri-City Herald* (Pasco, WA).

Pennsylvania Association for Retarded Citizens v. Commonwealth of Pennsylvania, Civil Action No. 71-42 (1971).

People First of California. (1984). *Surviving in the system: Mental retardation and the retarding environment*. Sacramento: State Council on Developmental Disabilities.

Perske, R. (1980). *New life in the neighborhood*. Nashville: Abingdon Press.

Perske, R. (1981). *Hope for the families*. Nashville: Abingdon Press.

Perske, R. (1984). *Show me no mercy*. Nashville: Abingdon Press.

Perske, R. (1985a, February). Writing a first novel. *The Writer*, pp. 33–34.

Perske, R. (1985b). A second look at neighbors. *TASH Newsletter, 11*, 2.

Perske, R., & Smith, J. (Eds.). (1977). *Beyond the ordinary: The preparation of professionals to educate severely and profoundly handicapped persons* (p. 3). Seattle: American Association for the Education of the Severely/Profoundly Handicapped.

President's Committee on Mental Retardation. (1977). *Mental Retardation: Past and Present* (pp. 105–106.3). Washington, DC: Author.

Stewart, R. (1979, August 16). Blood bank approves Joe Mayer as donor. *The Providence Journal* (Providence, RI).

UPI. (1984, December 16). Jason Kingsley stars in "Fall Guy." *The Nashville Tennessean*.

Walden, G. (1984, April 14). Mitchell Levitz creates his own miracle. *Westchester County Reporter Dispatch* (White Plains, NY).

Chapter 11

From Parent Involvement To Family Support
Evolution To Revolution

Ann P. Turnbull and Jean Ann Summers

An evolution has occurred in the nature of parent-professional relationships. This evolution or gradual change has moved the field from viewing parents as the cause of their child's problem to viewing them, in their roles as decision-maker and intervenor, as the major solution. However, in the authors' work and in their conversations with families and professionals, they are beginning to see that the forward movement of this evolution has been stalled and that things just are not working out as expected. They think that something a little more radical than gradual evolution is needed at this point: a revolution in thinking about families. To understand how they arrived at this conclusion, this chapter highlights major milestones of the evolution and then suggests how it might be transformed into a revolution.

RETROSPECTIVE VIEWS OF FAMILIES

Historically, the predominant view of parents was as the *cause* of their son or daughter's disability. Whether the problem was viewed as rooted in genetics (Goddard, 1912), in psychological dysfunction (Kanner, 1949), or just bad child-raising methods, parents were the scapegoats (Kirk & Gallagher, 1979). A quote from a professional reference book exemplifies this scapegoating:

> Parents, of course, often have valid cause when they complain, "you only treat the child, but we have to live with him." But while the parental plight is a difficult one, we must remind them that what the child is today is in most cases the result of years of faulty upbringing and the parent's inability to change even their most obvious attitudes toward the child . . . in fact, I have often marvelled at how many children change through treatment in spite of their parents. (Sperling, 1965, p. 303)

One mother shared with the authors a harrowing tale of being blamed by a psychologist for her child's hyperactivity and seizure disorders. Even the fact that she had five other perfectly normal children could not keep her from accepting this burden of blame and going through a long struggle with depression and guilt. Guilt, in fact, is an easy "trip" to lay on parents. Sometimes it is easier to accept blame for the birth of a child with a disability than it is to face the frightening prospect that events in the universe are random and essentially out of control (Gardner, 1971). For these and other reasons, parents today are frequently still willing to accept erroneous accusations and innuendoes from professionals that they are inadequate.

The research focus during the 1950s and 1960s, dominated by the work of Farber and his colleagues (Farber & Ryckman, 1965), was on the impact of the child on the family and the characteristics of families associated with positive adjustment. Family intervention focused primarily on the encouragement of institutionalization and on counseling to help assuage parental (more likely, maternal) anguish (Wolfensberger, 1970).

As the evolution moved forward, the role of the school was one of "rescuing" the child from his or her "bad" environment and his or her "bad" parents. In the 1960s, this perspective slid naturally into the idea that parents had to be involved *because* they had deficits. This is the cultural deprivation model, introduced to the disability field by the Head Start program. Head Start emphasized parent involvement at two levels (Zigler & Valentine, 1979). First, it provided training to improve parenting skills—to sharpen the ability of parents to provide early stimulation to their children. Second, Head Start emphasized parent control of the program. The idea here was that persons with cultural disadvantages have fewer opportunities for decision making and less access to resources. Parent involvement was seen as a way to empower this group, both in sharpening their decision-making skills and in giving them meaningful control of the program.

Running parallel to both the parents-as-scapegoat perspective and the correct-the-deficit perspective, was the view that parents should be service providers. This role was imposed more by a lack of action on the part of schools than by any conscious deliberation. Parents assumed this role when their children were excluded from school. They set up classes in church basements or anywhere they could, and they funded teacher salaries and materials from bake sales or from their own pockets. It was a response out of desperation; but, over time, the schools came to accept parent-provided services as the norm for students with disabilities. A parent was told only about 10 years ago by a director of special education, in response to a request for services for a 6-year-old child with moderate mental retardation, "If you can find six or eight other children whose parents are interested in having them in school, get a grant from the state department, and find a teacher, we can probably provide a room in the administrative building for a class." Just as shocking as it is that a director of special education made the request is the fact that the parents willingly complied. Imagine school personnel telling parents of children who do not have disabilities that they have responsibility for developing fifth grade. Yet, it was something school personnel could and did say to parents of children with disabilities, and something the parents could and did accept as their role.

But along about the beginning of the 1970s, parents began to view the evolution as stuck in a rut. Thus entered the age of parents-as-advocates. During this period, parents were not *offered* empowerment, as in the Head Start program. They *took* it—with a vengeance. Parent advocates spearheaded the series of court battles and other efforts, which culminated in 1975, in PL 94-142, the Education for All Handicapped Children Act. Samuel Kirk (1984), a distinguished special educator over the last 5 decades, characterized the impact of parent advocacy as follows: "If I were to give credit to one group in this country for the advancements that have been made in the education of exceptional children, I would place the parent organizations and parent movement in the forefront as the leading force" (p. 41).

PL 94-142 sets the stage for current values and assumptions regarding parent involvement, at the same time that it preserves the roots of past values and experiences. An analysis of congressional testimony suggested that Congress reasoned that parents were the best protectors of their children's rights and should, therefore, be given every opportunity to take a major decision-making role in the educational process (Turnbull, Turnbull, & Wheat, 1982). Second, those authors attended to the wealth of expert testimony and concluded that parents should be partners in the education process itself, coordinating what was learned at home with what was learned at school. This suggests a redefinition of the school's expectations for parents: that parents with children who experience disabilities should be partners both in decision-making and intervening.

How have these two expectations evolved?

EVOLUTION OF PARENT INVOLVEMENT

Parents as Decision-Makers

Considering the substantial amount of professional time and energy devoted to individualized education program (IEP) development (Price & Goodman, 1980) and the "lip service" given to the importance of the parents' role, it is disconcerting that such a limited amount of research has addressed the nature of parent participation in decision making. The limited number of studies that have been conducted indicate that the majority of parents take a passive role in IEP decision making (Goldstein, Strickland, Turnbull, & Curry, 1980; Lynch

& Stein, 1982; McKinney & Hocutt, 1982). One study, which used an observational methodology to code at 2-minute intervals the speaker and topics being discussed, found that parent contributions accounted for less than 25% of total contributions at IEP conferences (Goldstein et al., 1980). The mean length of the conferences was 36 minutes, and topics coded on the average of less than once per conference included placement, related services, legal rights and responsibilities, individual responsible for implementing goals and objectives, the child's health, future contacts between parents and professionals, and future plans for the child. One can conclude that, in general, parents do not take an active role in deciding what, when, or how their child will be taught.

There are a number of barriers that might explain the discrepancy between society's values and the reality of parent involvement in decision making. These include institutional and logistical barriers (time, paperwork), attitudinal barriers (leftover perceptions on the part of educators as to the questionable value of parent contributions, feelings of parental intimidation), and educational barriers (lack of information on the part of both educators and parents as to exactly what parents' rights are, how parents might meaningfully participate, and how parents can get the information on which to base intelligent recommendations for educational goals) (Turnbull, 1984).

But perhaps a more important issue on which to reflect is that many parents seem to be perfectly satisfied with the more passive role for a variety of reasons. As stated by one mother:

> Sometimes I get to the end of my rope and can't handle one more thing. The kids are crying, my husband is down-and-out with no job, the car is parked because we can't afford to run it, and the doctor tells me I'm pushing my luck to postpone surgery. About that time the teacher calls for me to come talk about Danny. I just can't hack it. She's a good lady and she's helped Danny. But I've got all I can handle at home. (Turnbull, Brotherson, & Summers, 1983)

The same studies assessing the nature and extent of parent participation also typically assessed parent preferences about participation and/or their satisfaction with the IEP. In the observational study previously described (Goldstein et al., 1980), the satisfaction data from parents, resource teachers, classroom teachers, and principals was overwhelmingly positive. Parents responded to eight satisfaction questions with a mean rating of 4.6 on a 5-point scale. One study (Lynch & Stein, 1982) found that nearly three-fourths of a sample of 400 parents perceived that they were "actively" involved in their child's IEP—active involvement being defined by them as expressing opinions and suggestions, working with and trusting the professionals, listening to and agreeing with the teacher's recommendations, and understanding what was going on. These findings led the authors to focus on the suitability of their original assumption about the value of parent participation in decision making for all families, as well as on the barriers that can prevent many parents from participating to the degree that they would like to.

Parents as Intervenors

Turning to the role of parents as intervenors, there is ample evidence in the empirical literature that parents can be effective teachers and trainers of their children. Parent training efforts typically focus on techniques for teaching skills to, or managing the behavior of, the child. Parents have been effective teachers of communication (Casey, 1978; Schumaker & Sherman, 1978), self-help skills (Adubato, Adams, & Budd, 1981; Fowler, Johnson, Whitman, & Zukotynski, 1978) academic skills (Blechman, Kotanchik, & Taylor, 1981; Wedel & Fowler, 1984), and socially appropriate behavior (Luiselli, 1978), to name a few.

One important issue is how long parents continue to teach their children after the training program is over. A follow-up study (Baker, Heifetz, & Murphy, 1980) of 95 families, 14 months after training, found that 16% of the families were still setting aside time for formal teaching sessions on a skill, and 22% were working on a behavior management program. Seventy-six per cent reported that they were using incidental teaching on one or more skills.

A common professional assumption is that, because child progress from parent intervention has been documented, parents should assume the intervenor role. Another assumption is that "good" parents not only intervene, but they do so frequently and with enthusiasm. Contrast this assumption with the view of a father of a child with a sensory disability (Winton, Turnbull, & Blacher, 1984):

> I believe that parents should love their handicapped children as they are and work with everything they've got to help them reach their highest potential. But there is a fine line involved in doing this, almost a paradox. To love them as they are might tempt parents not to encourage them to achieve their highest potential, but rather to be content. On the other hand, placing emphasis on the child's reaching his/her highest potential could lead parents to dwell on what they can't do. The result could be that it is harder to love them as they are. (p. 55)

This father is expressing a concern that his acting as a teacher might interfere with some of his other roles as a father, such as giving unconditional love and support. It might also give an implicit message to the child that being "less able" translates into being "less lovable." A child's positive self-esteem could hinge on "fixing broken parts." There is enough anecdotal evidence to show that his fears might be well justified. At the very least, one should examine, through research, the unintentional consequences of the parent serving as intervenor.

Other parents have expressed concerns about the effect of training programs on the family's quality of life. How much can we expect parents to sacrifice present peace and quiet for future gains? Here is an example:

> Rosalyn Gibson . . . still spoon-fed her blind three-year-old because the alternatives created such chaos. Meanwhile the teachers encouraged Nancy to feed herself at school and urged Rosalyn to follow their lead . . . they spoke of time saved in the long run. Rosalyn thought about the family meals ruined by flying food and recrimination, and the long hours of clean-up. Probably a child needs both perspectives: someone who cares for the realities of today, the quality of life in the present; and someone who pushes for change and growth (Featherstone, 1980, p. 29)

In a comprehensive review and critique of the literature on family involvement in intervention with children having severe disabilities, Snell and Beckman-Brindley (1984) identified the following limitations in the research reported to date: 1) the family's overall functioning has been tangential to the child's behavior change; 2) there has been a failure to assess whether the intervention is warranted in light of family priorities; 3) participants in the research have primarily been married, non-employed mothers with ambulatory children having moderate deficiencies; 4) generally no estimates of time and cost requirements are included; and 5) the generalized effects of intervention on the child and family are unknown. They argue for change in professional approaches to place greater emphasis on individualization and to provide real choices to families concerning whether they want to assume the intervenor role. Their position stands in stark contrast to the rationale for parent intervention stated in a classic review article by Johnson and Katz (1973): "The advantage of parents as change agents is that they constitute a cheap, continuous treatment resource which is able to augment existing therapeutic manpower capabilities and work conveniently within the home" (p. 181). From a parent's perspective, parent time is not cheap; parents do not necessarily value augmenting professional roles, and teaching a child at home can be highly inconvenient. Such a statement from professionals is a reminder that anything is possible to those with no responsibility for implementation.

FROM EVOLUTION TO REVOLUTION

All of these considerations about parents as intervenors lead back to the same question raised about parents as decision-makers. That is, should not the assumptions held about parent involvement be examined?

First, is not the assumption that parents should be intervenors a direct outgrowth of the older assumptions that parents have deficits to be corrected, and that parents should be service providers? Similarly, perhaps the assumption that parents should be decision-makers is a logical extension of the earlier assumptions that parents should be advocates for their children as well as service providers.

Second, the authors find it odd that one always speaks of parent involvement rather than family involvement. One of the more deeply embedded assumptions is that only parents—not brothers, sisters, aunts, uncles, grandparents, and cousins—are the ones who have an effect on, and are affected by, a child with a disability. In practice, professionals are even more circumscribed than that, because most of their research and interventions are focused on mothers. In the literature, the term "parent" usually means "mother," and "family" usually means "the mother-child dyad" (Benson & Turnbull, 1986).

In short, assumptions are not only rooted in the past, they come from a frightfully narrow perspective of what a family is. The authors are continually struck with how disappointed many service providers are that parents have not lived up to their expectations (e.g., eagerly invited them for weekly home visits, followed through on the home lesson plan, attended parent meetings and training sessions). Until service providers can break away from the past, they will continue to be plagued with problems and barriers that keep parents from filling the roles expected of them. Until service providers can develop a new perspective, they will continue to run short of creative options to serve the needs of families at risk, not just children at risk. A radical change in perspective brought about from within the system is needed. A revolution must occur.

The term "parent involvement" sums up the current perspective. It means parents should be involved in the system. It means the service delivery system is at the center of the universe, and families are revolving around it. It brings to mind an analogy about the old Ptolemaic view of the universe with the earth at the center. This view was useful for many centuries. It could predict movements of heavenly bodies; it was the established scientific approach; it was the right way. But over time, shifts in the heavens caused astronomers to develop a more and more complex formula to account for more and more exceptions. The system got top-heavy.

Copernicus came along and made a startling reversal—he put the sun in the center of the universe rather than the Earth. His declaration caused profound shock. The Earth was not the epitome of creation; it was a planet like all other planets. The successful challenge to the entire system of ancient authority required a complete change in the philosophical conception of the universe. This is rightly termed the "Copernican Revolution." The new perspective broke the logjam; it was easier to explain phenomena; it opened the way to new vistas.

Professionals could continue to act as if their service delivery system is the center of the universe and develop new incentives to whet the appetites of parents for their training programs. Likely they would continue to be frustrated with parents who do not eagerly pursue the opportunities. Many of the programs they would design would be useful. They would probably get more and more top-heavy with ideas and programs, less and less sure about what works and why.

Consider what would happen if there were a Copernican Revolution in the field of disability. Visualize the concept: the *family* is the center of the universe and the service delivery system is one of the many planets revolving around it. Now visualize the service delivery system at the center and the family in orbit around it. Do you see the difference? Do you recognize the revolutionary change in perspective? There would be a shift from an emphasis on parent involvement (i.e., parents participating in the program) to family support (i.e., programs providing a range of support services to families). This is not a semantic exercise—such a revolution leads the authors to a new set of assumptions and a new vista of options for service. The discussion that follows focuses on assumptions and options in the areas of family diversity, interaction, needs, and life-cycle changes.

Diversity

First, when looking beyond the mother-child dyad, it can be seen that families are infinitely diverse. Families vary in the number of parents, number of children, and number of extended family or friends who may be closely involved. They vary in ethnic background, religion, income level, occupation, and location. They vary in the values and beliefs they hold, and in the types of coping strategies they employ to reduce their feelings of stress (Turnbull, Summers, & Brotherson, 1984).

Further, the characteristics of families have changed substantially over the last 25 years and will continue to change in the future. Some interesting trends on families in the United States from 1960 to 1990 have been provided by the Joint Center for Urban Studies of MIT and Harvard University (Masnick & Bane, undated). Highlights relevant to this discussion include:

From 1960 to 1975, one-worker husband/wife households decreased from 43% to 25% of all households and they are projected to fall to 14% by 1990.

In 1978, over half the women with children were employed.

Since 1950, full-time women workers have earned only 60% of what men earn.

Between 1975 and 1990, over 75% of new households will be headed by persons who have never married, are divorced, or are widowed, rather than the traditional pattern of households headed by married couples.

By 1990, over 60% of all households will be childless.

An additional relevant issue, identified by Yankelovich (1981), is the increasing strong preference of adults to seek self-fulfillment, enjoyment, and new experience even at the expense of family responsibilities. He found, in a survey of the general population, that 66% of the parents indicated that

". . . parents should be free to live their own lives even if it means spending less time with their children" (Yankelovich, 1981, p. 74). Given the time and financial restrictions inherent in family life, many parents are not eager to expand their parental responsibilities.

A major implication of these trends is the role of families in attending to the needs of children and youth with disabilities. Families must not only be placed in the center of the universe, but that must be done with an accurate perception of the complexity and competing responsibilities of family life in the mid-1980s. Bernal (1984) warned about the socioeconomic and cultural bias of training parents to intervene with their children:

> My personal view of behavioral parent training is that it is best suited for white middle-and-upper class families, since it was developed for service to these families. Issues arise relevant to the match or mismatch between parent training (as well as parent trainers) and diverse populations, such as low-income and culturally or ethnically different families. The parent trainer who attempts to work with low-income families soon learns that the required appointments, homework, and monitoring of parent and child behavior are not family priorities when economic pressures and uncertainties disrupt schedules, plans, and availability of resources on a daily basis. These families may have needs for which a parent training approach may be inappropriate. (p. 488)

Through research and service programs, service providers must learn to individualize their responses to families according to their diverse characteristics and preferences. Some families clearly want to be decision-makers, others just as clearly do not. Some parents place priority on implementing home intervention programs, others do not. Some families might find comfort in support groups, others might prefer written self-help materials. In some families, the person who ought to be involved in the IEP conference might not be the mother, but the grandmother or the live-in boyfriend. There is a need to be flexible, and to have a wide array of options available for families to choose how much, who, and in what way they want to participate.

Interaction

Second, one must realize that families are an interactive system. When a group of people all live under one roof, they become very intricately interconnected. To a greater or lesser extent, what one person does affects everyone else in the family. The way families get along, without killing one another (usually!), is that they have certain unwritten rules. These rules govern how they communicate with each other, who makes decisions, who takes which roles and responsibilities. They also have their own particular style of cohesion—that is, how close or distant different subgroups within the family are to each other (Olson, Sprenkle, & Russell, 1978).

Service providers should view every point of contact with families as a potential intrusion into the delicate balance of the system. When a mother is encouraged to participate in school, how does that affect the rest of the family? If she becomes overly involved with her child with a disability, what happens to her other relationships? If a mother is engaged in a feeding training program that takes 2 hours a night, when does she talk to her teenaged daughter about her dating concerns? Who does the dishes? What happens to the pleasant dinner conversation the family might once have enjoyed? When does she spend some time with her husband? When does she set aside time just for herself? Service providers have to consider very carefully what it is they are asking families to do. Helen Featherstone's (1980) experience illustrated this beautifully:

> I remember the day when the occupational therapist at Jody's school called with some suggestions from a visiting nurse. Jody has a seizure problem which is controlled with the drug Dilantin. Dilantin can cause the gums to grow over the teeth . . . The nurse had noticed . . . this overgrowth, and recommended, innocently enough, that (his) teeth be brushed four times a day, for five minutes, with an electric toothbrush. The school suggested that they could do this once on school days, and that I should try to do it the other three to four times a day . . . This new demand appalled me . . . Jody . . . is blind, cerebral-palsied, and retarded. We do his physical therapy daily and work with him on sounds and communication. We feed him each meal on our laps, bottle him, change him, bathe him, dry him, put him in a body cast to sleep, launder his bed linens daily, and go through a variety of routines designed to minimize his miseries and enhance his joys and his development. (All this in addition to trying to care for and enjoy our other young children and making time for each other and our careers.) Now you tell me that I should spend fifteen minutes every day on something that Jody will hate, an activity that will not help him to walk or even defecate, but one that is directed at the health of his gums. This activity is not for a finite time, but forever. It is not guaranteed to help, but "it can't hurt." And it won't make the overgrowth go away but may retard it. Well, it's too much. Where is that fifteen minutes going to come from? What am I supposed to give up? Taking the kids to the park? Reading the bedtime story to my eldest? Washing the breakfast dishes? Sorting the laundry? Grading students' papers? Sleeping? Because there is no time in my life that hasn't been spoken for, and for every fifteen-minute activity that is added, one has to be taken away. (pp. 77–78)

Service providers need to be very sure that their recommendations are consistent with the families' priorities and are reasonable in light of the many competing time demands they face. Anything that families are asked to do—whether it is a school meeting or a home training program—must be important enough to be worth their valuable time. Service providers also need to be sure that anything they ask is efficient and designed to be accomplished with a minimum of time and effort.

Addressing family interaction also means broadening one's view from the mother-child dyad to a total family perspective. An excellent model for consideration is the Supporting Extended Family Members (SEFAM) Program directed by Rebecca Fewell at the University of Washington. This project has developed relevant and supportive interventions for fathers (Meyer & Fewell,

1985), brothers and sisters (Meyer, 1983), and grandparents (Vadasy, Fewell, & Meyer, in press).

Future research and intervention need to address strategies for supporting families in establishing balance in their interactions with each other. Assisting families to place no single member at the center of their family universe, but to be sensitive to the needs of all members, is an important future direction.

Needs

Third, service providers need to understand that families have a number of functions to meet their individual and collective needs (Turnbull, Summers, & Brotherson, 1984). Some families' needs are tangible, such as those related to economics, physical caregiving, education, and vocational development. Other needs are much more intangible. They include needs for rest and recuperation, socialization, affection and intimacy, and developing a sense of self-identity and self-direction. When one begins to list all the things that families must do for themselves and each other, one begins to get a feeling of wonder that families survive at all. Janet Bennett (1985), the mother of a daughter with Down syndrome, described the flow of her daily responsibilities when her child was born and the pressure she felt to add one more—participation in the ARC:

> At the time of Kathryn's birth I also had to manage the school schedules of Amanda, who was in the sixth grade, and Peter, in the second grade; both were timed to overlap and consequently conflict with Martha's kindergarten hours. Between 11:30 and 12:30 each day I had to feed one child, pick up two, drop off one, feed three, drop off two. Kathryn's naps had to fit in whenever they could; breast-feeding was an interesting challenge. I was recovering from a combined Caesarean delivery and hysterectomy and, while trying to manage my own lunches along with the others, unwittingly encouraged attacks from a developing hernia.
>
> If I had had an unretarded baby, I'd never in a million years have thought of volunteering for anything during that period. Now that I had Kathryn, why in the world would I be expected to do anything of the kind? Yet in the face of minimal help from the organization, it was telling me I should help it. And numb from shock and diminished self-confidence, I did my best to comply. (p. 164)

Families with children and youth with disabilities have always been expected to do more and to involve themselves in the service delivery system with enthusiasm and gusto. Recently, the authors joined with a couple of colleagues in planning a series of problem-solving workshops for families with adolescents with disabilities. The authors believe that developing problem-solving skills is important because one can help families learn to identify needs and set priorities, brainstorm a variety of options, and take action using the option suited to their own preferences and resources. Thus, they were excited about making this training available to families. However, after publicizing the workshop broadly, very few families indicated an interest. One family member, who had elected not to participate, shared his reason with the authors: "We are gung-hoed out on workshops. We have been going to them for years and we are tired of it. No more." Can not everyone identify with being "gung-hoed out"? It is a fact of life for anyone when he or she is constantly busy and can never seem to get everything done. Why does the myth still exist that families with a member experiencing a disability have extra time in their day for extra tasks? The authors do not have extra time; families do not either.

As an alternative, the authors developed a self-instructional problem-solving guide for parents with basic information on family system and problem-solving concepts, vignettes of families, and exercises to apply to their own family situation. This kind of packaging allows families to read it if and when they choose—in the bathroom, 15 minutes before the kids wake up in the morning, or while waiting in the doctor's office.

In reality, it is usually mothers rather than families who are expected to perform in a heroic (or "sheroic"!) manner in attending to the extraordinary needs of children with disabilities and the expectations of the service delivery system. But the reality of family life must not be overlooked. How many employed mothers have extra time on their hands? Consider the fact that American women with families have been found to have a 70-hour work week (Gauger, 1973). How can service providers possibly ask for more?

Future research should identify time-efficient strategies for responding to an array of family needs. One interesting line of research would be to identify a sample of families who consider themselves at least reasonably successful in responding to the needs of their members. Time-in-motion studies could be conducted on these families to discern their methods for allocating responsibilities and the resources they use.

The impact of disability on the family's ability to meet its needs is a complex phenomenon. Research appears to be based on a negative, deficit-oriented view of the member with a disability. Research is needed on the positive and negative contributions to families of children or youth with disabilities as compared with the positive and negative contributions in families where children and youth do not experience disabilities. It is an erroneous assumption that raising a child with a disability is all problems and a child without a disability is all fun and games. A mother of eight children, the youngest of whom had Down syndrome, shared with the authors that she felt some relief when she came to grips with the fact that her child had Down syndrome, because she knew she did not have the coping skills for another normal adolescence.

Further, children and youth with disabilities make positive contributions to their families (Turnbull, Summers, & Brotherson, 1984). It is an over-looked fact in research; yet, families consistently describe such contributions in anecdotal accounts (Turnbull, Summers, & Brotherson, 1984; Turnbull &

Turnbull, 1985). A father of a 12-year-old daughter with severe disabilities and life-threatening medical complications shared his view:

> Twelve years ago I didn't know God's purpose for our situation. I do now. If I could live those years over and had my choice about what would happen, I wouldn't change anything. Sarah has taught us more about unconditional love than we ever could have known otherwise. She has never asked for anything; only given freely to us of her love. Metal is never purified until it goes through the heat. We have learned and grown and loved as a family. (Turnbull, Brotherson, & Summers, 1983)

Obviously, Sarah has made profound, positive contributions to the way this family meets their needs for affection and self-definition. Qualitative research is needed to enable families to define their own experience as a basis for constructing ecologically valid research instruments. In short, families deserve the right to define their own needs rather than to have researcher biases limit their choices on preconceived instruments.

Changes

The fourth and last assumption derives from the observation that families change over time. Families with young children meet their needs in much different ways than families with older children. For instance, one shows affection to young children by hugging, cuddling, and tucking them into bed. One shows affection to teenagers by listening to them, respecting them, and trusting their independence. Families also have different needs at different times. For example, with young children with disabilities, families must deal with "breaking the news" to relatives and friends and adjusting to an altered kind of parenthood. But families with young adults with disabilities must deal with the seemingly endless vista of parental responsibility for an individual who may always be dependent in some ways. And they must make plans to enhance security after they become too old to assume responsibility or die.

Researchers need also to recognize that the transitions to a new stage in life are the times of greatest stress (Terkelsen, 1980). When a child enters school and when he or she leaves it, are times of vulnerability in many families. For families with children and youth with disabilities, transitions are usually more difficult, because changes are delayed and hard to come by. Families establish routines to keep stress more manageable (Birenbaum, 1971), and disruptions in routine may mean a corresponding increase in stress.

How can researchers support families through transitions? First, they can give ample warning and advance information about changes to come. Consider that children who do not have disabilities move to a new classroom every year, and when they are in junior high school, they move every hour. They get used to changes, and so do their parents. But children and youth with disabilities in special class placement may stay in the same class, with the same teacher, for several years. They may never change schools, get a driver's license, go through high school graduation, get married, or leave home— the significant marker events that life moves on. Thus, they become accustomed to routine, and so do their families. Routine is, perhaps, one of the hardest habits to break.

Second, researchers should develop intervention strategies to assist families and service providers in looking ahead to the future environment the child will occupy. What skills will the child need to function successfully in the next class placement? In adult services programs? Are those skills being taught? What information do families need about the adult residential and vocational programs, and where can they go to find it? Where can families go to find out about guardianship? Wills and trusts? Social security? Options for expressing sexuality?

In a recent research study completed by one of the authors' colleagues (Brotherson, 1985), interviews were conducted with 48 parents of sons and daughters at the stage of transition from secondary school to adult services. She investigated the families' frequency of future planning and their satisfaction with the process they had used. Parents who reported a greater frequency of future planning also reported higher levels of family satisfaction. The area of greatest need for parents was for residential placements for their children. The next most important areas of need were socialization and leisure opportunities for persons with mental retardation and employment or vocational opportunities for persons with physical disability. Families rated reframing (i.e., interpreting stressful situations in a more positive way so that stress is minimized) as the most important coping strategy they used in future planning. Consultation with professionals ranked equally with alcohol, cigarettes, and TV, and only slightly above medication as the most important coping strategy. These findings should cause all professionals to pause and reflect on their meaning.

The authors are excited about an intervention program in which they are presently involved that assists families with adolescents with moderate and severe disabilities in transitional planning from secondary school to adulthood (Turnbull et al., 1984). This model incorporates three training phases. The first phase involves working with families to select options for residential living and vocational preparation for their son or daughter. Strategies include assisting families in identifying the quality of life criteria that are important for their adolescent and for themselves, strategies for helping to identify the preferences of their son or daughter, guidelines for conducting ecological inventories of community programs, guidelines for evaluating alternatives against quality of life criteria, and procedures for establishing priorities. The second phase focuses on the IEP conference as a forum for preparing for the future. Specifically, family members are helped to identify the critical skills needed by their son or daughter to be admitted to the residential and vocational programs they prefer. Families are provided with information on strategies for participating in IEP conferences to ensure that objectives addressing critical skills are included in the IEP. The third phase involves conducting a series of life-planning seminars with families on legal and ethical issues, such as estate planning, financial resources, sexuality, right to treatment, and case management. Each phase is being evaluated thoroughly as the basis of revising all materials for national dissemination through the Association for Retarded Citizens of the United States.

It is very difficult to think about the future, because it is unknown. Some families find it especially difficult, because they cope with stress simply by "taking things one day at a time." For those who are not interested in engaging in future planning, service providers need to be even more certain that the instructional goals developed are relevant to the child's future. Individualization means that some families can opt out of future planning. Further, important as professionals think transition planning is, they should recognize that it is primarily a WASP value (McGoldrick, 1982).

SUMMARY

Current attempts at parent involvement may be working less than perfectly because the wrong perspective is being used. Families are the ones needing help, not the service delivery system. Using this perspective, the authors have borrowed four assumptions from family systems theory to suggest a new approach. These recommendations are:

1. Because families are all different, service providers need to individualize their responses, respect families' preferences, and provide an array of options for participation from which families can choose.
2. Service providers need to make certain that their interventions do not upset the delicate balance of the family system, by making certain that what they ask is both important and efficient, and by recognizing the legitimate interests of all family members.
3. Service providers need to recognize the competing responsibilities of families, to support them in setting priorities according to their values, and to help focus attention on the positive contributions that a child with a disability makes to meeting family needs.
4. Service providers need to be supportive to families as they move through the life cycle. This is, after all, a joint mission of service providers and families—to prepare the child, to the best of his or her ability, to become a successful adult.

The authors know that what they are suggesting is not easy. Revolutions never are—just ask Copernicus. But it has exciting possibilities for "realness.'' Let us get on with the revolution with our best Kennedy imitations, by posing the challenge: ''Ask not, what families can do for the service delivery system, but what the service delivery system can do for the families.''

REFERENCES

Adubato, S. A., Adams, M. K., & Budd, K. S. (1981). Teaching a parent to train a spouse in child management techniques. *Journal of Applied Behavior Analysis, 14,* 192–205.

Baker, B. L., Heifetz, L. J., & Murphy, D. (1980). Behavior training for parents of retarded children: One year follow-up. *American Journal of Mental Deficiency, 85,* 31–38.

Bennett, J. M. (1985). A ten o'clock scholar. In H. R. Turnbull & A. P. Turnbull (Eds.), *Parents speak out: Then and now* (pp. 175–183). Columbus, OH: Charles E. Merrill.

Benson, H., & Turnbull, A. (1986). Approaching families from an individualized perspective. In R. H. Horner, L. M. Voeltz, & H. D. B. Fredericks (Eds.), *Education of learners with severe handicaps: Exemplary service strategies* (pp. 127–157). Baltimore: Paul H. Brookes Publishing Co.

Bernal, M. E. (1984). Consumer issues in parent training. In R. F. Dangel & R. A. Polster (Eds.), *Parent training* (pp. 477–503). New York: Guilford Press.

Birenbaum, A. (1971). The mentally retarded child in the home and the family cycle. *Journal of Health and Social Behavior, 12,* 55–65.

Blechman, E. A., Kotanchik, N. L., & Taylor, C. J. (1981). Families and schools together: Early behavioral intervention with high-risk students. *Behavior Therapy, 12,* 308–319.

Brotherson, M. J. (1985). *Parents' self-report of future planning and its relationship to family functioning and stress in families with disabled sons and daughters.* Unpublished doctoral dissertation, Department of Special Education, University of Kansas, Lawrence.

Casey, L. (1978). Development of communicative behavior in autistic children: A parent program using signed speech. *Devereux Forum, 12,* 1–15.

Farber, B., & Ryckman, D. B. (1965). Effects of severely mentally retarded children on family relationships. *Mental Retardation Abstracts, 2,* 1–17.

Featherstone, H. (1980). *A difference in the family.* New York: Basic Books.

Fowler, S. A., Johnson, M. R., Whitman, R. L., & Zukotynski, G. (1978). Teaching a parent in the home to train self-help skills and increase compliance in her retarded daughter. *AAESPH Review, 13,* 151–161.

Gardner, R. A. (1971). The guilt reactions of parents of children with severe physical disease. In R. L. Noland (Ed.), *Counseling parents of the ill and the handicapped.* Springfield, IL: Charles C Thomas.

Gauger, W. (1973, October). Household work: Can we add it to the GNP? *Journal of Home Economics,* 2–23.

Goddard, H. H. (1912). *The Kallikak family: A study in the heredity of feeblemindedness.* New York: Macmillan.

Goldstein, S., Strickland, B., Turnbull, A. P., & Curry, L. (1980). An observational analysis of the IEP conference. *Exceptional Children, 46,* 278–286.

Johnson, C. A., & Katz, R. C. (1973). Using parents as change agents for their children: A review. *Journal of Clinical Psychology and Psychiatry, 4,* 181–200.

Kanner, L. (1949). Problems of nosology and psychodynamica of early infantile autism. *American Journal of Orthopsychiatry, 19,* 416–426.

Kirk, S. A. (1984). Introspection and prophecy. In B. Blatt & R. J. Morris (Eds.), *Perspectives in special education: Personal orientations* (pp. 25–55). Glenview, IL: Scott, Foresman.

Kirk, S. A., & Gallagher, J. J. (1979). *Educating exceptional children* (3rd ed.). Boston: Houghton Mifflin.

Luiselli, J. K. (1978). Treatment of an autistic child's fear of riding a school bus through exposure and reinforcement. *Journal of Behavior Therapy and Experimental Psychiatry, 9,* 169–172.

Lynch, E. W., & Stein, R. (1982). Perspectives on parent participation in special education. *Exceptional Education Quarterly, 3*(2), 45–63.

Masnick, G., & Bane, M. J. (undated). The nation's families: 1960–1990: A summary. Cambridge, MA: Joint Center for Urban Studies of MIT and Harvard University.

McGoldrick, M. (1982). Ethnicity and family therapy: An overview. In M. McGoldrick, J. K. Pearce, & J. Giordano (Eds.), *Ethnicity and family therapy* (pp. 3–30). New York: Guilford Press.

McKinney, J. D., & Hocutt, A. M. (1982). Public school involvement of parents of learning-disabled children and average achievers. *Exceptional Education Quarterly, 3*(2), 64–73.

Meyer, D. J. (1983). A sibshop for siblings. *Sibling Information Network Newsletter, 2*(1).

Meyer, D., & Fewell, R. (1985). *Supporting extended family members (SEFAM) program: A handbook for fathers.* Seattle: University of Washington Press.

Olson, D. H., Sprenkle, D. H., & Russell, C. (1978). Circumplex model of marital and family systems: Cohesion and adaptability dimension, family types and clinical applications. *Family Process, 18,* 3–28.

Price, M., & Goodman, L. (1980). Individualized education programs: A cost study. *Exceptional Children, 46*(6), 446–458.

Schumaker, J. B., & Sherman, J. A. (1978). Parent as intervention agent: From birth onward. In R. L. Schiefelbusch (Ed.), *Language intervention strategies* (pp. 237–315). Baltimore: University Park Press.

Snell, M. E., & Beckman-Brindley, S. (1984). Family involvement in intervention with children having severe handicaps. *Journal of Speech and Hearing, 3,* 213–230.

Sperling, M. (1965). Psychoanalytic aspects of discipline. In M. J. Long, W. C. Morse, & R. G. Newman (Eds.), *Conflict in the classroom* (pp. 126–145). Belmont, CA: Wadsworth.

Terkelsen, K. B. (1980). Toward a theory of the family life cycle. In E. Carter & M. McGoldrick (Eds.), *The family cycle: A framework of family therapy* (pp. 21–52). New York: Gardner Press.

Turnbull, A. P. (1984). Parental participation in the IEP process. In J. A. Mulick & S. M. Pueschel (Eds.), *Parent-professional participation in developmental disability services: Foundations and prospects* (pp. 107–123). Cambridge, MA: Ware Press.

Turnbull, A. P., Brotherson, M. J., Bronicki, G. J., Benson, H. A., Houghton, J., Roeder-Gordon, C., & Summers, J. A. (1984). *How to plan for my child's adult future: A three-part process to future planning.* Unpublished manuscript, University of Kansas, Lawrence.

Turnbull, A. P., Brotherson, M. J., & Summers, J. A. (1983). [Qualitative studies of families with a member with a disability]. Unpublished raw data, University of Kansas, Bureau of Child Research.

Turnbull, A. P., Summers, J. A., & Brotherson, M. J. (1984). *Working with families with disabled members.* Lawrence, KS: University Affiliated Facility.

Turnbull, A. P., & Turnbull, H. R. (1985). Developing independence in adolescents with disabilities. *Journal of Adolescent Health Care, 6*(2), 108–119.

Turnbull, H. R., Turnbull, A. P., & Wheat, M. (1982). Assumptions about parental participation: A legislative history. *Exceptional Education Quarterly, 3*(2), 1–8.

Vadasy, P. F., Fewell, R. R., & Meyer, D. J. (in press). Supporting extended family members' roles: Intergenerational supports provided by grandparents. *Journal of the Division for Early Childhood.*

Wedel, J. Q., & Fowler, S. A. (1984). "Read me a story, mom." A home-tutoring program to teach prereading skills to language-delayed children. *Behavior Modification, 8*(2), 245–266.

Winton, P. J., Turnbull, A. P., & Blacher, J. (1984). *Selecting a preschool: A guide for parents of handicapped children.* Baltimore: University Park Press.

Wolfensberger, W. (1970). Counseling the parents of the retarded. In A. A. Baumeister (Ed.), *Mental retardation: Appraisal, education, and rehabilitation* (pp. 329–400). Chicago: Aldine.

Yankelovich, D. (1981). New rules in American life: Searching for self-fulfillment in a world turned upside down. *Psychology Today, 14*(11), 35–91.

Zigler, E., & Valentine, J. (Eds.). (1979). *Project Head Start: A legacy of the war on poverty.* New York: Free Press.

Response

A Mother's Perspective

Claire D. Canning

✦✦✦

To cope with the changing picture of the family of today, and the family of the future, Turnbull and Summers have suggested, rather than increased parental involvement beyond the scope of parental energies, a diverse and increased family support system to aid the entire family of the child with disabilities. They believe that a revolution must occur, with a focus on the diversity of families, mutual interaction of families, and individual needs and changing needs of the family as the child goes on to different stages. I prefer to think of the process as evolution without revolution.

While the observations are most commendable and far reaching, in my opinion this would work only in Utopia, and it is simply not consistent with the tremendous national deficit which must be addressed. But although unlimited funding and a limitless increase in trained personnal do not seem to be on the horizon, consider for a moment just how far services, support systems, and families have come. The past decade has seen more progress and legal mandates for our children than any other time in history, and many more parents are taking part in planning and decision making.

Economic pressures will remain a reality, the structure and complexity of the family will change, unbelievable demands will be made on people, but one day at a time, one small step at a time, we will insist on continuing progress for our children. And we will *not ever* turn back and accept less. Through increased scientific expertise, training and dedication of empathetic professionals, and loving devotion of families of children with disabilities, we have come a long, long way together. What we need to do now is learn how to do more for people with disabilities, but to do it more innovatively.

Despite the unspeakable sorrow the parent of a handicapped child knows, Turnbull and Summers are so right when they say that less able does not mean less loveable. As the mother of five wonderful children, I can say that no child has ever brought more love than our child with Down syndrome, and the quiet joys of each day more than compensate for the occasional tears. As we are told, some of the greatest learning takes place in pain and despair.

Our daughter, Martha, who is now 14, is still struggling with learning to tie her shoes and secure buttons; she is weak in fine motor skills. But she swims, hikes in the woods, rides a horse, bowls, sets a beautiful table, consistently does chores, and is the only one of our children who knows how to hang up her clothes! She is learning to play the organ, and reads on a fourth grade level. She never forgets to say "Thank you," and feels a love for us that I just cannot describe in words. She is our only child who calls her father "sweet pal." She is a good and thoughtful neighbor who helps neighborhood children with their paper routes, and even sells Girl Scout cookies. She loves her toddler nieces and nephews and is extremely gentle with them. She is a young woman who handles menstruation beautifully. She wants to be mature and help plan her own future. We want her to develop her potential as fully as possible. No child has ever helped us more to put our values in proper perspective, and she has drawn our family closer with an awe and appreciation for the many tiny wonders of life we once took for granted. She has created a special bond of unity among her siblings. When they were younger, it took careful planning to achieve the delicate balance of giving each family member his or her own special time, but the rewards have more than compensated for the efforts.

What do I feel I can do to help Martha, and other children with disabilities? First, I must realize that families are as infinitely diverse as are children with disabilities, as are coping strategies. But most parents do want to help their child, so I can try to instill confidence in the abilities of the mothers and fathers I meet. They must learn never to say "I am only a parent." Training will help overcome barriers that prevent many parents from participating. One simple example: Our local educational advisory committee sponsored, with excellent parental response, an evening to teach parents to take a more active part in planning their child's educational program. They must learn not to be intimidated by jargon, but to have confidence in their knowledge of their own child and goals for him or her.

In 1984, for the first time, our own evolution nearly became a revolution when our special education director and my husband and I could not agree on Martha's IEP. We had to threaten mediation on a state level to satisfy a very legitimate demand. Fortunately, it has turned out amicably and extremely well. But we must teach others not to be afraid to be persistent, to be peaceful advocates and not adversaries. In all things, parents must be taught to be partners in the decision-making process for their children.

As Turnbull and Summers have so well stated, I, too, see burn-out as a very real problem for parents of children with disabilities. If our daughters want to be in Girl Scouts, we are asked to start a new troop. If my child plays the organ, I must practice with her for the extra help she needs. Extra help is needed for so many little things. Beyond the home, this expands to the community, where parents of children with disabilities must serve on boards of directors for parent organizations, educational advisory committees, school monitoring of special education programs, human rights committees, all types of awareness programs, and advocacy roles that parents of so-called normal children never dream of. Respite care for parents who never get away from daily pressures is a very real necessity. And we must never condemn anyone who no longer has the energy to continue to work for the cause, but we must educate younger parents to carry on.

Also, just as normal children eventually leave home, I see planning for semi-independent living in a group home as the most essential of our plans for the future for every family of a person with disabilities. Preparing the groundwork for acceptance in neighborhoods is a gigantic task in itself. Our local parent group now operates 12 group homes in our community. The inadequacy of programs and underfunding are a great concern for the future, if life is to be stable and secure for adults with disabilities.

Let me tell you about very dear friends of ours, a couple with four children: two are National Merit scholars, two are mentally retarded persons. One is profoundly brain-damaged, and the other is a young man with Down syndrome. The mother holds a full-time position managing an office. Yet, one morning, after preparing her family for the day and before going to work, she hosted a breakfast for local legislators to point out to them the human disasters that would result from cutting the funds that provide services to local young adults with disabilities. When this woman's son could not comprehend why he could not drive a car, she and her husband compensated by allowing him to buy a dirt bike, which he is content to ride in the many fields near his home. When the son earned his first paycheck working at minimum wage in a plant in the community, his parents took him to the bank and asked that his check be cashed in one dollar bills so he could understand on his own terms the enormity of his very important work. This young man saves at a local small branch of a bank near his home where, with minimal help, he keeps his checking account. He is a taxpayer and a happy, satisfied, contributing member of society.

The wonder of all of this is that there are similar families across the country. There are professionals, too, across the country and around the world, people we would never have had the privilege to know were it not for our child with Down syndrome. Together, we have the unique honor of working to make this a better world. Until that magical day when funding will be available for unlimited services for our children, remember that each of us can be the small pebble that, dropped on the water, causes many ripples and succeeds in effecting change. Together, let us press for every human service that will help our children and young adults develop to their fullest potential, whatever that may be.

Chapter 12

Psychosocial Development in Persons with Down Syndrome

Carol Tingey

Although each individual develops in his or her personal, almost private, mysterious way, it has been possible through the observation of the development of many different individuals over time to see that there are certain skills and a certain order of development that occurs for most individuals. This order of development has been described by various scientists. A discussion of the theories of Erikson, Piaget, and Bandura follows.

THE ORDER OF DEVELOPMENT

Development Described By Erikson

Erikson (1963) saw the development coming as the individual struggles with the growing and expanding conflicts that are presented during the biological life cycle. As Erikson described it, much of this order of development correlates with the physical development of the individual and the development of a body that is physically mature and capable of reproduction. As the body develops autonomy through controlled movement capabilities, the child moves away from the parent and to more independent interaction with others. As the body becomes capable of reproduction, these interpersonal relationships become more significant, and they guide the individual into a selection of life companionship. When a life companion is found, it is possible for the reproductive cycle to start another phase. Since human infants are not able to survive without extended care, part of maturity is the ability to develop the skills of nurturing a new generation either by producing and rearing children or by providing for the needs of the offspring of others. After a new generation has reached a level of some independence, the parenting individuals can move to another stage of psychological development. Erikson sees the "struggle" in each of these stages as:

Infancy: basic trust versus mistrust
Toddler: autonomy versus dependency
Early childhood: initiative versus shame or doubt
Middle childhood: industry versus inferiority
Adolescence: identity versus identity confusion
Young adult: intimacy versus isolation
Adulthood: generativity versus stagnation
Maturity: ego integrity versus despair

The individual faces these struggles as he or she faces the changes due to the development of his or her body and the expectations of others. It is assumed that maturation occurs as a result of the work of the struggle.

Development Described By Piaget

Piaget (Flavell, 1963) saw the child's social behavior as dependent, at least in part, on the child's cognitive maturity. The infant who has not yet been able to learn that objects exist when he or she cannot see them is limited in social interchange to interaction with only those things present in the immediate time and place. Later, the young child is able to put together a prediction of what should be happening in a particular situation because he or she has been able to observe and remember the activity through repeated participation in the situation. The child develops a "social schema" and with this conceptional framework is able to know the world and how to interact in it. In the beginning, the child's whole world is the sensorimotor interaction with the primary caregiver, usually the mother. As the child experiences interaction with individuals other than the primary caregiver, patterns for social interaction become more complex. Social/emotional development is achieved by increasingly complicated cognitive understanding of the situations and events around the individual.

Piaget has defined cognitive development by observing the methods of gathering information that individuals use throughout development (Flavell, 1963):

Period of sensorimotor intelligence (birth–2 years): The child develops from a neonatal, reflex level of self-world to a practical organization of his or her immediate environment.
Period of preparation for and organization of concrete operation (2–11 years): The child comes to grips with symbols (2–7 years); the child develops concrete grouping of concepts (7–11 years).
Period of formal operations (11–15 years): The child develops new and final organization and reorganization and is able to think abstractly.

Development Described By Bandura

Still others argue that increasingly complicated behavior occurs because the individual is able to learn by observing others and being complimented or otherwise rewarded for doing the things that the others are doing (Bandura, 1977). This description of development is called social learning theory since it is assumed that private thoughts and feelings cannot be observed and, therefore, cannot be quantified. Development, according to Bandura, can only be understood by directly observable events. Changes in behavior, according to this theory, are related to the rewards and punishment received for exhibiting the behavior. Bandura and co-workers (Bandura & Walters, 1959; Bandura, Ross, & Ross, 1963) suggested that individuals observe and interpret the behavior of others and then choose to repeat the behaviors of those who are admired or whose behavior draws wanted attention. The individual, therefore, learns to do what is expected in the society because the individual can imitate the behavior of others who are "successful." In this way, it is seen that the child will grow up to be like the successful people in his or her environment by doing what he or she sees others being rewarded for doing (Bandura, 1969, 1977). Although the child will most likely repeat those behaviors that he or she sees most frequently in public places, even behaviors observed on TV appear to be modeled by children. Children who receive inconsistent responses from parents are more likely to produce antisocial behaviors. Bandura explains the process as: 1) observing the behaviors of others, 2) coding and storing the event or events, and 3) repeating the performance at selected times and places.

DEVELOPMENT IN PERSONS WITH DOWN SYNDROME

Erikson's, Piaget's, Bandura's and other theoretical explanations for development may not represent the developmental life cycle of an individual with Down syndrome. The description of the development of adolescence and maturity as development of the ability to nurture another generation as well as adding to the well-being of society, as suggested by Erikson, may not be comprehensive enough to explain the situation that occurs when the individual is not able to move from adolescent sexual development into full-blown adult sex roles. In the process of studies of the biological aspects of Down syndrome, it has been found that very few individuals with Down syndrome move into that stage of development as described by Erikson. One review of the literature, describing reproductive capacity of individuals with Down syndrome, found that it was difficult to determine if some of the cases described were indeed different cases or additional descriptions of the same case. Nevertheless, that search was able to identify only 24 females and no males with diagnosed cases of Down syndrome who had reproduced (Jagiello,

1981). Nine of these infants had Down syndrome, two were retarded, and three were stillborn. The other infants were normal. It is not known whether the earlier and subsequent developmental crises occur when the path toward "maturity" lacks a completely developed adult sex role. It is also not known if the apparent lack of ability to develop the internal sense of independence or the financial state of independence inhibits the ability to move into the stage of young adulthood in which the individual strives to make a personal, individual, concrete, mature, unique contribution to the family, the neighborhood, and society in general. Certainly contributions made in these areas could be altered, perhaps to include perspectives on value system rather than economic and social leadership contributions. Seigel (1974) indicated that the ability to earn one's own living is probably the single most valid indicator of adequate adjustment. In order to make statements about the adult life role of individuals with Down syndrome, and the earlier steps to that adult role, it would be necessary to observe a number of individuals in order to determine if the descriptions of "normal" development toward "normal maturity" are comprehensive enough to explain the differences that occur when it is not possible to attain the mature adult sex role.

Inhelder (1968), who worked with Piaget, described early concrete learning experiences as being typical of the long-term needs for those who have difficulties in learning. The time, space, and number systems that Piaget described as being learned by the developing child are some of the same concepts that educators have seen to be difficult for the school-age child with Down syndrome to learn (Hallahan & Kauffman, 1978). Although it has been found that mental development for individuals with Down syndrome continues into the third and fourth decade of life (Berry, Groeneweg, Gibson, & Brown, 1984), there is little evidence of adult education for individuals with Down syndrome. It is not known how the difficulty attaining these understandings affects social development. If it is difficult to understand time, is it more difficult to project understanding and develop schema for events in the future? Is it more difficult to see how the actions of the present time set the stage for interaction at a later time? If numerical relations are difficult to develop, is it more difficult to learn the importance of management of money and the skills to develop this management? If these skills are difficult to develop, how do they affect not only the ability to perform skills, but also the ability to "feel good" about one's self and be confident about the ability to face a new challenge without help? In order to see how the individual with Down syndrome faces these developmental challenges and what psychological/social skills and concepts the individual develops, it would be necessary to observe individuals with Down syndrome throughout the life cycle, to document how the cognitive difficulties affect the development of social autonomy. If Piaget's theory of development of social skills through the development of cognitive ability is accurate, it could be assumed that the difficulties in development for the individual with Down syndrome might cause altered steps and differing developmental achievements.

In his early discussions of persons with Down syndrome, J. Langdon Down, a physician, described the ability of the individual with Down syndrome to imitate what others were doing (Benda, 1969). This ability to do what others are doing has been observed by almost anyone who has had contact with individuals with Down syndrome. The imitative intent of this behavior has not, however, been studied by those who investigate human behavior. Bandura (1977) described the young child's imitation as a strategy for developing adult skills. The intent of the imitation by the child with Down syndrome is not clear. It appears from time to time that the imitation may be repetition without understanding or a form of entertainment rather than a method of practicing a new skill. It is also important to realize that the studies of spontaneous environmental imitation undertaken by Bandura (1977) show that the child reflects the behaviors of the immediate environment. This would appear to make the study of the immediate environment of the individual with Down syndrome extremely important. It would be important to study the development of individuals with Down syndrome in institutional settings to describe the behaviors of ''adults'' who were raised with a limited amount of ''mature'' behaviors being displayed (presumably these behaviors were being demonstrated by the staff, but probably not as frequently by friends and peers, which are a rich source for most individuals during the developmental period). It would also be important to study the details of natural home and community environments. If development can be explained for individuals with Down syndrome as a matter of what they imitated, then the exact elements of the day-to-day environment become of vast significance because that will determine the body of available behaviors. It would also be important to ask whether it would be appropriate for individuals with Down syndrome to imitate spontaneously all behaviors seen in a typical home, school, or neighborhood environment, such as driving a car, arguing with a family member, running away from home, or eating a third piece of pie—without the skills to execute the sophisticated cognitive monitoring of the performance expected of individuals without disabilities, or assistance to compensate for the lack thereof.

Concepts of development and definitions of maturation used to describe the process of development and the steps toward maturation achieved by the general population may have limited relevance in describing the development of individuals with Down syndrome. Certainly the medical field has indicated that there are a number of physiological differences in the individual with altered chromosomal structure that go beyond the mere description of the cellular structure. Such differences cause variations in health status and physical capabilities. Perhaps because these physical symptoms are easily observable not only by the medical professsion but also by the public, it has been natural to assume that the study of development of individuals with Down syndrome should be spearheaded by medically oriented research (Brian, 1984). Findings from the medical research can be used to postulate a description of psychosocial needs, but it would be shortsighted to assume that a more thorough study of maturation with focus on interactional and cognitive behaviors is not required for descriptive understanding. When the study of human development of nonhandicapped individuals is undertaken, the study of the physiology of development is considered as background information for the beginning of identifying areas of personal-social interaction that warrant scientific scrutiny. For the individual with Down syndrome, it would be fruitful to have well-designed observations of social maturation in infancy and early childhood, in the school years, and in post-school experiences, as seen in the situations listed in Table 1. These selected situations are not meant to be exhaustive, but detailed enough to represent pertinent areas for descriptive exploration.

Methods of Investigation

Human behavior cannot be studied solely in examination rooms or laboratory experiments. For human behavior to be understood, it must be studied in the setting in which it occurs, since it is that setting that partially determines the appropriateness of the behavior. For example, at some point in time and under certain circumstances, it is appropriate to pick one's nose, take off one's clothes, and go to sleep. None of these behaviors would be considered to be appropriate at a banquet. To know that an individual is capable of performing these acts is of little consequence unless it is also known whether the individual actually performs these acts at a time and place that is appropriate, and whether the individual can determine the appropriateness of the situation and initiate and terminate the behavior without assistance. Although it is interesting to have the reports of others concerning the behaviors exhibited, as is customary in many of the social development scales used with handicapped populations (Cain, Levine, & Elzey, 1963; Doll, 1953) these reports are most valuable if used as preliminary identification of areas to be observed rather than documentation of behavioral achievements. Although psychometric testing can be valuable in determining how the individual compares to the behaviors and skills of the large normal population, the testing situation limits the ability to generalize findings to natural settings. For the understanding of social competence, therefore, developmental scales and other testing results are only initial findings rather than data to evaluate interactional competence.

To determine behaviors that occur in natural interactional settings, it is necessary to observe those interactions as they occur. Techniques described by Junker (1960), in which the observer is immersed in the setting, appear to be most fruitful. Research with this participant observation technique is classified by degree of participation: 1) complete participation, in which the

Table 1. Selected social interactional situations for observation

Situation	Variables
Infancy	
Mother; child interaction	Age
Father; child interaction	Age
Sister; child interaction	Age; birth order
Brother; child interaction	Age; birth order
Interaction with extended family members	Relationship; amount of contact
Interaction with babysitters	Occasional; in-home; day care, nursery school; nanny
Early childhood	
Response to other infants	Age; size of group; amount of contact
Response to nonhandicapped children	Age; size of group; amount of contact
Interaction with others with Down syndrome	Age; size of group; amount of contact
Interaction with non–Down syndrome handicapped children	Age; size of group; amount of contact
Play behavior	Solitary; parallel; group; large and small play objects
Development of self-care skills	Quality of response; autonomy
Interaction with visitors in home	Frequency; children; teen; adult friends of self; friends of sibs; friends of parents
Interaction with household employees	Housekeeper; gardener; appliance repairperson
Relationship to neighbors	Proximity; children; teen; adults
Relationship to church congregation	Age; sex; role status
School years	
Relationship to students in same class	Age; sex; achievement
Relationship to students in other special class	Age; sex; achievement; proximity
Relationship to students who share same bus	Age; sex; pick-up points
Relationship to students in regular class	Attending same school; friends of sibs
Relationship to students in same extracurricular class	Swim, music, dance, etc.; sex; handicapped; Down syndrome; public; private
Relationship to others in Special Olympics program	Administrators; coaches; other players; age; sex; location; skill in activity
Relationship to others in school and church socials	With family; with class; with self; age; sex
Community recreation events	With group; with family; by self
Same sex friend	Age; classroom placement

(continued)

Table 1. (*continued*)

Situation	Variables
Opposite sex friend	Age; classroom placement
Pets	Personal; family; care duties; relationship with
Spending money	Earns own; handles independently; makes purchases by self
Teen and adult years	
Socials planned by others	School; church; family; recreation; age; sex; alone; group intergrated/ segregated by sex, by handicapping condition; day or overnight
Socials planned by self	As above
Group dates or dances	Planned by outside group, family, self
Long-term relationships	Sex; age; location; parent support
Informal interaction with others	Phone; mail; public transportation for social activities
Responsibility for own living area	Cleans own room or living area; assists with moving furniture, painting, minor repairs
Attends post–high school training	Lives at home, in dorm, in apartment
Has steady boy/girl friend	Engagement; marriage; children
Purchases own transportation	Bicycle; motor bike/cycle; car
Pays for living quarters	Rent; purchase
Plans own meals	Menu; purchase; prepare; clean up
Chooses own clothing	From closet; from store
Worksite	
Competitive employment	Secures own job; has rehab support; relationship to supervisor
Sheltered employment	Training; supervision; age; sex; health; academic skill
Work relationships	Other workers—handicapped or non-handicapped; lunch and break patterns; transportation
Amount of earnings	By task/hour; quality of work

observer takes the role identical to those whom he or she is observing, and others in the setting do not know that observations are being made; 2) participation in which the participant takes the role of those being observed, but all parties know of the study; 3) participation in which an observer goes to the site and spends a day or two interviewing and observing, but is not immersed in the life experiences of the group; and 4) complete observation, in which there is no interaction between those being observed and the observer, and the identity of the observer is withheld (by one-way mirrors or by staying at a distance). This technique has been used to study interactions on the worksite of mentally retarded workers. A form of participant observation has also been used as a technique to develop an understanding of the life situations of mentally retarded persons by having nonretarded individuals live with them (Wolfensberger & Vanier, 1974). A situation similar to observer as a participant has been suggested by Michaelis (1980), in which observers are sent into the homes of handicapped children in order to "follow the child" through a 12-hour period and quantify the interactional patterns. More thorough data of this type are necessary in order to make a description of the behaviors that are occurring and the frequency of those behaviors. Participant observation techniques have not been used to complete advantage in order to study the life of the individual with Down syndrome.

Another technique that could be used to advantage to study the social maturity of the individual with Down syndrome would be to study language interaction patterns in a natural setting. Recorded and transcribed language samples can be used to determine the cognitive developmental level and the linguistic sophistication (Brown, 1973; Michaelis, 1976). Schiefelbusch (1981) postulated that since language is a social tool used to interact with others, competence in language can be used as an index for social competence. He believes that the evaluation of language as an interaction/communicative process is a valuable measure of the social competence of the individual. Transcribed language samples (Michaelis, 1976) of individuals with Down syndrome indicate a difference in cognitive structure of language. It is quite possible that an investigation of the social/interactional components of language in the natural setting would yield further understanding of the social maturity of individuals with Down syndrome (Pickett & Flynn, 1983). Some study has occurred with the social language patterns of some mentally retarded individuals which indicates that speech patterns are altered depending on the status of the person to whom the individual is speaking (Michaelis, 1976). These data appear to indicate that in order to study communicative competence, it would be necessary to examine that competence in several interactive situations. It is quite possible that the person with Down syndrome has competent communicative skills with family and neighbors, but has a great deal of difficulty with clerks in stores and supervisors at the job site (Crapps, Langone, & Swaim, 1985; Gaule, Nietupski, & Certo, 1985). This would seem to be a natural developmental sequence, as most children are able to interact more effectively with those in the home than they are with others outside the immediate intimate circle. It may be that this difficulty with interaction with "strangers" is prolonged for the individual with Down syndrome. It is difficult to measure communicative competence without more naturalistic language data.

Another method of investigation is to ask the individual what he or she thinks, feels, and wants. If these questions were to be posed to the individual with Down syndrome, more accurate data could be gathered if the questions were used in interview format. Particularly due to communication difficulties mentioned above, it would probably be most effective to have the interviewer be someone who has had experience communicating with individuals who have Down syndrome. This technique can be used with specific questions that have open-ended responses or questions that specify multiple choice responses. Orlansky and Heward (1981) used this technique for open-ended interviews with handicapped persons. Unfortunately, none of these interviews was conducted with an individual with Down syndrome. Perske (Nathan, 1976), in materials prepared for the President's Committee on Mental Retardation, interviewed several individuals with Down syndrome. Materials presented in the *National Down Syndrome Congress Newsletter* and *Sharing Our Caring* indicate that life adjustment occurs in more than isolated cases. Although these anecdotal case data are interesting, they cannot be used as a basis for description of how a large majority of individuals with Down syndrome are conducting their personal/social lives, nor can they be used as a description of the usual development for most individuals. It is necessary to gather data on a sizeable representative sample of individuals with Down syndrome living in various life situations in order to make any kind of generalized statements about typical life experiences.

Comparison to normal maturational stages and to normal "rites of passage" may be of interest in explaining the depth of the handicapping condition; but to describe the psychological maturity of the individual with Down syndrome, it would be much more productive to approach the study with a tabula rasa and to see what is actually there, not in comparison to what is there in the lives of others. It would be productive to observe the selection and use of various objects, of clothing, of food, of companions, and of recreational facilities. In the observational data collected by observations in homes, for instance, it was found that handicapped children living at home watch an unusually large amount of television and that television viewing is usually done without other members of the household present (Michaelis, 1980).

Evaluation Battery for Individuals with Down Syndrome

Frequently, when psychological evaluation is made, the purposes of the tests being administered are forgotten and the scores are reported as if they represented more than the test was designed to measure. For example, intelligence tests were first developed in France to identify children who would have difficulty in the school classroom, if no individual adjustments were made (Flavell, 1963). Current intelligence tests have been somewhat altered and changed to deal with more current information and for ease of administration (Berry & Gunn, 1984; Chronbach, 1970; Rice, 1979); however, the purpose is still the same (Klein, 1977). In many cases, the results of an intelligence (psychological) examination is redundant to information already known by parents and teachers. Most parents and teachers already know that the child with Down syndrome will not be successful in the regular classroom unless some adjustments are made. What is not known is what the child is able to do well, or exactly how regular classroom work needs to be adjusted in order to meet the needs of the child, or how work stations or work settings need to be designed in order for the individual to be productive. It is already known that the individual with Down syndrome will need some adaptations. What is not known is exactly what these adaptations should be.

Important questions not currently being addressed are: "What are the strengths of individuals with Down syndrome?" "What types of situations are most successful for them?" It has not been determined, except by personal case observations, that the individual with Down syndrome is indeed the "loveable child." And if that child is loveable, what happens to that loveable child when the child becomes an adult? It is also not known if being loveable is indeed a productive response in all situations. It would appear that being loveable may not always be the most mature response and that, at times, the individual with Down syndrome would show more maturity by being angry or hostile. (From the observation of the behavior of individuals with Down syndrome, society might begin to ponder the maturity represented in laws and courts and wars.)

Physical conditions examined repeatedly by medical evaluation show up, of course, in atlantoaxial instability (Howard, 1985) and in fine motor difficulties (Elliott, 1985), but how are these related to the development of significant skills? What do they mean to the learning of games and other recreational activities? How do they affect the development of grooming skills? Do they interfere with the individual use of the telephone, shower, or the sewing machine, or make it more difficult to count change? Most of the data on learning relate to school-oriented tasks. It would be important to know if physical conditions determine or limit the development of skills usually thought to be produced by socially mature individuals. Certainly the oral structures of persons with Down syndrome make the producing of speech sounds more difficult (Cromer, 1974; McDonald, 1980). How does this relate to confidence in social communication? It appears that there are neurological differences in the processing of auditory information for individuals with Down syndrome (Lincoln, Courchesne, Kilman, & Galambos, 1985). It is not known how these differences relate to reception of language and social interaction.

Perhaps of most importance in the evaluation of social development is the ability to react quickly and efficiently in problem-solving situations. Is it difficult for the individual with Down syndrome to find an adequate way to perform in a new situation? How much difficulty does the individual with Down syndrome have in meeting new people and in speaking to individuals who are directing service situations? How much difficulty does the individual with Down syndrome have in requesting assistance when the solution does not seem to be readily available?

Other important questions are: In what social situations are most individuals with Down syndrome successful? Is it important to have regularly schedules activities, or can individuals with Down syndrome enjoy spontaneous, spur-of-the-moment activities? How can individuals with Down syndrome learn to plan, and to execute those plans? How do individuals with Down syndrome relate to other handicapped persons? Is relating different if those other persons have Down syndrome, too? Do individuals with Down syndrome like to be with nonhandicapped persons more than they like to be with handicapped persons? Who are the "best friends" of persons with Down syndrome? Does that change as the person gets older?

Results of the Evaluation

The observation and evaluation should be in the form of a procedure that is designed not to see where deficiencies occur, but to see what characteristics are actually present. It is important to know what characteristics are present in order to nurture socially appropriate behavior. It is also possible that this information may broaden the concepts of what constitutes significant developmental steps in the general (larger) population as well. It is highly possible that the investigation could find that persons with Down syndrome possess characteristics that demonstrate not the usual kind of maturity, but a deeper, more holistic respect for human worth. Certainly these characteristics have been described anecdotally by parents, families, and others who have had the opportunity to know individuals with Down syndrome personally. Parents describe changes in their perspective, their value systems, and their mode of life after the birth of a child with Down syndrome (Michaelis, 1977; Tingey-Michaelis, 1985). Siblings can grow with a sense of giving and purpose that cannot be described by the usual order of developmental sequences (Edmunson, 1985; Grossman, 1972; Michaelis, 1980).

Obviously, of course, these growth patterns represent struggle. This struggle to understand and develop and grow toward a maturity, faced by the individual with Down syndrome and the family of that individual, may not be represented in the stages described by Erikson, Piaget, or Bandura. An observational study may develop a way of looking at another maturity, a maturity represented by genuine compassion and warmth toward others regardless of perceived talents, capabilities, and possessions. Perhaps this perspective could describe a richer, fuller maturation unmarked by the typical "rites of passage," levels of struggle, cognitive steps, imitative sequences, and established definitions of maturity. Perhaps the "new" maturity is marked by the distinct lack of egocentricity and by the intensity of desire on the part of the individual with Down syndrome to be actively participating with and caring for those who share the life space.

Harris (1967) described a life space in which individuals provide unconditional love toward one another, given not because something is expected in return, or in order to be granted favors, but given from a desire to give. It may just be that this type of maturity is reached sooner for the individual whose life struggle must include the necessity to understand, but without the usual cognitive capacities to facilitate understanding. The struggle to understand when understanding is more difficult may result in the understanding of things that are not explainable by cognitive examination.

ATTITUDES ABOUT INDIVIDUALS WITH DOWN SYNDROME

It is more acceptable for a person with Down syndrome to appear in public than it was a few years ago, or so one is told. Although it is important to know if the individual is newsworthy, it is perhaps more important to know exactly how that person is treated as he or she interacts in the everyday world with everyday neighbors when he or she is doing ordinary everyday things.

Although it may be exciting for a few minutes to be carrying the Special Olympics Banner in the parade and later cross the screen on the evening news, it may be far more important to be able to carry a serving tray unnoticed in the line at McDonald's. Although it is exciting to be a poster child and have a printed picture appear in the local shopping mall, having a comfortable share of informal pictures in the school yearbook and the family photo album can be far more important.

Dybwad (1985) has indicated that some professionals tend to evaluate the individual with Down syndrome as less than a person. Although there is no indication that such an attitude is widespread, advocates may well take notice in order to discover why, under certain conditions, some professionals in the field may be unwilling to allow full personhood to the individual with Down syndrome.

If one is to deal effectively with attitudes in relation to Down syndrome, those attitudes must be separated into at least two categories: 1) the attitudes of others toward those with Down syndrome, and 2) the attitudes of persons with Down syndrome toward themselves. There has not been systematic collection of data for either of these topics.

Attitudes of Others Toward Individuals with Down Syndrome

Information about the attitude of a wide variety of people is needed in order to make any statements about the progression toward making daily life activities at home and in public comfortable (Beckman, 1984). Information is also needed about everyday life events of people with Down syndrome. There is a need to know the life events of those who share home and life space with individuals who have Down syndrome. Moses (1985) has described a pain that comes to the family of an individual with Down syndrome and has indicated that the family must adjust to the loss of the dream of a "perfect child." There is, therefore, a need to know the impact of the adjustment on the family.

It is, of course, significant to have conferences about, special days/ months dedicated to, and fundraising for, the "condition" of Down syndrome. That, however, is not enough. To understand how inadequate it is to deal with those who have Down syndrome with only a special focus, think of being able to go out only when someone is willing to take you somewhere. For most adults, this prospect is indeed a limiting one. Most adults are used to being able to do what they want, when they want, and how they want. They are used to being looked at when they want and to be alone when they want, and not having their personal desires subordinated to decisions made by others. It is not enough to know that some special things are happening. It is important to know what ordinary things are happening to individuals with Down syndrome and to those who love them. (A selected sample of attitudes of others that need to be observed and described is presented in Table 2.)

Attitudes Toward Themselves

It is also highly important to know what individuals with Down syndrome think about themselves. In his delightful description of events in his life, Nigel Hunt (1967) showed a close attachment and love toward his parents and a confident feeling about his ability to write about himself and the things that he had been doing. Later, after both parents had died, Nigel was no longer as confident about his ability to interact with others. Individuals with Down syndrome as children may have different attitudes about themselves and their capabilities than they do as they get older. One has only to think of one's own childhood to remember when, it was believed, anything was possible. Certainly individuals with Down syndrome would make more realistic evaluations of their potential as they become older. It is not known just what this evaluation is. Although it has sometimes been assumed that a disabled person of necessity must have what the general public thinks of as a "low self-concept", it is not known if this is true. Those who understand the mental health field are very much aware of differences in individual ability to tolerate stress. If we define stress as a situation that requires more attention and effort than the ordinary (Selye, 1956), then certainly the condition of Down syndrome and its concurrent learning difficulties can be categorized as a stressor (Intagliata & Doyle, 1984). It would seem that, although the condition is a stressor for the individual who has it, there is no evidence to indicate that the condition produces the same amount of stress for all who have it. Certainly concurrent physical problems and the treatment necessary for those conditions cause additional stress, but even that may not affect different individuals in the same way.

It is not only important to know how individuals with Down syndrome

Table 2.   Selected attitudes of others to investigate

General public
  Neighbors
  Family friends
  Cultural leaders
  Civic leaders/personnel
  Political figures
General service delivery personnel
  Public transportation
      Air; city bus; cross-country bus; train
  Police; guards
  Firefighters
  Ticket takers
      Parks; sports events; theaters; concerts
  Checkout clerks
      Variety stores; grocery stores
  Clerks
      Department stores; banks; music stores
  Food service
      Owner/manager
      Waiter/waitress
      Fast food; cafeteria; formal dining
  Medical
      Doctor; dentist; nurse
      Private practice; public service
  Librarian
      City library; children's library; school library
  Recreation personnel
      City parks; amusement parks; national parks; campgrounds; swimming pools;
        gymnasiums
  Business personnel
      Locally owned; neighborhood; shopping mall; corporation; chain store
  Hotel/motel
      Major city hotels; small hotels; suburban motels; chains
  Advertising
      National advertisement; local advertisement
      TV; radio; newspaper
  Child care personnel
      Day care; nursery schools; babysitters; nannies
  School system
      Students; teachers; administrators; custodial staff
Specific service delivery personnel
  Specialized residential
      Geriatric; mental illness; substance abuse; developmental
  Social service personnel
      Administration; direct care workers
  Special education
      Administrators; support personnel; teachers; students; custodial

feel about themselves, but also, perhaps to a lesser degree, how they feel
about others who have Down syndrome. To have accurate answers to these
questions, it will be necessary to have descriptions of attitudes such as those
shown in Table 3.

Table 3. Selected attitudes of individuals with Down syndrome for observation

Attitude	Variables
Toward self	Age
Toward others of same sex	Age; proximity; handicap
Toward others of opposite sex	Age; proximity; handicap
Toward various family members	Age; birth order; sex
Toward individuals in service delivery system	Teachers; directors; social workers

Methods of Investigation

Methods of investigation for attitudes and beliefs are more representative of the actual behavior of the individual if a specific behavioral question is phrased, for example, "If you got on a bus and there were two seats left, one by the door and one by a person with Down syndrome, which seat would you take?" rather than a question that asked, "Would you be uncomfortable sitting on a bus next to a person with Down syndrome?" (Jones & Davis, 1965). It would seem that such a system of inquiry could represent the attitudes of others toward the individual with Down syndrome much more thoroughly than what is acceptable to print in the newspaper or show on the television screen. Although this form of inquiry could be used to assess the attitudes of the individual with Down syndrome toward himself or herself, it would need to be facilitated by investigators who are familiar with the speech/communication patterns of individuals with Down syndrome, as free and open discussion with strangers is usually somewhat difficult for many individuals with Down syndrome (Cardoso-Martins, Mervis, & Mervis, 1985; Davies & Rogers, 1985). Another method of investigation would also be necessary for young children. Methods similar to those used in sociograms (Kuhlen & Collister, 1952) could be adapted to request whom they would share a toy with, or simply to observe how play patterns naturally occurred (e.g., When given a choice, will a young child with Down syndrome choose to play with another child with Down syndrome, a child with a different handicap, or a child with no handicap? Of course, in each of these situations, it is extremely important to know if the child was an acquaintance or a stranger.).

FAMILIES OF INDIVIDUALS WITH DOWN SYNDROME

Frequently, data about families of handicapped children are lumped together as if to indicate that the response of a family to one kind of condition is similar to the response to another condition (Allen & Affleck, 1985; Chinn, Winn, & Walters, 1978; Noland, 1970). Highly skilled researchers are taught to examine each of the variables (reasons) separately to be certain that the conclusions drawn are, in fact, related to the condition being studied. Data about families of handicapped children have not been kept separate, and statements made by and about families of children with one kind of problem have been generalized to families with children who have other problems. Although this contributes to a simple, descriptive picture of parenting handicapped children for use by professionals, the data are so poorly categorized as to be not only of little scientific importance, but actually contributing to unwarranted conclusions. For example, families of children with muscular dystrophy face very few of the same concerns of families of children with learning disabilities. The care of and emotional response to an autistic child has very little in common with the care of a child who has spina bifida. There are also differences in diagnostic situations. Children with hearing problems may not be identified for a year or two, but infants with Down syndrome are usually identified in the delivery room or shortly thereafter. In order to make descriptions of the family system where there is a child with Down syndrome, as Turnbull and Summers suggest (Chapter 11, this volume), it will be necessary to look at each variable in that system carefully. There is a long list of variables about conditions and families that have not been investigated separately.

Some of these that specifically relate to the family of the child with Down syndrome are:

What is the impact of immediate identification on concurrent and later family adjustment?

What kinds of additional adjustment problems do families of children born with heart and other health problems face?

Do siblings of children with Down syndrome have certain adjustments to make, and are those adjustments different if the child is older/younger? same/different sex?

What kind of adjustments do professional, blue collar, and lower class families who have children with Down syndrome face?

Does family income affect the adjustment of the family?

Do members of families with children with Down syndrome participate more in the planning of the child's individualized education program (IEP) than parents of children with other disabilities?

How much are various family members involved as intervenors in the implementation of school-related goals?

Exactly how much do various members of families with children with Down syndrome participate in the training of life-related goals at home?

Exactly what do these family members do for the child and how do they feel about doing it?

There is also a series of other questions about the family that need to be understood. Since it is a condition that is present at birth, are there more

Table 4. Selected family relationships for observation in birth family

Family members	Variables
Mother	Time spent; closeness
Father	Time spent; closeness
Maternal grandparents	Time spent; closeness
Paternal grandparents	Time spent; closeness
Maternal aunts and uncles	Time spent; closeness
Paternal aunts and uncles	Time spent; closeness
Maternal cousins	Birth order; age
Paternal cousins	Birth order; age
Sisters	Birth order; age
Brothers	Birth order; age
Brother or sister from multiple birth	Health; sex; handicap

concerns about the possibility of additional children in the family being born handicapped? There are also some general concerns that need to be investigated in relation to having a child with Down syndrome in the family (Gath & Gumley, 1984). Some of these would be the characteristics and attitudes of other family members, such as those shown in Table 4.

Family constellations are not always "traditional" (i.e., father, mother, and natural children). The relationships developed through caregiving situations in families do not describe the total variables that may be significant in understanding the family. When he was striving for status on a little league team, one 11-year-old told the team members that his brother, 3 years older, who has Down syndrome, was adopted (N. Michaelis, personal communication, June, 1971). This statement was apparently necessary not to remove the day-to-day interaction with the brother, but to take away the possibility of the taunting that his sister was getting from a boy up the street. "If your brother is retarded, you must be, too!" (T. Michaelis, personal communication, January, 1970). Certainly, families who adopt a child with Down syndrome do not need to be subjected to the emotionally painful genetic counseling experience. A step-parent is also not held "responsible" for the condition. These and other differences need to be investigated separately. Some of these variables are:

Step relationships
Relationships due to marriage
When the child is adopted
If other children in the family have died
If the child has uncorrected heart problems
If the child has corrected heart defects

If the child has other concurrent handicaps (vision, epilepsy, cerebral palsy, etc.)

In addition to descriptive situations, it is also necessary to make some observations of exactly what is occurring in the home. There have been some observations of mother and child interaction to explain language, but unfortunately, these are largely conducted only when the child is young. Older children interacting with the mother or children of any age interacting with other family members have not been studied. Although self-report is important in the identification of domains for study, it must be supplemented by observational data.

It would also seem important to investigate the family's attitudes about the advice, counseling, and service that has been provided to the family. Although this could be examined by questionnaire, it is important that open-ended descriptions also be gathered so that parents and other family members have an opportunity to respond according to their own feelings and mind-set. Although a negative response set should not be developed, it may be necessary to encourage honest responses rather than the sugar-coated "best thing that has happened to our family" or the typical "wonderful person" responses that many "accepting" people have come to be expected to say (Grossman, 1972). No child, handicapped or nonhandicapped, is "wonderful" all of the time. No parent, and no brother or sister should be expected to enjoy any child *all of the time*. To attempt to do so would be unrealistic. One brother of a boy with Down syndrome summed it up during a frustrating table conversation by coolly asking his brother: "Do you have to be retarded all the time?" (N. Michaelis, personal communication, February, 1975). Unfortunately, the answer is "Yes." It would be unrealistic to assume that mental retardation is not at times frustrating—to everyone, particularly to those who share day-to-day intimate interaction!

What is not known about having Down syndrome all of the time is exactly how that predicts or is correlated with developmental events, attitudes, and family life. If definite statements about psychosocial development in Down syndrome are to be made, scientific investigation must occur. Perhaps society has now developed to the point that the stigma has been set aside enough to no longer fear observing and describing the significant variables in the lives of individuals with Down syndrome and their families.

REFERENCES

Allen, D. A., & Affleck, G. (1985). Are we stereotyping parents? *Mental Retardation, 23*(4), 200.

Bandura, A. (1969). *Principles of behavior modification.* New York: Holt, Rinehart & Winston.

Bandura, A. (1977). *Social learning theory.* Englewood Cliffs, NJ: Prentice-Hall.

Bandura, A., Ross, D., & Ross, S. A. (1963). Imitation of film-mediated aggressive models. *Journal of Abnormal and Social Psychology, 66,* 3–11.

Bandura, A., & Walters, R. (1959). *Adolescent aggression.* New York: Ronald Publishers.

Beckman, P. J. (1984). Perceptions of young children with handicaps: A comparison of mothers and program staff. *Mental Retardation, 22*(4), 176–181.

Benda, C. E. (1969). *Down's syndrome: Mongolism and its management* (rev. ed.). New York: Grune & Stratton.

Berry, P., & Gunn, P. (1984). Maternal influence on the task behavior of young Down syndrome children. *Journal of Mental Deficiency Research, 24*(4), 269–274.

Berry, P., Groeneweg, G., Gibson, D., & Brown, R. I. (1984). Mental development of adults with Down syndrome. *American Journal of Mental Deficiency, 89*(3), 252–256.

Blacher, J. (1984). Sequential stages of parental adjustment to the birth of a child with handicaps: Fact or artifact? *Mental Retardation, 22*(2), 55–68.

Brian, S. (1984). Down syndrome: "These our beloved children." *Early Child Development and Care, 15*(4), 281–289.

Brown, R. (1973). *A first language.* Cambridge, MA: Harvard University Press.

Cain, L. F., Levine, S., & Elzey, F. F. (1963). *Manual for the Cain-Levine Social Competency Scale.* Palo Alto, CA: Consulting Psychologists Press.

Cardoso-Martin, C., & Mervis, C. B. (1985). Maternal speech to prelinguistic children with Down syndrome. *American Journal of Mental Deficiency, 89*(5), 451–458.

Cardoso-Martin, C., Mervis, C. B., & Mervis, C. A. (1985). Early vocabulary acquisition by children with Down syndrome. *American Journal of Mental Deficiency, 90*(2), 177–184.

Chinn, P., Winn, J., & Walters, R. H. (1978). *Two-way talking with parents of special children.* St. Louis: C. V. Mosby.

Chronbach, L. J. (1970). *Essentials of psychological testing.* New York: Harper & Row.

Crapps, J. M., Langone, J., & Swaim, S. (1985). Quantity and quality of participation in community environments by mentally retarded adults. *Education and Training of the Mentally Retarded, 20*(2), 123–129.

Cromer, R. F. (1974). Receptive language in the mentally retarded: Processes and diagnostic distinctions. In R. L. Schiefelbusch & L. L. Lloyd (Eds.), *Language perspectives: Acquisition, retardation, and intervention* (pp. 237–268). Baltimore: University Park Press.

Davies, R. R., & Rogers, E. S. (1985). Social skills training with persons who are mentally retarded. *Mental Retardation, 23*(4), 186–196.

Doll, E. A. (1953). *A manual for the Vineland Social Maturity Scale: The measurement of social competence.* Minneapolis: Educational Test Bureau.

Dybwad, G. (1985, April). [Response to: Perske, R. *Attitudes, acceptance, and awareness*]. Paper presented at the Down Syndrome State-of-the-Art Conference, Boston.

Edmunson, K. (1985). The "discovery" of siblings. *Mental Retardation, 23*(2), 49–51.

Elliott, D. (1985). Manual asymmetries in the performance of sequential movement by adolescents and adults with Down syndrome. *American Journal of Mental Deficiency, 90*(1), 90–97.

Erikson, E. (1963). *Childhood and society.* New York: Norton.

Flavell, J. (1963). *The developmental psychology of Jean Piaget.* Princeton, NJ: D. Van Nostrand.

Gath, A., & Gumley, D. (1984). Down syndrome and the family. *Developmental Medicine and Child Neurology, 24*(4), 500–508.

Gaule, K., Nietupski, J., & Certo, N. (1985). Teaching supermarket shopping skills using an adaptive shopping list. *Education and Training of the Mentally Retarded, 2*(1), 53–59.

Greenberg, R., & Field, T. (1982). Temperament ratings of handicapped infants during classroom, mother, and teacher interaction. *Journal of Pediatric Psychology, 7*(4), 387–405.

Grossman, F. K. (1972). *Brothers and sisters of retarded children.* Syracuse, NY: Syracuse University Press.

Hallahan, D. P., & Kauffman, J. M. (1978). *Exceptional children: Introduction to special education.* Englewood Cliffs, NJ: Prentice-Hall.

Harris, T. A. (1967). *I'm OK, you're OK.* New York: Harper & Row.

Howard, W. D. (1985). Atlanto-axial instability in Down syndrome: The need for awareness. *Mental Retardation, 23*(4), 197–199.

Hunt, N. (1967). *The world of Nigel Hunt: A diary of a mongoloid youth.* New York: Garrett Publications.

Inhelder, B. (1968). *The diagnosis of reasoning in the mentally retarded.* New York: John Day Co.

Intagliata, J., & Doyle, N. (1984). Enhancing social support for parents of developmentally delayed children: Training in interpersonal problem solving skills. *Mental Retardation, 22*(1), 4–11.

Jagiello, G. (1981). Reproduction in Down syndrome. In F. F. de la Cruz & P. S. Gerald, (Eds.). *Trisomy 21 (Down Syndrome)* (pp. 151–162). Baltimore: University Park Press.

Jones, E. E., & Davis, K. E. (1965). From acts to disposition: The attribution process in personal perception. In L. Berkowitz (Ed.), *Advances in social psychology* (Vol. 2, pp. 219–266). New York: Academic Press.

Junker, B. (1960). *Field work: An introduction to the social sciences.* Chicago: University of Chicago Press.

Klein, S. D. (1977). *Psychological testing of children: A consumer's guide.* Boston: Exceptional Parent Press.

Kuhlen, R. G., & Collister, E. C. (1952). Sociometric status of sixth- and ninth-graders who fail to finish high school. *Educational Psychology Measurement, 12,* 632–637.

Lincoln, A. J., Courchesne, E., Kilman, B. A., & Galambos, R. (1985). Neuropsychological correlates of information processing by children with Down syndrome. *American Journal of Mental Deficiency, 89*(4), 403–414.

McDonald, E. T. (1980). Early identification and treatment of children at risk for speech development. In R. L. Schiefelbusch (Ed.), *Nonspeech language analysis and intervention* (pp. 49–80). Baltimore: University Park Press.

Michaelis, C. T. (1976). *The language of a Down syndrome child.* Unpublished doctoral dissertation, University of Utah, Salt Lake City.

Michaelis, C. T. (1971). *Concepts of Piaget as a basis for productive thinking activities for the retarded.* Unpublished master's thesis, University of Utah, Salt Lake City.

Michaelis, C. T. (1977). Merry Christmas Jim, and Happy Birthday. *Exceptional Parent, 7*(3), 6–7.

Michaelis, C. T. (1980). *Home and school partnerships in exceptional education.* Rockville, MD: Aspen Systems.

Moses, K. (1985, April). *Socialization and maturation.* Paper presented at the Down Syndrome State-of-the-Art Conference.

Nathan, R. (Ed.) (1976). *Report to the president on mental retardation: A century of concern.* Washington, DC: President's Committee on Mental Retardation.

Noland, R. L. (1970). *Counseling parents of the mentally retarded.* Springfield, IL: Charles C. Thomas.

Orlansky, M. D., & Heward, W. L. (1981). *Voices interviews with handicapped people.* Columbus, OH: Charles E. Merrill.

Pickett, J. M., & Flynn, P. T. (1983). Language assessment tools for mentally retarded adults: Survey and recommendations. *Mental Retardation, 21*(6), 224–247.

Rice, B. (1979). Brave new world of intelligence testing. *Psychology Today, 13*(9), 15.

Rosine, L., & Martin, L. (1983). Self management training to decrease undesirable behavior of mentally handicapped adults. *Rehabilitation Psychology, 28*(4), 195–205.

Schiefelbusch, R. L. (1981). Development of social competence and incompetence. In M. J. Begab, H. C. Haywood, & H. L. Garber (Eds.), *Psychosocial influences in retarded performance* (pp. 179–196). Baltimore: University Park Press.

Selye, H. (1956). *The stress of life.* New York: McGraw-Hill.

Siegel, E. (1974). *The exceptional child grows.* New York: E. P. Dutton.

Tingey-Michaelis, C. (1985). *Research and practice in Down syndrome: First annual conference report.* Logan: Utah State University.

Wolfensberger, W., & Vanier, J. (1974). *Growing together.* Richmond Hill, Ontario, Canada: Daybreak Publications.

SECTION IV

LIFE
IN THE COMMUNITY

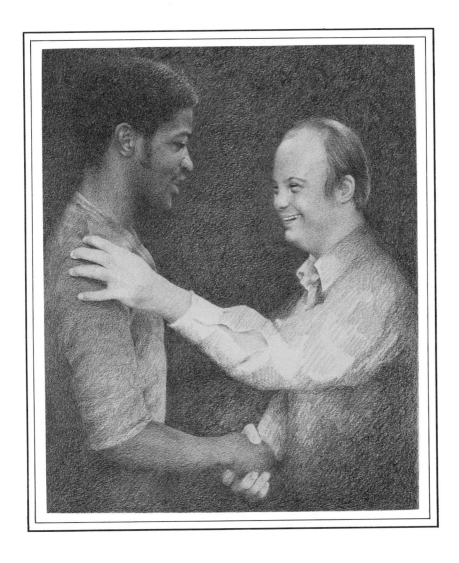

Introduction

Siegfried M. Pueschel

✦✦✦

The foregoing chapters have clearly demonstrated the significant progress that has been made over the past few decades relating to Down syndrome. Scientific advances in medicine, in particular in cardiovascular surgery and in the prevention and treatment of infections, as well as new concepts of general medical care have resulted in a marked increase in the life expectancy of persons with Down syndrome. Consequently, large numbers of youngsters with Down syndrome are now reaching adulthood. Moreover, achievements in developmental psychology and special education have had a significant impact upon the lives of individuals with this chromosome disorder so that many of them are presently better prepared when they enter the worlds of work and community living.

Of course, there are numerous concerns and questions about what individuals with Down syndrome may encounter once they leave school, "when the umbilical cord is cut" and they leave their family. The discussions by Edwards and by Karan and coauthors in this section of the book attempt to answer some of these questions.

In Chapter 13, Edwards explores various living arrangements available for persons with Down syndrome. She points out that the principle of normalization, the establishment of a home-like atmosphere in living quarters, and integration into community life are improvements over the distasteful institutional placements of yesteryear. She emphasizes that interrelated factors such as work and recreation need to be part of community living. She indicates that living arrangements in the community, whatever they may be, must have a built-in developmental continuum that assures the potential for optimal growth of the individual with Down syndrome.

In Chapter 14, Karan, Berger Knight, and Pauls focus on vocational opportunities for persons with Down syndrome and discuss the dynamic "Pathways Model" to employment. This model recognizes the fact that both maturing individuals and working circumstances may change over time. Karan et al. emphasize that persons with Down syndrome may need varying degrees of assistance to maximize their employment potential and that social support systems and other community activities must become integral parts of the world of work.

Although only two important areas of adult life (living arrangements and vocational opportunities) are featured in this section of the book, there are other aspects that should be considered in order to portray a realistic picture of the total person with Down syndrome. Some of these aspects have been discussed in previous sections of this volume, and others cannot be detailed here because of limited space.

In spite of the progress made in past decades, more research efforts and expansion of opportunities and services are needed to lead to a better quality of community life for persons with Down syndrome in future years. Such new developments should also help individuals with Down syndrome develop their own identity and autonomy. The rights and privileges of persons with Down syndrome, as citizens in a democratic society, must be protected in order to preserve their human dignity.

Chapter 13

Living Options
for Persons
with Down Syndrome

Jean Edwards

✦ ✦ ✦

Over the past 20 years, there has been a strong movement toward providing more normal experiences for persons with Down syndrome and other forms of mental retardation. This movement is based largely on the normalization principle, which emphasizes "making available to the mentally retarded patterns and conditions of everyday life which are as close as possible to the norms and patterns of the mainstream of society" (Nirje, 1969a, p. 181).

Services for persons with mental retardation in Scandinavia, where the normalization principle is more firmly embodied in their ideology, have become a model for developing services for persons with Down syndrome in North America. Smaller "integrated" residential facilities have been developed in conjunction with deinstitutionalization programs, and school systems have adopted "integration" and "mainstreaming" policies. Federal mandates have opened up equal education opportunities for persons with mental retardation, and efforts are being made to provide nonsheltered employment for persons with Down syndrome and other forms of mental retardation.

Consistent with this trend toward policies of normalization and integration, advocacy for comprehensive services for children and adults with Down syndrome has been increasing. Envisioned is a continuum of services that would provide an individual from infancy on with an interrelated series of educational, recreational, vocational, and residential programs. Although it is difficult to separate the sphere of residential services from the other three, it can be argued that one's residence should form the basis of any service delivery system (Kugel & Wolfensberger, 1969). When a person with Down syndrome no longer lives with his or her parents and is not yet able to live on his or her own, social agencies customarily intervene to provide some other place to live. This chapter, then, dicusses the emerging residential alternatives to the institution-oriented practices of the past. It focuses primarily on residences for adults.

The current renaissance of community-based services for persons with Down syndrome and other forms of mental retardation has been spurred largely by the principle of normalization. The dominant view today is that young people with Down syndrome should enjoy the residential setting of family homes, be integrated into neighborhoods, and make use of generic community resources. This view results from an increasing distaste for segregated institutions, and a reaction against the separation and depersonalization frequently associated with large institutions.

NORMALIZATION

There are several definitions of normalization. This chapter discusses just two of the major ones.

The first is credited to Bank-Mikkleson who defined normalization as "letting the mentally retarded obtain an existence as close to normal as possible" (Nirje, 1969b, p. 181). This sums up the principle very simply. Unfortunately, it may be too simple. Often, staff members working with persons with mental retardation interpret the definition as requiring only "common sense" thinking. The problems usually emerge from the phrase "as close to normal as possible." It is often easy for staff members of residential programs to think that they and their residents have come as close as possible to normal, because common sense tells them that persons who are mentally retarded have a lot of limitations.

Traditionally, most people have had very low expectations for persons with Down syndrome and they, in turn, have often lived up to those low expectations. The challenge of normalization is to try to set aside old stereotypes, and traditional expectations and approaches, and to treat persons with Down syndrome in the same manner that one treats anyone else.

In order to understand normalization, one needs to take a look at the word "normal." In Bank-Mikkelson's definition, normal denotes that which is considered typical by the general society. For example, it is considered normal for adults to work. Although there are exceptions, it is customary to think that normal adults will support themselves, their families, and the community by being members of the work force. In this sense, "normal" does not imply value or quality, but instead reflects what is considered the norm, or what is typical, by others.

When normalization is applied to a residential setting, many areas of an individual's life are affected. A resident is expected to learn how to act, to look appropriate, and to engage in normal behaviors. The group with whom the resident lives must be one for whom there exists a comparative normal group in the mainstream of society. For example, it is typical for young adults to live together, but it is not normal for a young person to live in a nursing home. The way in which the staff members interact with the residents should typify the way in which they interact with other, nonhandicapped people.

The second definition of normalization, developed by the Accreditation Council for Services for Mentally Retarded and Other Developmentally Disabled Persons (ACMRDD), emphasizes "the principle of helping individuals who are developmentally disabled to obtain an existence as close to normal as possible, by making available to them patterns and conditions of everyday life that are as close as possible to the norms and patterns of the mainstream of society" (McCarthy, 1980, p. 23).

This definition provides more direction. It implies that the models to be followed in delivering services to persons with mental retardation are to be sought in the community, and that desired behaviors are those being displayed by successful members of the community and neighborhood.

Normal patterns and conditions of everyday life include experiencing the same daily, weekly, and yearly routines that most people do; normal conditions mean living in the same type of housing as do other people of the same age. For children with Down syndrome, this means being part of a family; for adults it can mean living on their own, living with a friend, or living with a group of friends.

Normal routines and rhythms need to be made available. This may mean rising when their neighbors do, eating breakfast with those they live with, and then going to work. Ideally, work would be in the community, in a restructured or modified job, or it would be in a sheltered workshop or activity center. This establishes the fact that just as most adults work, so should most adults with Down syndrome.

In that most people work five days and have two days off, this normal weekly rhythm must also be a part of residential living for persons with Down syndrome. Individualized training programs are needed to teach young people how to develop a hobby. It is important that staff members take an objective look at the routines existing in the group home and ask themselves whether they would find these same routines occurring with the same frequency and intensity in a normal house across the street. If the answer is "no," then these routines should be examined to ascertain whether they are based on valid, programmatic rationale, or whether these non-normalized routines are occurring for some other reason. For example, many group homes have chore charts that indicate someone is to wash the kitchen floor daily. Realistically, no one washes floors daily in a typical home. However, if a resident is engaged in learning this skill, he or she may need to practice it daily; but if the floor is washed daily by people already possessing the skill, then a non-normalizing routine has been established that does not benefit the resident and it should be eliminated.

THE DEVELOPMENTAL MODEL

The developmental model is based on the belief that all individuals are capable of growth and development. This growth occurs in a sequence, and this sequence can be modified. Accordingly, developmental programs focus on what people can do and in which direction they will go next. The developmental model sees the person with Down syndrome as a developing person and, therefore, offers the most opportunities for change.

Down syndrome is not viewed as an inability to learn, but rather as a slowed rate of learning. The physical setting, along with normalizing approaches, is used to obtain normal behavior in the individual. In the past, models had a common element: persons with Down syndrome and other forms of mental retardation had no control over what happened to them. The developmental model, then, encourages the person with Down syndrome to interact with the environment and to exercise some control over it. There are, however, no built-in safeguards to eliminate all elements of risk.

In a group home setting, it is appropriate for residents to choose with whom they room, what they wear, and how they spend their free time. They should be able to choose whether to sit in the living room or outside on the porch—everyday choices that most people take for granted, but choices often denied to persons with mental retardation.

The developmental model emphasizes the development of the individual's human qualities. Residents are seen as individuals, not as labels or stereotypes. This emphasis is indicated by the use of individualized educational and training plans and the absence of undue regimentation in the home. Rules are not used to control all possible situations and circumstances. Restrictions on behavior are individualized, and are only used to accommodate the needs of a specific person. The developmental model, coupled with the notion of normalization, results in a home that allows for individual differences. There are opportunities and space for the residents to experience privacy. There are doors on the bedrooms and bathrooms. Residents are encouraged to acquire personal possessions and to apply decorative touches to the living areas.

Because the developmental model assumes that the resident possesses abilities and is a capable person, he or she is encouraged to accept more responsibility in order to achieve a more independent life-style. Residents are viewed as active members of their own habilitation teams. Habilitation itself is seen as a process one undergoes, rather than as a product that one is given.

The most critical element of a home-like design is the presence of normal risks and challenges. As a part of normal development, human beings are expected to learn to cope, thereby developing resourcefulness, judgment, and courage. To help persons with Down syndrome achieve these goals, developmental challenges must be aimed "one notch" higher than the level on which the person is functioning. The environment is not made to be totally safe and accident-free. Protection is provided in the group home, but it is consistent with each person's actual need.

The sincere belief that each person can learn is demonstrated through programs that prepare persons with Down syndrome for subsequent steps or goals in his or her individualized developmental plan. These programs were originally aimed at facilitating growth, movement, and progress. The system then accommodates growth and development with program options that take into account the individual's growth—by providing less structure, more integration into the community, and more normalized conditions in which to learn, work, and live.

RESIDENTIAL MODELS

All community residences are characterized by a group of persons with mental retardation living under staff supervision in a facility outside their parents' home. In the author and her colleagues' research for the state-of-the-art in residential programs for young persons with Down syndrome, they accessed the national data bank on long-term care maintained at the Center for Residential and Community Services at the University of Minnesota, and the Utah State University Affiliated Facility's 1985 report on adult service options for persons with mental retardation and developmental delays (Fifield & Smith, 1985). These data resulted in findings showing that, while there are currently a variety of placement options in the residential services system, the most common residence for people with developmental disabilities is still their natural or family home. Their review included data related to small group homes serving 10 or fewer persons; medium-sized group homes serving 11–20 residents; large group homes serving 21–40 persons; mini-institutions serving 40–80 persons; nursing homes serving 40–100 elderly persons, but with a group of 10–20 persons with mental retardation intermixed; ICFs/MR (intermediate care facilities for the mentally retarded) providing intensive nursing care; foster family arrangements serving 5 or fewer persons; sheltered villages providing a segregated, self-contained community for adults with mental retardation and a live-in staff in a cluster of buildings usually located in a rural setting; and semi-independent adult residences and mid-step apartment programs.

Deinstitutionalization efforts, which have resulted in both the prevention of individuals with mental retardation from entering large institutions and the movement of many out of institutions into the community, have spurred a rapidly changing service system. Generally, these changes lead in four main directions (Fifield & Smith, 1985): 1) from large to small facilities, 2) from public to private agency–operated facilities, 3) from isolated to integrated community environments, and 4) from self-contained to community-dependent resources and generic services. It is currently estimated that young people with mental retardation are leaving large public institutions at a rate of about 6,000 per year (Bruininks, Hill, Lakin, & White, 1985).

An overview of community residential options reveals differences between the models. The more recently developed models (e.g., semi-independent, small group homes, and mid-step apartment programs) are most often based on philosophies of normalization, are more apt to serve young residents, provide a higher degree of autonomy, follow a developmental model plan, ensure daytime work placement, and strive toward the goal of resident involvement in the community. As group homes become larger, however, life within them is apt to become less normalizing. Facilities for more than 45 residents were found to offer considerably lower levels of autonomy, work involvement, and opportunities for developmental movement. Sheltered villages, foster family homes, and nursing homes were more likely to be permanent placements.

Utah's UAF residential services technical report suggested a growing consensus among professionals that the most appropriate care for people with developmental disabilities, regardless of their level of impairment, is provided in smaller, community-based residences (Fifield & Smith, 1985). The author of this chapter also recommends that, in addition to the opportunity for normalized living (i.e., participation in community life and involvement in social, economic, and other developmentally beneficial activities), the smaller the residence, the greater the opportunity for the implementation of the developmental model of training.

No single type of program can provide an appropriate setting for all young people with Down syndrome, since young people with Down syndrome vary as much as any heterogeneous population. Therefore, to facilitate each individual's living as close as possible to the mainstream of society, every region must develop a comprehensive developmental system of residences so that each person with Down syndrome will have the opportunity to grow and to move to the facility most nearly matched with his or her expected maximum level of independence. Bruininks et al. (1985) have suggested that, although numerous community-based care centers exist and provide a continuum of care and have, in doing so, overcome "virtually every identified barrier to obtain the least restrictive placement" (p. 30), it nonetheless remains the case that neither is there much useful information disseminated about these programs, nor are there sustained efforts at replicating their more successful features.

Perhaps the best known comprehensive system is ENCOR, the Eastern Nebraska Community Office of Retardation, which operates 10 developmentally graded models for young people with mental retardation. The ten steps in the ENCOR comprehensive system include: 1) children's hostels, 2) adolescent hostels, 3) adult training hostels, 4) adult family care homes or board-and-care homes, 5) apartment clusters, 6) supervised living units, 7) co-resident apartments, 8) independent living, 9) behavioral development residential hostels and 10) development maximization units. The strengths of the ENCOR model are its commitment to the belief that all of its residents are capable of growth and development, and the day-to-day efforts of each staff person at each residential level to ensure that training is oriented toward maximizing that growth.

DECIDING ON A HOME

Deciding on the most appropriate placement for a young person with Down syndrome is difficult, since it represents a change in life-style both for the person with Down syndrome and for their parents. It will mean new friends, a new home, and perhaps a new neighborhood, presenting new responsibilities and expectations. For the parents, there will be changes relating to their separation from their son or daughter.

The most important question regards who decides what is best for the child. It will be possible, even practical, for some young people with Down syndrome to make their own decisions. However, regardless of how much the young person may be involved in the final decision about a community residence, it needs to be acknowledged that frequently the needs of the parents and those of their adolescent or adult child do not precisely coincide. Conflicts often arise over independence versus protection, proximity to resources versus the quality of the neighborhood, and integration versus separation.

Recommendations for Parents

The following recommendations are made to parents looking at residential options for young people with Down syndrome:

1. Evaluate programs on the basis of their potential to enhance your son's or daughter's strengths, and attempt to identify an atmosphere that best promotes personal growth and development.
2. Visit community residences and talk with staff members, board members, parents of residents, residents themselves, and neighbors.
3. Take your child to visit the residence to solicit feelings, and observe current residents' reactions to him or her.
4. Investigate a variety of residences to get some idea of the diversity among, and the differences between, residences and the services they provide.
5. Spend an evening and eat dinner with the residents and staff so that you can observe firsthand the quality of life at the home.
6. Be familiar with your state's plan for community residences and evaluate how a particular residence fits into the comprehensive picture.
7. Solicit advice from your state's Association for Retarded Citizens or Department of Mental Health, mental retardation section.

This process may be long and involved, so families need to get started early.

Things to Look For

First, note the location of the facility. Does its location afford access to the normal patterns and conditions of everyday life? The area should provide opportunities to use a variety of public centers for shopping, entertainment, recreation, and other growth-stimulating experiences. With these opportunities, a person can learn the daily tasks essential to increasing independence. As persons with Down syndrome expand their realm of interaction, they need to learn how to move around in the larger community. In this way, they gain greater autonomy. Further, by constantly testing their abilities through their interaction with their community, they increase their level of independence.

Second, the physical structure of the building should be appropriate to the physical needs of the individual. Are there architectural barriers? Does the building blend physically with the surrounding neighborhood? The physical structure should in no way isolate the residence from others in the neighborhood. A community is more likely to respond favorably to residences that do not contrast dramatically with other residential structures in the neighborhood.

Third, the residence should provide a program and a setting that allow for a normal daily rhythm. The resident should awaken, eat meals, work, and sleep at the same times as other members of the community. The facility should establish a normal rhythm for the week, that is, allow for leaving the place of residence to go to work or training, to recreational activities, or to perform other normal tasks on a schedule similar to that for the rest of society. This requires separating functions, since it is not normal in our society for people to live and work in the same setting, or to spend all of their leisure time in their residence. Even those who experience severe disabilities must be afforded these considerations.

While working with agency personnel to find the right residence, the author suggests developing with staff members a written agreement which includes a statement of goals, a written plan of action, a commitment to training times, and an enumeration of family responsibilities. This agreement can then serve as a guide for planning and training. It should be discussed frequently, revised periodically, and one should at all times be aware of the implementation status of these plans.

What options, then, are available when, after visiting many programs, one is still unable to decide what is most suitable for the young person's special needs? Unfortunately, there is to date no legislation ensuring the right of all young adults to leave their parents' home and move into an appropriate community residence. This leaves parents in a position where they must either admit their son or daughter into a program that only approximately, and perhaps inadequately, meets his or her needs; keep their child at home; or marshal forces with other parents to develop and create new and more appropriate services. Sometimes it is necessary for parents to initiate services themselves through the auspices of local, private, nonprofit organizations. Advocacy is certainly an option.

A CLOSER LOOK AT RESIDENTIAL OPTIONS

Group Homes

Although group homes vary greatly, most are characterized by a group of persons with mental retardation residing in existing community dwellings that are staffed with supervisors and/or trainers who help them cope with the exigencies of daily life. The concept of group homes grew out of an aversion to enormous, impersonal, and isolated institutions. Consequently, there has grown up advocacy for the alternative of small, family-like dwellings located most often in existing communities, or new homes built in residential neighborhoods. The emphasis in most group homes is on "living as others do."

States vary in their guidelines prescribing the number of residents such homes can accommodate. New York, for example, defines a group home as accommodating 7–12 people; Massachusetts limits a group home to 9 residents; Washington State defines a group home as lodging 20 or fewer persons, and Oregon, 12 or less.

Life in group homes varies not only in size and numbers, but also with the building, the availability of privacy, and the kinds and quality of training available. Usually, group home residents share daily responsibilities, have a private place of their own, and enjoy some of the pleasures of independence. Certainly their lives are still unlike those of most other people, yet for many it may be as near to independence and normalization as is possible.

Larger group homes (13–25 residents) have potential drawbacks, since their larger size may lead to the impersonality, restrictiveness, and custodialism of the institutions they seek to replace. Yet these larger programs can sometimes provide benefits as well, for example, with more differentiated and specialized staff roles.

Small Intensive Care Home

A small intensive care home usually serves five or less residents whose physical, emotional, and social needs are great. An intensive care home provides the maximum level of supervision and support services. Criteria for admission is minimal, and it is assumed that residents in these homes are at basic, beginning levels, and that they require intensive care and support services in order to take the initial steps toward independence. Some areas categorize homes as small care homes simply on the basis of their small size (6–10 residents); however, these homes should not be confused with small *intensive* care homes. An intensive care home is a home that provides comprehensive care and support services, such as speech therapy, occupational therapy, individualized skills training, 24-hour supervision, and an appropriate day program.

ICF/MR

An ICF/MR is another option for persons with mental retardation who require attendant care, but of a lesser degree than those who need to live in an intensive care home. Many of the young people needing this option do not necessarily have major medical needs, but instead require attendant care in the areas of dressing, eating, toileting, bathing, and other self-care activities. Most of these people are capable of attending outside day programs, but they need a high level of supervision and assistance during nonprogram hours. (Certification as an ICF/MR permits reimbursement with federal Medicaid funds.)

Often, families of these young people must opt for geriatric care facilities when no ICF/MR is present in their area. Sometimes an ICF/MR is no more than one wing of a geriatric care facility; in these cases it generally has its own program, but shares staff and administration with the larger facility.

Residential Training Home

A residential training home is a group home that serves nine or fewer persons. Like an intensive care home, it provides skills training, but a prerequisite to living in this type of home is that residents must be toilet-trained, independent in eating, and must have other basic self-help skills, such as dressing with minimum assistance. Residents learn housekeeping skills, grooming, and money management.

An Illustrative Example Sandy is 40 years old and lives in a beautiful new residential group home owned and operated by Good Shepherd Lutheran Homes of the West, Inc., in Hillsboro, Oregon. This home, built to serve 10 persons with mental retardation, strives to achieve normalization. A staff of five serves the home 24 hours a day with skill training occurring in the home along with the daily activities of cooking, cleaning, bed-making, laundry, and personal hygiene.

Sandy left her family at age 31 to enter a larger residential facility run by the same nonprofit corporation. She lived in this larger facility for six years. This home, which served 84 residents, provided Sandy with the individualized training that was needed to prepare her for the more independent living she now experiences in the residential training home.

Adult Foster Care

Foster family care is the most difficult of the options to describe. It is heavily influenced by the idiosyncratic philosophies of the operators. The model of adult foster care, also known as family care homes or board-and-care homes, has a long history and varies from state to state.

Adult foster care can be defined as the placement of one to five persons with mental retardation in an existing family residence. A goal of foster family care is to integrate the resident into the existing family constellation, with the expectation that "in the normal environment, with understanding foster homemakers, he will learn to conduct himself in ways which will make him acceptable to those with whom he must live and work" (Dorgan, 1958, p. 418). Adults with Down syndrome are not kept as children, although adult foster care is often viewed that way.

One of the weaknesses of this option is that the model can sometimes become overly protective. Many foster care operators are not knowledgeable about mental retardation and, therefore, treat residents as adult-age children, overprotecting and isolating them. For others, however, adult foster care can be a great step toward independence and greater decision-making abilities, especially in cases where moving to a semi-independent apartment is not a possibility.

An Illustrative Example Candy lived 14 years of her life in the state residential institution for persons with mental retardation. In 1975, she left that institution and moved to a highly structured and supportive training group home. There she mastered most of her independent living skills: she learned to cook, clean, care for her own needs, and travel in her limited community. However, she did not learn to handle budgeting or to make medical or personal decisions without staff supervision.

At this point, it would have seemed appropriate for Candy to move on to an apartment training program and more independent living, but this was impossible. Yet, Candy had progressed steadily and was certainly ready for more independence. Adult foster care provided this option for Candy. Today, she lives in an adult foster care home with four other former group home residents and a foster care provider. The level of responsibility is high and the opportunity for independence greater. The chance for privacy and freedom is greater, but there is also supervision and support for the areas in which Candy still experiences difficulty.

Semi-Independent Apartments

A unique characteristic of institutions, group homes, and many foster care facilities is 24-hour supervision of residents. The semi-independent model is different because the amount of supervision can be variable. Other factors that can vary are the level of mental retardation, autonomy, home responsibilities, and employment of the residents. While all semi-independent community programs provide less supervision than other models, the pattern varies greatly. In some programs, staff members live with the group or in an adjoining apartment, but work directly with the residents for only a specified number of hours. In others, staff members live elsewhere and come into the residents' home or apartment on an "on call" basis or for a weekly appointment. The most common models are as follows.

1. The apartment cluster is composed of several apartments near one another, functioning to some extent as a unit, and supervised by staff members who reside in one of the clustered apartments. Apartment cluster living allows residents to make their initial step to independence in a supported environment with a minimum of risks. Residents can demonstrate their competence and readiness for greater independence, and staff can gather data to support the decisions that later need to be made relative to maximum levels of independence.

2. The single co-resident apartment is for one or two adult staff workers (often college students) and two or three mentally retarded persons, living together as roommates and friends.

3. The single maximum independence apartment is occupied by two or three persons with mental retardation, with supervision and assistance being supplied on an "on call basis" by a citizen advocate, a case worker, or a staff person from a sponsoring agency.

Regardless of the staffing variation, the pervasive theme of such programs is normalization, characterized most dramatically by a greater degree of risk taken on the part of the staff and supporting agency, and a greater amount of independence given to the residents. The high-potential, high-risk nature of this program often frightens many families.

An Illustrative Example   Mary is 31 years old. She attended a public high school and lived at home until she was 25. At 25, she took her first step of independence and moved to a group home a few miles away from her family. There she learned to care for herself, cook, clean, bank, budget, and seek out her own recreation. Today, Mary lives in a semi-independent training apartment with Kathy, her roommate. During the early phases of this experience, Mary had a skill trainer who came daily to provide training and support in money management, household cleaning, and grocery purchasing. This trainer also provided support for working out relationships with roommates and neighbors.

After 2 years in this program, Mary is more capable and needs less support from the skill trainer, who now only visits when Mary calls or by appointment once or twice a week. Soon Mary can enter the independence phase of the program where only occasional follow-up will be necessary. Follow-up and support will always be available should Mary need more training or assistance.

DETERMINING THE LEAST RESTRICTIVE ENVIRONMENT

As parents and program planners ponder the best living alternatives for a particular person with Down syndrome, there are four aspects of planning that need to be considered: analysis of behavioral repertoire, family readiness, communitization training and availability of residential options.

Analysis of Behavioral Repertoire

In order to plan for the movement of a given person with Down syndrome to the least restrictive environment possible, one must establish the behavioral characteristics needed and select the appropriate assessment measures. Based on these criteria, one may determine a given person's readiness for a community-living residence. Each of the aforementioned residential options maintains a prerequisite baseline skills level for admission to its program.

Essential to ascertaining the behavioral repertoire of the person with Down syndrome, effective assessment measures must be coupled with acute observational skills. The assessment measures are most often drawn from published procedures, checklists, or other forms developed by community-based residential facilities. Families as well as program planners need to be careful when choosing these assessment tools, as many commercial assessments have been standardized on nonretarded populations and may focus on children rather than adults. A summary of some other considerations and concerns that are significant in planning for movement and training programs follows.

> What is the setting in which the assessment is going to take place? Young people with Down syndrome are often other-directed. This discourages autonomous behaviors. The person has often been in a school or institutional program that has not been nurturing self-expression and so he comes to the assessment process desiring to conform and please rather than to demonstrate his competence. What is the level of the individual's verbal communication ability? Age, experiences, and expectations of significant others in their lives greatly affect the assessment process. What is the level of the person with Down syndrome's intellectual functioning? While intelligence and adaptive behavior are only moderately correlated, intelligence can affect the ability to respond to assessment tools. What degree of emotional adaptation does the person demonstrate? This factor is important since emotional problems often interfere with coping behavior and in that way affect the measurement of adaptive behavior. (Robinson & Robinson, 1976, p. 444)

The solution to these questions rests in making sure that the assessment process is comprehensive and that it includes a battery of tests and observations that are spread out in both time and place. They should begin early and should progress over time. They should document learning rates as well as behavioral changes.

Observational methods need to be part of the formal measures of adaptive behavior. Evaluators need to work hard at observing the person with Down syndrome in naturalistic environments (least structured and life-centered environments). Fact gathering by observation should be a daily event so that the individual is observed in different settings, by different people, and at different times of the day and evening. This forms the ideal in observation technique. Observers look, listen, and record, mindful of their possible biases and cautious to remain free of interpretive comments.

Family Readiness

Families are often reluctant to relocate a person with Down syndrome to the least restrictive environment, for doing so means changes for the family. In a sense, it may mean the loss of a "job" for the parent. While this job may have been a difficult one, giving up the paternal role and loosening attachments is hard. Parents have worked very hard at rearing their child. The process has been time consuming, often wearying. The "pay" is small, and the compensation has often been the Down syndrome person's semi-dependence on the parents. Families need support early in the process. Ideally, retraining should begin when the child enters elementary school. Families need to be oriented early on to the developmental model and normalization. Without this orientation, families may not take the first step toward exploring the options of independence.

Communitization Training

Program planners and helping professionals must help families develop attitudes that nurture community involvement, community exploration, and community experiences for the person with Down syndrome. Part of the communitization process includes learning about the rights of adults with mental retardation: the right to leave their mother and father and live in the least restrictive environment, the right to "risk" (Perske, 1972), the right to marry, the right to own property, and all the other rights enumerated in the "Declaration of General and Special Rights of the Mentally Retarded" adopted by the United Nations General Assembly in 1971.

Part of the communitization process also includes learning about normalization and the principles of individuation. The connotation of normalization as both process and product (both community movement and integration) must be clarified and coordinated with persons' rights to make choices about where they live, the work they do, their sexuality, and their leisure activities. Communitization includes familiarization with homemaking and home management. Finally, communitization means locating leisure and recreational activities outside of the residence and in the community, where they will serve the dual purpose of supplying enjoyment and providing training for independence.

Availability of Residential Options

Bruininks et al. (1985) found that almost every state has residential programs for persons with Down syndrome and other forms of mental retardation, and that most of these include options for persons with medical and behavioral problems as well. The problem, though, is that not every option is available in every community and/or state. Comprehensive systems are few in number, and no central coordinating agency or other mechanism exists to pull the fragmented system of private, not-for-profit, and state-funded programs into a coordinated whole. Furthermore, there are several obstacles that prevent this from ever happening. For example, the lack of funds as well as recent heavy bonding by states for capital outlays both to improve institutional settings and to enhance efforts at deinstitutionalization, have severely limited the development of programs aimed at those persons who are coming from their natural families into community living arrangements. The latter program has suffered in the interests of the former two. Priorities are established, the funds are committed—but redirecting priorities toward residential options and setting up a coordinated system of making those options available to persons in need is as difficult as it is important. One sees, then, that the barriers to a true continuum of services are still great.

SUMMARY

Three interrelated factors are relevant to the quality of life for persons with Down syndrome: where they live, where they work, and where they spend their leisure time. For many years, institutionalization was the preferred living arrangement option for families when their child with Down syndrome reached adulthood. Only when normalization as a policy became trenchant was a strong incentive against institutionalization as an option introduced. As a consequence of this, community-based living arrangements, comprehensive systems, and services within the developmental model are being developed throughout North America today.

Still, however, parents and professionals frequently differ strongly about which living arrangement provides the most normalizing environment, that which is least, restrictive and "as close as possible to the norm of society" (Nirje, 1976, p. 3). Young people with Down syndrome have themselves become advocates in this process.

Two varieties of alternative living arrangements continue to exist: community-based residences, such as group homes and apartments, and the more restrictive sheltered villages. While models for community-based living arrangements vary, the developmental continuum that assures family-like living arrangements and the opportunity for maximum growth and development still offers those with Down syndrome the greatest chance for living in the "least restrictive environment." The other type of residential arrangement, the sheltered village, provides a more protective environment, usually in a country or otherwise rustic setting away from the mainstream of the community. These villages vary in their degree of containment, types of housing arrangements, and their orientation toward resident skills training; but they are generally oriented toward the reference group in the community and not toward the urban or cultural expectations of the mainstream of society.

Young people with Down syndrome who live in urban community-based living arrangements are better prepared for accommodating cultural expectations more closely tied to societal norms. Their process of communitization is directed to the larger aspects of their community: their neighbors, tradespeople, and recreational and leisure organizations.

Normalization has led to more home-like living options with a developmental orientation. As part of the normalization continuum, the families of children with Down syndrome serve as the first (and normal) link in the process leading to a less restrictive environment for their children.

Determining the least restrictive environment and locating persons with Down syndrome in accordance with their developmental needs require cooperation between the families and professionals in assessing the behavioral repertoire of the individual, their family's readiness, and the communitization process that has taken place. Observational skills and standardized measures must be used to accumulate the data needed to make appropriate decisions. Methods of observation should operate on the entirety of the continuum between the most naturalistic and least structured and controlled, on the one hand, and the least naturalistic and most structured and controlled (experimental testing method) on the other.

To facilitate the move to the least restrictive environment, professionals need to start working early with families, educating them about normalization and developmental models. Educational and informational meetings are needed to address issues relating to independence, the rights of persons with Down syndrome, normalization and individuation, behavior management, homemaking, health and safety measures, and leisure-time training. But professional efforts of a more general and comprehensive nature are in order as well.

> Currently, funding patterns for residential services support agencies rather than individuals. Research and demonstration projects are needed on voucher systems and/or contracts for services in which designated funds follow the client to pay for services based on the assessment of individual needs. Very few residential programs provide acceptable client-based assessment. Without such assessment, planning and evaluation of services is difficult if not impossible. (Bruininks et al., 1985, p. 33)

The report (Bruininks et al., 1985) goes on to address "the primary gap between the state-of-the-practice and the state-of-the-art in residential services" (p. 31), indicating that the number of "state-of-the-art" programs are indeed limited in "quality, quantity, and variety" (p. 31). For example, families indicate a willingness to care for developmentally disabled persons at home, but are dissuaded from doing so by an appalling lack of necessary support services (e.g., crisis intervention, referral services, respite care options, assistance in making necessary modifications in the physical environment). In order to close the gap in residential services, a concerted effort needs to be made at:

. . . (a) identifying and overcoming significant financial disincentives, (b) modifying attitude barriers of both professionals and parents, (c) overcoming self-interest advocacy by those who benefit from the status quo, (d) increasing research and the dissemination of information on exemplary programs, and (e) providing adequate training and career incentives for staff to provide appropriate programming. (pp. 31–32)

Their final plea is further research—"research to study case management, funding practices and incentives, reimbursement methods, and client development and program monitoring systems" (p. 32).

The task, then, is for professionals and parents to form a partnership early on, each of them maximizing their concern for their specialized points of view, the former with an eye toward disability service systems and treatment practices, and the latter with an eye toward selecting the most appropriate and opportunity-enhancing alternative living situation for their child's special needs. It is only then that young adults with Down syndrome will be able to take the very normal and natural step of leaving their parents. This is their right every bit as much as it is the right of their parents to have them grow up and leave home.

REFERENCES

Bruininks, R. H., Hill, B. K., Lakin, K. C., & White, C. (1985). *Residential services for adults with developmental disabilities.* Logan: Utah State University, Developmental Center for Handicapped Persons.

Dorgan, J. (1958). A new home. *Canadian Journal of Public Health, 49*(10), 411–419.

Edwards, J. P. (1976). *Sara and Allen: The right to choose.* Portland, OR: Ednick Communications.

Edwards, J. P. (1983). *My friend David: A sourcebook about Down syndrome.* Portland, OR: Ednick Communications.

Fifield, M. G., & Smith, B. C. (1985). *Executive summary of technical reports.* Logan: Utah State University, Developmental Center for Handicapped Persons.

Kugel. R., & Wolfensberger, W. (Eds.). (1969). *Changing patterns in residential services for the mentally retarded.* Washington, DC: President's Committee on Mental Retardation.

McCarthy, J. (1980). Residential and hospital service delivery models. *Mental Retardation, 2*(6), 67.

Nirje, B. (1969a). The normalization principle and its human management implications. *Journal of Mental Subnormality, 16,* 62–70.

Nirje, B. (1969b). The normalization principle and its human management implications. In R. B. Kugel & W. Wolfensberger (Eds.), *Changing patterns in residential services for the mentally retarded* (p. 122–232). Washington, DC: President's Committee on Mental Retardation.

Nirje, B. (1971). Toward independence: The normalization principle in Sweden. *Déficience Mentale, 21,* 2–7.

Perske, R. (1972). *New directions for parents of persons who are retarded.* Nashville, TN: Abingdon Press.

Robinson, N. M., & Robinson, H. B. (1976). *The mentally retarded child: A psychological approach* (2nd ed.). New York: McGraw-Hill.

Tymchuck, A. (1984). *Steps to success training guide for group homes*. Portland, OR: Ednick Communications.

Tymchuck, A. (1985). *Effective decision making*. Portland, OR: Ednick Communications.

United Nations. (1971). *Declaration of general and special rights of the mentally retarded*. New York: Author.

Wolfensberger, W., Nirje, B., Olshansky, S., Perske, R., & Roos, P. (1972). *The principle of normalization in human services*. Toronto: National Institute on Mental Retardation.

Chapter 14

Vocational Opportunities
An Exploration of the Issues

Orv C. Karan,
Catherine Berger Knight, and Donna Pauls

In October, 1984, a national conference was convened in Boston that brought together most of the leading authorities in the country in the area of employment of persons with mental retardation and other developmental disabilities. The conference, a book of proceedings (Kiernan & Stark, 1986), and the model that provided the basis for the presentations and discussions were all called "Pathways to Employment for Adults with Developmental Disabilities." That model, as illustrated in Figure 1, represents current thinking in the employment area. Within this model, employment refers to activities for which one receives compensation, including both sheltered and nonsheltered work.

There are several interesting features to the Pathways Model. First, it is dynamic. It recognizes that both individuals and conditions change, and as they do, what may have been acceptable employment at one point in time may not be acceptable at another point.

The Pathways Model also recognizes that individuals with developmental disabilities, including those with Down syndrome, require different levels of assistance to maximize their employment potential. Thus, some persons with Down syndrome, by using the generic resources available to everyone, such as newspaper classified ads, employment services, or word-of-mouth contacts, are perfectly capable of finding employment on their own. Others may require time-limited services such as those provided by state agencies of vocational rehabilitation, whereas still others require lifelong support. Due to the severity of their disabilities, this latter group would not ordinarily receive vocational rehabilitation services. In response to this service gap, the Office of Special Education and Rehabilitative Services (OSERS) is promoting the

This work was supported in part by the Research and Training Center Grant #G008300148 from the National Institute of Handicapped Research, Department of Education, Washington, D.C. 20202

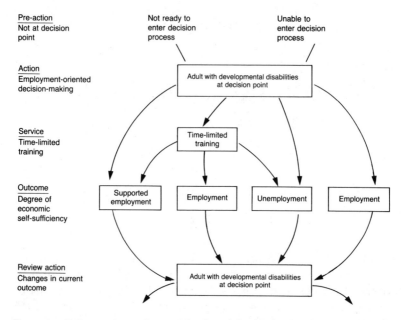

Figure 1. Pathways to employment for the adult with developmental disabilities. A habilitation model. (From: Kiernan, W. E., & Stark, J. A. [1986]. *Pathways to employment for adults with developmental disabilities* [p. 106]. Baltimore: Paul H. Brookes Publishing Co.)

concept of "supported employment" (Will, 1984), which combines an emphasis on the full range of normal job benefits with provisions for ongoing support at the worksite for those for whom competitive employment is unlikely (Bellamy, Rhodes, & Albin, 1986; Bellamy et al., 1984; Mank, Rhodes, & Bellamy, 1986; U.S. Department of Education, 1984; Wehman & Kregal, 1985).

Finally, the model recognizes that unemployment is an event that may occur either through circumstances or choice. It may simply be a stage in one's life entered while moving from one employment situation to another; or it may be that one is doing volunteer work; or it may be a decision made after weighing the alternatives and deciding that unemployment is the right choice at a particular point in time. As conditions, interests, and opportunities change so may the state of unemployment.

That it even considers employment options and possibilities for change are probably the most important features of the Pathways Model. Typically, one's employment options are limited to the positions available within one's community. For the overwhelming majority of individuals with mental retardation and other developmental disabilities, the options are usually restricted to segregated sheltered environments. Conventional wisdom guides these services and sustains the misconception that competitive employment can only be considered after one acquires certain prerequisite skills. Presumably, individuals who demonstrate their competence advance, that is, "flow" (Bellamy, Rhodes, Bourbeau, & Mank, 1982), through a continuum of sheltered work settings on their way to competitive employment. In reality, those with the more severe handicaps are usually placed at the bottom levels of the continuum (Bellamy et al., 1982), where less than 3% ever advance to the sheltered workshops, let alone into nonsheltered employment (U.S. Department of Labor [DOL], 1979). In fact, the average placement of persons into nonsheltered employment is less than 10% annually from sheltered workshops and almost nonexistent from other programs within the continuum (National Association of Developmental Disabilities Councils [NADDC], 1985; U.S. Department of Health and Human Services [DHHS], 1981; DOL, 1979). Based on these movement data, the annual likelihood of nonsheltered placement for individuals who have been in sheltered programs longer than 2 years is only 3% (Moss, 1979). In all fairness, though, these private nonprofit voluntary facilities continue to operate under a number of fiscal and programmatic constraints that have inhibited their ability to advance people through the continuum.

In spite of its many flaws, the "flow through" model is still the standard of vocational services in most parts of the United States. In fact, it was never seriously challenged until well into the mid 1970s, when national outcome data began illustrating the inherent limitations of this approach (Greenleigh Associates, Inc., 1975; Whitehead, 1979). Shortly thereafter, several innovative demonstration projects (Moss, 1979; Rusch & Mithaug, 1980; Schneider, Rusch, Henderson, & Geske, 1981; Wehman, 1981) started to yield impressive outcomes by circumventing the flow through model completely, and proceeding directly to training at the site of employment. By achieving successful nonsheltered placement with individuals whose only prior vocational experiences were derived from sheltered environments, these demonstrations provided convincing evidence that one's lack of productivity could be more a function of the program than of the individual (Beebe & Karan, 1986).

These and other more recent innovative programs continue to demonstrate that many individuals can benefit from employment services provided directly in the community. Furthermore, the benefits to society are frequently observable through indicators such as increased social skills by the participants (Hill & Wehman, 1983), more individualized program options (Beebe & Karan, 1986), and reduced program costs (Rudrud, Ziarnik, Bernstein, & Ferrara, 1984; Schneider et al., 1981). Other noteworthy benefits of providing services directly in the community include less need for retraining on the job and positive influences on both staff and consumer morale, since real movement can be seen (Rudrud et al., 1984). Further, the natural interaction opportunities in community-based employment programs enable both handicapped and nonhandicapped individuals to learn from each other (Rudrud et al., 1984).

In most cases, whereas it is simply not possible to offer a wide array of vocational choices in segregated settings, the opportunities and choices that exist in the community are practically endless. The Pathways Model represents an exciting and optimistic look at what could be in terms of employment, choice, and change. Obviously, as a model, it remains insulated from many of the realities that still prevent the full vocational normalization of most persons with mental retardation. For this reason, the following discussion is devoted to identifying guidelines, which, in the authors' opinion, must be considered in bringing the Pathways Model to its full potential, meaning that individual choice and more employment options become a reality for most persons with Down syndrome.

GUIDELINE ONE

All mentally retarded and other developmentally
disabled adults, including persons with Down syndrome,
are not the same, or "different strokes for different folks."

It is very much "in" today to serve individuals who are "severely handicapped" or "severely disabled." In fact, the Rehabilitation Act of 1973 even made vocational rehabilitation services a priority for such individuals. In spite of this, many persons with mental retardation and other developmental disabilities cannot even get into the vocational rehabilitation system, particularly if their IQ score is less than 50 (Karan, Porubcansky, & Gardner, 1976). They are often deemed unable to benefit from vocational rehabilitation services (Kiernan & Stark, 1986). In fact there are only a limited number of adults with mental retardation who are even served by state vocational rehabilitation agencies (NADDC, 1985; U.S. Department of Health, Education, and Welfare [DHEW], 1978), and persons with mental retardation and developmental disabilities tend to be rejected from these services at a higher than average rate (NADDC, 1985).

In all fairness, any review of state vocational rehabilitation services needs to recognize the limitations under which it operates. For one thing, its service model was never intended to accommodate the sometimes complex and continuing needs of persons with mental retardation and other developmental disabilities. In addition, the agency has multiple responsibilities to a wide array of individuals with handicaps; the combination of its federal and state funding is inadequate and there is usually a lack of suitable resources in most communities.

This does not, however, excuse the basic fact that there is too much "mixing of apples and oranges" in the terminology. When the employment potential of adults with mental retardation and other developmental disabilities is discussed, it must be remembered that these persons have a wide range of abilities, interests, and life experiences. Just because two individuals both have Down syndrome should, in no way, imply that they are both the same. Unfortunately, for a whole host of political, ideological, historical, and other reasons, this basic point is often lost.

Today's young adults with mental retardation, who have been exposed to educational opportunities that were unavailable a decade ago, are a qualitatively different group of persons than the generations that preceded them. Generally speaking, this new breed of young adults, at all levels of handicap, have more skills, more normalized life experiences, and more potential than their earlier counterparts (Brown, 1984). Both they and their parents rightfully expect the same opportunities for further education and jobs that are available to their nonhandicapped peers (Valera, 1982).

As these recent graduates push the adult system from one end, residents of large public institutions, who are slowly being returned to the community, are pushing it from another end. Many of these adults grew up before the passage of Public Law 94-142 and, therefore, missed training opportunities that are today all but taken for granted. Community service providers have not had much experience serving these adults, nor have these adults been well represented in any of the impressive nonsheltered employment demonstrations to date.

Then there are those individuals who have lived at home with their families all their lives. Most of these adults are middle-age or older, and because of the age, health, and/or death of their parents are just now coming to the attention of the adult service system.

And of course, there are those who have both mental retardation and mental health difficulties. It has been estimated that there are 50,000–80,000 of these dually handicapped individuals, including those with Down syndrome, in the United States (Menolascino & Stark, 1984).

Many, if not most, of those from any of these four groups could reasonably be called "severely handicapped." Without question, the life experiences of each member of each group will contribute to conditions that in no way can be fully appreciated or understood within one generic label, be it "severely disabled," "developmentally disabled," or even "the lowest 1% of the population." What instead may be more useful in communicating effectively about individuals with such diverse backgrounds and skills is to describe the extent of job adaptations and levels of support/supervision needed to sustain their employment opportunities. For just as there may be those with "severe handicaps" who require minimal supervision, there will also be those with "mild handicaps" who need intensive supervision to maximize their employment potential.

GUIDELINE TWO

*Predictions about the employment potential
of the person with Down syndrome cannot be made
on the basis of standardized vocational assessment instruments
or his or her performance within a sheltered work environment.*

Traditionally, the purpose of vocational assessment for persons with mental retardation has been to identify specifically what an individual is capable of doing and then to identify with equal specificity a job that matches the person's capabilities (Peterson & Jones, 1964). This approach to evaluation attempts to make predictions, and considerable research has been devoted to developing vocational assessment instruments that can measure those employee skills thought relevant to employment success (Karan, 1976; Mayeda, Pelzer, & Magni, 1979; Mithaug, 1981).

In spite of the relatively low predictive validity of such instruments (Pelzer & Mayeda, 1980) and a growing feeling that the currently prevalent assessment techniques tend to underestimate abilities and emphasize limitations (Bates, 1981), vocational assessment procedures originally developed for less cognitively impaired individuals are still being applied invalidly to those with mental retardation (Karan, 1977; Schalock & Karan, 1979).

It is interesting how willing people are to accept the responsibility when a particular employment program succeeds. But where does the responsibility fall when the person is unsuccessful? For example, as noted earlier, persons with Down syndrome and other developmental disabilities are often denied vocational rehabilitation services or rejected from services presumably because they lack interest, motivation, or capability. Focusing the blame for failure on the individual, however, provides an all too comfortable rationale for the person's lack of progress.

A related issue is that many of the judgments made about how people will cope with nonsheltered employment settings and conditions are often based on impressions made of them in sheltered settings. In such programs, some persons will spend months, years, and even lifetimes trying to learn prerequisite skills—and never advance. In effect, they may be permanently trapped (Karan & Schalock, 1983), learning skills that may never be acquired or needed, and that actually bear little resemblance to the needs of real jobs in the real world.

Such practices can no longer be accepted without question since there have been simply too many demonstrations in which individuals with mental retardation, whose only previous employment experiences were in sheltered settings, have been shown to be capable of working in a full range of employment settings (Bellamy et al., 1984; Brickey & Campbell, 1981; Clarke, Greenwood, Abramowitz, & Bellamy, 1980; Maurer, Teas, & Bates, 1981; Rusch, 1986; Schutz & Rusch, 1982; Sowers, Thompson, & Connis, 1979;

Wehman, 1981; Wehman et al., 1982) and of receiving reasonable wages for their work (Wehman & Hill, 1982).

Vocational assessment should no longer be used as an exclusionary mechanism, but rather must be viewed for what it is—namely, the beginning point of programming (Schalock & Karan, 1979). Vocational assessment must be based on actual work situations, and data need to be obtained while the person is in such an environment. These data can then provide feedback about the quality of one's work and can help identify useful areas in need of remediation. Interventions can then focus on enhancing both the skills of the individual and the strengths of the organization and community in order to maximize the fit and reduce the discord between people and their vocational environment. Although such an assessment takes time, it can be easily justified because it provides direction for modifying environments and for developing individualized training sequences and strategies that can contribute to better person-job matches (Karan & Schalock, 1983).

GUIDELINE THREE

The vocational life of the person with Down syndrome cannot be separated from all the other events, activities, and experiences to which he or she is exposed on a 24-hour basis.

Being employed means more than simply doing a set of specific tasks for a set period each day. Each of us is enmeshed in a complex social system or ecology, as both a giver and receiver in transactions with other individuals in a variety of roles and settings both vocational and nonvocational (Kauffman, 1981). Failure to realize the intricacies of these relationships often results in an underestimation of their influences.

Figure 2 provides a conceptual model to illustrate the reciprocal relationships between individuals with Down syndrome and the multiplicity of persons, places, and things with which they interact. Since there is so much evidence to suggest that the major reason such persons fail vocationally is due to social interpersonal difficulties (Crawford, Aiello, & Thompson, 1979; Edgerton & Bercovici, 1976; Foss & Bostwick, 1981; Greenspan & Shoultz, 1981; Niziol & DeBlassie, 1972; Richardson, 1978; Rosen, Clark, & Kivitz, 1977; Rusch, 1979; Sowers et al., 1979; Wehman, 1981), the model balances the individual's social interpersonal behaviors on a rather precarious base to convey how fragile these are and how easily they can be shifted.

A careful consideration of the model has important implications for determining the appropriateness of the work environment of the individual with Down syndrome. Thus, not only is it necessary to consider various employment benefits when examining the appropriateness of a particular job for an individual but these must also be balanced on the basis of different personal

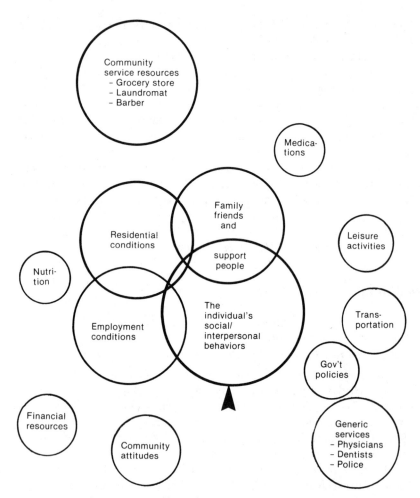

Figure 2. Reciprocal relationships between the person with Down syndrome and a multiplicity of other persons, places, and things. (From: Karan, O. C., & Knight, C. B. [1986]. Training demands of the future. In W. E. Kiernan & J. A. Stark [Eds.], *Pathways to employment for adults with developmental disabilities* [p. 258]. Baltimore: Paul H. Brookes Publishing Co.)

values, interests, opportunities, and conflicts in other non–job-related areas as well. What happens on the job may have ramifications outside the job, and simultaneously, an individual's nonvocational life may have both direct and indirect implications on his or her vocational life. Because of this, one must be careful to consider the "bigger picture" when considering the "right job" for a particular individual. For example, although a reduction in opportunities for integration with nonhandicapped persons can be viewed as a negative working condition, this may be balanced with higher pay which provides the personal resources to participate in integrated leisure activities during nonwork hours (Bellamy et al., 1984).

A consideration of the "bigger picture" also has implications for improving vocational assessment practices, particularly if an individual with Down syndrome is having difficulty functioning effectively on the job. Once the scope of inquiry is broadened to include person/environment interchanges occurring outside the employment setting, these may be found also to influence the person's job (Gardner, Karan, & Cole, 1984). It may be necessary to observe the individual across settings and time to identify both immediate and distant events that may be influencing the person and affecting his or her ability to function effectively on the job.

GUIDELINE FOUR

The social support provided within community environments is crucial to the vocational success of the person with Down syndrome.

Environments are characterized by the demands they make on individuals and the resources available to meet those demands. In employment settings where retention has occurred, the authors believe that there have been good matches between persons and their environments, and the environments have provided sufficient support to help the individuals meet the demands placed on them (Karan & Knight, 1986).

Social support has been cited in numerous studies as a major factor in the successful community adjustment of mentally retarded persons including those with Down syndrome (O'Connor, 1983), and its importance is no less critical in the area of employment. Individuals with social ties have been found to show less vulnerability to stress and to be more socially adjusted. Social support appears to be a vital ingredient for good mental and physical health (Heller, 1979; Mitchell, Billings, & Moos, 1982).

Clearly a social life and interactions with others are important for persons with Down syndrome (Baker, Seltzer, & Seltzer, 1977; Bercovici, 1981; Bjaanes & Butler, 1974; Butler & Bjaanes, 1977; Edgerton, 1967; Edgerton & Bercovici, 1976; Heller, Berkson, & Romer, 1981; Landesman-Dwyer & Berkson, in press; Weiss, 1974). Peer relationships play a critical role in the successful adjustment of adults with mental retardation in community settings (Romer & Heller, 1983), and there is evidence that individuals with greater degrees of peer contact are more likely to: 1) remain in the community (Gollay, Freedman, Wyngaarden, & Kurtz, 1978), 2) transfer to less restrictive settings, 3) demonstrate independence in self-care skills (Heller & Berkson, 1982), 4) earn more money, and 5) transfer out of sheltered workshops for positive reasons (Melstrom, 1982).

After reviewing the literature on the social adaptations of persons with mental retardation, Romer and Heller (1983) concluded that: "we should consider the possibility that the social mileu is as powerful a determinant of social adjustment as an individual's social skills are" (p. 311). As yet, though, with the exception of recent findings that nonhandicapped workers were generally indifferent toward the placement of mentally retarded workers in their settings (Wehman et al., 1982), the role of the larger community of nonhandicapped adults in promoting the adjustment of adults with mental retardation has not really been examined (Romer & Heller, 1983).

Supervision and support are critical elements in enhancing the employment potential and opportunities of persons with mental retardation. Many individuals, including professionals, both generic and specialized, parents, paraprofessionals, community service providers, the person on the street, all play important direct and indirect roles in providing this support. In this respect, there is a need to engage in better public relations and training to maximize the helpful participation of such a wide variety of potential supporters. For example, efforts to better utilize the generic service system should be expanded. Better training of mental health service providers (Reiss & Trenn, 1984; Szymanski & Grossman, 1984), whose biases currently limit their services (Alford & Locke, 1984), certainly ranks as a high priority given that the prevalence of psychopathology among persons with mental retardation is 4–5 times that of the normal population (Matson, 1984). Bus drivers, police officers, firefighters, barbers, and taxicab drivers, among others, all need to become more familiar with the special characteristics and needs of individuals with Down syndrome, while simultaneously becoming desensitized to their own fears, biases, and stereotypes that interfere with their serving such individuals as part of their daily clientele.

The family is obviously an important part of the support network of the person with mental retardation, and the role family members play in the successful employment of mentally retarded individuals is receiving increasing attention. As Wehman (1981) noted, "By helping to overcome transportation problems, working out SSI limitations, and providing strong moral support to their son or daughter in the job placement, parents can make a competitive placement successful or completely block it" (p. 7).

Movement toward integrated nonsheltered employment in the community is often resisted by some parents who are justifiably concerned about the security, stability, and safety that is provided in sheltered employment settings, but which may not be available in an integrated community employment environment (Hill, 1984; Whitehead, 1979). Recent studies have even shown a positive correlation between the parents' desire to see their family member remain in a noncompetitive setting and the level of severity of the person's handicap (Hill, 1984; NADDC, 1985).

Unfortunately, most parents have not been prepared for the employment potential of their children, even though they are usually in the best positions to serve as their children's advocates. Because of their lack of information about adult service availability and resources and their limited knowledge of what can be accomplished, they are often at a distinct disadvantage when it comes to working effectively with the service delivery system. However, through effective training, parents and/or significant others can become the ''glue'' that reduces the system fragmentation so notorious in adult services and can ultimately contribute to the best employment options for their family member. Greater emphasis in the area of parent training is now reflected in several programs that are attempting to provide parents with ongoing support and information to help them provide their child with the support they need (Wehman et al., 1982), and, simultaneously, deal with the stress they experience as their son or daughter moves into greater levels of independence (Intagliata & Doyle, 1984).

Finally, the social support provided by those who directly assist the individual with mental retardation in maintaining employment is also a critical component. In this respect, paraprofessional training will be particularly important to the successful implementation of more integrated nonsheltered employment since those who assist mentally retarded adults in such settings will not need advanced degrees.

During the late 1960s and well into the 1970s, while research in the vocational habilation area emphasized teaching technologies and provided the foundation for most current employment practices with adults with mental retardation and other developmental disabilities, little attention was paid to the importance of human interactions. Behavioral technology was king then. Now, however, terms like personal relationships, bonding, warmth, and respectfulness are some of the defining characteristics of effective supportive relationships between service providers and consumers (Karan, 1982; Stark, Baker, Menousek, & McGee, 1982). As these relationships develop, it is essential that ways to keep the providers in the field are found. Given that paraprofessonals represent the overwhelming majority of individuals with whom mentally retarded individuals have daily contact, the need for incentives to keep such persons in the field is great. High turnover rates of critical support persons can wreak havoc on the employment continuity and stability of a person with mental retardation.

Thus, contemporary approaches to employment will depend not only on trained personnel who can develop good supportive relationships with employees with mental retardation, but who themselves will be able to receive the support, resources, security, and job opportunities they need to sustain them in these important roles. In this respect, a significant question that is frequently overlooked in the support literature is: What provisions of support are available to those who provide support?

Figure 3 provides a conceptual illustration of the interface between the

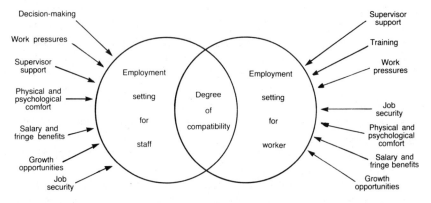

Figure 3. The mutuality of needs of both vocational support persons (staff) and workers with mental retardation (consumers). (Adapted from: Karan, O. C., & Knight, C. B. [1986]. Training demands of the future. In W. E. Kiernan & J. A. Stark [Eds.], *Pathways to employment for adults with developmental disabilities* [p. 260]. Baltimore: Paul H. Brookes Publishing Co.)

mutuality of needs of vocational support persons and workers with mental retardation. In this figure, the employment setting of the individual with mental retardation is also an employment setting for the support person. The setting could be either a sheltered or nonsheltered work environment, but in either case, the support person has some responsibility for promoting a social milieu that contributes to a successful employment adjustment for the person with mental retardation. Such individuals also have their own employment needs which, if not met, will dilute the energy they can direct toward promoting a healthy social environment for the individual with mental retardation.

As more efforts are made nationally toward more integrated employment options, it will become increasingly important to find ways to support the support persons. This will be particularly true when the level of support required to sustain a person with mental retardation on the job is intensive and the bond between the supporter and the supported is strong and meaningful. In fact, many of the current initiatives toward "supported employment" could be seriously compromised if the high staff turnover rates that pervade community residential services start to appear in the employment area as well.

GUIDELINE FIVE

The success of the employment potential of the person with Down syndrome will rest on the creation of employment opportunities that enhance that potential.

The many demonstrations of employment success suggest that the primary barrier to employment is not readiness for pay, but rather the presence of an opportunity to perform real work (Bellamy et al., 1984). There is simply too much evidence to show that skill deficiencies, transportation logistics, communication problems, and physical difficulties are not viable enough reasons to exclude persons with mental retardation from integrated employment (Brown et al., 1984). This evidence helps one to appreciate employment problems better for what they really are, not a lack of a person's potential or readiness, but rather a lack of appropriate employment services and opportunities (Bellamy et al., 1984).

The process of creating nonsheltered employment opportunities includes three essential ingredients: 1) to find job openings; 2) to train for these jobs; and 3) as noted in the last guideline, to provide continuing support so as to resolve immediate and potential problems.

To locate job openings, one has to survey the labor market within the specific community where employment will be sought (Mithaug, 1981). Some of the more specific methods for conducting a job market survey include reviews of help wanted ads, telephone surveys, questionnaires, professional referrals, personal contacts, and mailed surveys (Rusch & Mithaug, 1980; Wehman, 1981). Other resources include the state employment service, the chamber of commerce, the city assessor, the vocational rehabilitation agency, voluntary agencies, professional associations, unions, and political parties (Mithaug, 1981). As a general rule, one would want to access generic resources whenever possible (Beebe & Karan, 1986). Wehman et al. (1982) recommended advocating with employers to gain their support. This has also been shown to be a good way to identify their expectations, to educate them on the financial benefits of hiring employees with mental retardation, and even to solicit their assistance in convincing other employers.

Once potential jobs have been identified, a comprehensive job analysis is usually conducted to include a consideration of the personal, social, and actual job skill requirements important to employment success (Belmore & Brown, 1978; Schalock & Harper, 1978). This information helps identify the training objectives that specifically relate to successful completion of a job in a specific environment (Karan, 1982; Wehman, 1981). In conducting a comprehensive job analysis, it is also necessary to consider any special conditions that occur (Bates, 1981) and to include this information in the job training program. Mithaug (1981) recommended identifying information about the nature of the job, such as: 1) its main function, 2) its organizational climate, 3) its physical characteristics, 4) its psychological and social considerations, 5) its conditions affecting the required work, and 6) its practices affecting the makeup of its workforce.

As nonsheltered employment becomes more of a reality for more persons with mental retardation, the need for inexpensive modifications of the job sites and tasks will become of greater importance, particularly for those individuals with physical limitations. Through creative yet practical job modifications, it is not unrealistic to minimize the list of restrictions that limit the available employment choices. Providing inexpensive yet functional special materials or devices, modifying the job tasks without simultaneously affecting either the quality or the quantity of the work, providing ongoing assistance, and even attempting to modify the social attitudinal environment (Wehman et al., 1982) are all forms of job modifications that have proven useful.

Existing sheltered facilities may have more difficulties creating non-sheltered employment opportunities than do newly developing employment programs. Some of the newer programs devoted exclusively to placement in nonsheltered employment have been able to use more of their resources for direct supervision since a smaller portion of their budget is allocated for building and maintenance costs (Beebe & Karan, 1986).

GUIDELINE SIX

Vocational normalization for persons
with Down syndrome will require proactive systems changes.

There are obviously major gaps in the service delivery systems for adults with mental retardation and other developmental disabilities. The two major gaps most often identified in the literature (Bellamy et al., 1984; Elder & Magrab, 1980; DHHS, 1981; DOL, 1979) are: 1) the lack of central coordination of service delivery and 2) the lack of a single resource for long-term funding and employment-related services. These have been addressed in national studies (NADDC, 1985; DHHS, 1981; DOL, 1977, 1979) without resolution.

The service needs of persons with mental retardation cut across the lines of authority and responsibility of several agencies, both public and private. For example, the employment-related services needed for a student leaving school and attempting to enter the employment market could involve the local school, special education and vocational education programs, the local office of the state vocational rehabilitation agency, and private rehabilitation facilities, such as a sheltered workshop. Such agencies are rarely well coordinated. Furthermore, most of these key agencies are simply not doing their share in terms of maximizing the vocational potential of persons with mental retardation. Schools are not enabling students to make the transition from the classroom to the workplace. Studies have shown that only 30% of the individualized education programs (IEPs) evaluated included training for post-school employment as a goal (Schalock, 1986). In particular, those students who have severe impairments are often restricted to nonvocational programs in the school curriculum and often do not have access to school services such as career counseling and job placement assistance (NADDC, 1985). In spite of the fact that the Vocational Education Act of 1968 as Amended contained provisions to earmark 10% of the federal allocation to states for special programs for handicapped students (Public Law 90-576) and that recently enacted amendments (Public Law 98-524) included even stronger requirements, programs for students who have handicaps have not included many accommodations for those with mental retardation and other developmental disabilities (NADDC, 1985).

For most adults with Down syndrome there is no entitlement to employment services, and eligibility requirements permit wide discretion on the part of case managers and counselors (Hawley & Whitehead, 1981). The time-limited involvement of state vocational rehabilitation agencies makes it difficult, if not impossible, for those with greater service needs to benefit. And, although state mental retardation/developmental disabilities (MR/DD) agencies administer a broad array of services, sometimes on a lifetime basis, they tend to expect state vocational rehabilitation agencies to provide employment services. This same reasoning is seen in some of the provisions of the Title XIX Home and Community Care Waivers in which vocational services are not funded since, at the federal level, it is assumed that such services can be obtained through the state vocational rehabilitation agencies.

The Jobs Training Partnership Act (JTPA), the successor legislation of the Comprehensive Employment and Training Act of 1982, funds training and employment services. The act grants greater power to the local private industry councils (PICs) and also specifically provides for participation by state and private rehabilitation agencies. Yet, reports from the PICs indicate that only higher functioning mentally retarded persons seem to be receiving services. Few persons who have greater experiential, cognitive, and social deficits receive the benefits of JTPA funding (President's Committee on Employment of the Handicapped, 1984).

Many states' services are provided through state appropriations and/or through other federal/state funding combinations such as Title XIX and state appropriations. Unfortunately, such supplemental service programs often provide for the maintenance of individuals where they are rather than moving them up and out. Programs specifically focused on upward movement are almost nonexistent (NADDC, 1985). State MR/DD agencies, for example, are often able to fund or provide transportation, residential, and social recreational services almost indefinitely as part of an array of services within a community-based rehabilitation facility. But these same agencies may not be able to pay for such services if an individual's earnings exceed a certain level due to employment within the competitive sector. Thus, the incentive to remain in the sheltered work environment may be strong because the wage earnings of the competitively employed worker may not be sufficient to pay for needed services, which are available at no cost as long as the person remains in the sheltered setting (Whitehead, 1979).

An additional factor is the threat of loss of assistance and benefits provided under the Social Security Act. The structure of this program is such that persons with mental retardation are discouraged from entering the non-sheltered employment market. Although Congress has made numerous attempts to remove disincentives (the Social Security Disability Amendments of 1980, PL 96-265, and the Social Security Disability Benefits Reform Act, PL 98-460) the implementation of these changes often fails to extend to the state or local Social Security offices and/or is misinterpreted by the field offices (NADDC, 1985).

Without question, the lack of coordination among the state agencies; the competition among service providers; the lack of reliable data on program benefits and effectiveness; the multiple planning bodies with inadequate control and responsibilities; the multiple funding sources without financial coordination; the overlapping legislation and lack of a clear national policy; and the lack of adequate resources, including facilities, technology, and experienced trained staff are central concerns that stand in the way of vocational normalization for many persons with mental retardation. Strong and well-directed advocacy is needed to peel away these multiple layers of obstruction.

Yet, in spite of these overwhelming disincentives and obstacles, there are some incentives that have been shown to work. These include employer incentives, agency incentives, and even employee incentives (NADDC, 1985). Examples of employer incentives include such things as targeted jobs and tax-credited programs that offer employers a tax credit of up to 50% of the first $6,000 the worker earns in wages the first year and 35% of the first $6,000 in the second year. There are also on-the-job training programs administered by the ARC-US that pay 50% of the entry wage for the person's first 4 weeks and 25% of the entry wage for the second 4 weeks. In other cases, employers receive stipends and other cash incentives under some of the models of supported employment now operating in various states including Virginia, Washington, New Jersey, and Massachusetts. On a more limited scale, employer incentives also include on-site supervision, job coaching, and follow-along provided by the referring agency without cost to the employer (NADDC, 1985).

A few states, including Michigan, have experimented with the payment of bonuses for competitive job placement by sheltered workshops and other vocational rehabilitation facilities. In other cases, sheltered workshops, adult training centers, and other community-based facilities are encouraged by the state vocational rehabilitation agency to place people into competitive employment and often are rewarded for successful closure through increased fees (NADDC, 1985).

For the individual, incentives to move toward integrated competitive employment include higher wages, reduced dependency, enhanced self-worth, and the freedom to live and work with people who are not handicapped (NADDC, 1985).

SUMMARY AND CONCLUSIONS

The employment area within the mental retardation field is now receiving more deserved attention. Changing conditions are common, and they are being radically influenced by recent ideologies, technologies, priorities, and opportunities.

Obviously, the goal is not simply sheltered or nonsheltered employment, but rather choice and quality of life. Some individuals with Down syndrome may be quite content with placement within a sheltered environment. Not only is this their right, but given their particular circumstances it may also be the right choice as well. However, they should also have the opportunity to experience employment in integrated nonsheltered environments so that they can be better informed and wiser about the choices they make.

Creating more employment opportunities will require comprehensive policy changes to resolve many of the thorny issues that continue as obstacles (Bellamy, Sheehan, Horner, & Boles, 1980). Problems of wages and other disincentives to competitive placement in the community, and inherent problems of a fragmented adult services system are some of the critical issues that must be addressed. Such problems are especially complicated by ineffective program strategies as well as the difficulty of attempting to operate programs within unsupportive policies, rules, regulations, and resources. Resulting conflicts create tensions that affect service delivery and minimize opportunities. Yet as these issues are resolved, enhanced employment opportunities are possible. Based on where the field is today, the authors state the following conclusions:

1. Persons with Down syndrome who have a wide range of abilities and previous life experiences are capable of productive paid work.
2. A variety of work options should be available to these individuals.
3. The most appropriate working environment for any individual can only be determined after weighing all potential advantages and disadvantages a given setting affords the individual, and balancing these so as to be in the person's best interests.
4. Work is only part of an individual's day and needs to be examined in terms of how it affects the individual's quality of life around the clock.
5. How successful an individual is in maintaining a job is largely influenced by a cluster of variables that, taken together, constitute the individual's social support network.
6. Employment problems are not necessarily due to the lack of individual potential or readiness, but rather to the lack of appropriate employment services and opportunities.

If one treats persons with Down syndrome as they are, they will remain as they are. But if one treats them as if they were what they could be, by creating opportunities for them to participate in normal life experiences, by teaching them appropriate skills and behaviors to benefit from these experiences, and by providing continuing support so as to resolve immediate and potential problems, they will begin to realize their potential.

REFERENCES

Alford, J. D., & Locke, B. J. (1984). Clinical responses to psychopathology of mentally retarded persons. *American Journal of Mental Deficiency, 89,* 195–197.
Baker, B. L., Seltzer, G. B., & Seltzer, M. M. (1977). *As close as possible: Community residences for retarded adults.* Boston: Little, Brown.
Bates, L. A. (1981). *Vocational evaluation of severely physically impaired individuals: Considerations and technique.* Menomoniee: University of Wisconsin-Stout, Stout Vocational Rehabilitation Institute, Research and Training Center.
Beebe, P. D., & Karan, O. C. (1986). A methodology for a community-based vocational program for adults. In R. H. Horner, L. H. Meyer, & H. D. B. Fredericks (Eds.), *Education of learners with severe handicaps: Exemplary service strategies* (pp. 3–28). Baltimore: Paul H. Brookes Publishing Co.
Bellamy, G. T., Rhodes, L. E., & Albin, J. M. (1986). Supported employment. In W. E. Kiernan & J. A. Stark (Eds.), *Pathways to employment for adults with developmental disabilities* (pp. 129–138). Baltimore: Paul H. Brookes Publishing Co.
Bellamy, G. T., Rhodes, L. E., Bourbeau, P. W., and Mank, D. M. (1982, March). Mental retardation services in sheltered workshops and day activity programs: Consumer outcomes and policy alternatives. Paper presented at the National Working Conference on Vocational Services and Employment Opportunities, Madison, WI.
Bellamy, G. T., Rhodes, L. E., Wilcox, B., Albin, J., Mank, D. M., Boles, S. M., Horner, R. H., Collins, M., & Turner, J. (1984). *Quality and equality in employment services for adults with severe disabilities.* Unpublished manuscript, University of Oregon-Eugene.
Bellamy, G. T., Sheehan, M. R., Horner, R. H., & Boles, S. M. (1980). Community programs for severely handicapped adults: An analysis of vocational opportunities. *TASH Review, 5*(4), 307–324.
Belmore, K., & Brown, L. (1978). Job skill inventory strategy for use in a public school vocational training program for severely handicapped potential workers. In N. Haring & D. Bricker (Eds.), *Teaching the severely handicapped* (Vol. 3). Columbus, OH: Special Press.
Bercovici, S. M. (1981). Qualitative methods in cultural perspectives in the study of deinstitutionalization. In R. H. Bruininks, C. E. Meyers, B. B. Sigford, & K. C. Lakin (Eds.), *Deinstitutionalization and community adjustment of mentally retarded people* (Monograph No. 4, pp. 133–144). Washington, DC: American Association on Mental Deficiency.
Bjaannes, A. T., & Butler, E. W. (1974). Environmental variation in community care facilities for mentally retarded persons. *American Journal on Mental Deficiency, 78,* 429–439.
Brickey, M., & Campbell, K. (1981). Fast food employment for moderately and mildly mentally retarded adults: The McDonald's project. *Mental Retardation, 19*(3), 113–116.
Brown, L. (1984, September 22). Keynote address at the State Vocational Planning Conference, Madison, WI.

Brown, L., Shiraga, B., York, J., Kessler, K., Strohm, B., Rogan, P., Sweet, M., Zanella, K., VanDeventer, P., & Loomis, R. (1984). Integrated work opportunities for adults with severe handicaps: The extended training option. *Journal of the Association for Persons with Severe Handicaps, 9*(4), 262–269.

Butler, W. E., & Bjaannes, A. T. (1977). A typology of community care facilities and differential normalization. In P. Mittler (Ed.), *Research to practice in mental retardation: Volume 1. Care and intervention* (pp. 337–347). Baltimore: University Park Press.

Clarke, J. Y., Greenwood, L. M., Abramowitz, D. B., & Bellamy, G. T. (1980). Summer jobs for vocational preparation of moderately and severely retarded adolescents. *The Journal of the Association for the Severely Handicapped, 5,* 24–37.

Crawford, J. L., Aiello, J. R., & Thompson, D. (1979). Deinstitutionalization and community placement: Clinical and environmental factors. *Mental Retardation, 17,* 59–63.

Edgerton, R. B. (1967). *The cloak of competence: Stigmas in the lives of the mentally retarded.* Berkeley: University of California Press.

Edgerton, R. B., & Bercovici, S. M. (1976). The cloak of competence: Years later. *American Journal of Mental Deficiency, 80,* 485–497.

Elder, J. O., & Magrab, P. R. (Eds.). (1980). *Coordinating services to handicapped children: A handbook for interagency collaboration.* Baltimore: Paul H. Brookes Publishing Co.

Foss, C., & Bostwick, F. (1981, December). Problems of mentally retarded adults: A study of rehabilitation service consumers and providers. *Rehabilitation Council Bulletin.*

Gardner, W. I., Karan, O. C., & Cole, C. L. (1984). Assessment of setting events influencing functional capacities of mentally retarded adults with behavior difficulties. In A. S. Halpern & M. J. Fuhrer (Eds.), *Functional assessment in rehabilitation* (pp. 171–185). Baltimore: Paul H. Brookes Publishing Co.

Gollay, E., Freedman, R., Wyngaarden, M., & Kurtz, N. R. (1978). *Coming back: The community experience of deinstitutionalized mentally retarded people.* Cambridge, MA: ABT Books.

Greenleigh Associates, Inc. (1975). *The role of the sheltered workshop in the rehabilitation of the severely handicapped* (Report to the Department of Health, Education, and Welfare, Rehabilitation Services Administration). New York: Author.

Greenspan, S., & Shoultz, B. (1981). Why mentally retarded adults lose their jobs: Social competence as a factor in work adjustment. *Applied Research in Mental Retardation, 2,* 23–28.

Hawley, I., & Whitehead, C. (1981). Rights and entitlements of the handicapped: An issue for public and private service providers. *Journal of Rehabilitation Administration, 5*(2).

Heller, K. (1979). The effects of social support: Prevention and treatment implications. In A. P. Goldstein & F. H. Kanfer (Eds.), *Maximizing treatment gains* (pp. 353–382). New York: Academic Press.

Heller, T., & Berkson, G. (1982, April). *Friendship and residential relocation.* Paper presented at the Gatlinburg Conference on Research in Mental Retardation, Gatlinburg, TN.

Heller, T., Berkson, G., & Romer, D. (1981). Social ecology in supervised communal facilities for mentally retarded adults, VI: Initial social adaptation. *American Journal of Mental Deficiency, 86,* 43–49.

374 / Karan, Knight, and Pauls

Hill, J. (1984). *Survey of parent attitudes.* Richmond, VA: Rehabilitation Research and Training Center.

Hill, M., & Wehman, P. (1983). Cost benefit analysis of placing moderately and severely handicapped individuals into competitive employment. *The Journal of the Association for the Severely Handicapped, 8,* 30–38.

Intagliata, J., & Doyle, N. (1984). Enhancing social support for parents of developmentally disabled children: Training in interpersonal problem solving skills. *Mental Retardation, 22,* 4–11.

Karan, O. C. (1976). Contemporary views on vocational evaluation practices with the mentally retarded. *Vocational Evaluation and Work Adjustment Bulletin, 9*(1), 7–13.

Karan, O. C. (1977). The use of extended evaluation for mentally retarded clients. *Vocational Evaluation and Work Adjustment Bulletin, 10,* 20–26.

Karan, O. C. (1982). From the classroom into the community. In K. P. Lynch, W. E. Kiernan, & J. A. Stark (Eds.), *Prevocational and vocational education for special needs youth: A blueprint for the 1980s* (pp. 169–181). Baltimore: Paul H. Brookes Publishing Co.

Karan, O. C., & Knight, C. B. (1986). Developing support networks for individuals who fail to achieve competitive employment. In F. R. Rusch (Ed.), *Competitive employment issues and strategies.* Baltimore: Paul H. Brookes Publishing Co.

Karan, O. C., Porubcansky, R. E., & Gardner, W. I. (1976, January). *An investigation of mentally retarded clients both rehabilitated and nonrehabilitated or rejected by Wisconsin DVR during fiscal year 1974* (Progress Report No. 16P-56811/5-11; pp. 83–93). Madison, WI: Regional Rehabilitation Research and Training Center in Mental Retardation.

Karan, O. C., & Schalock, R. L. (1983). Who has the problem? An ecological approach to assessing vocational and community living skills. In O. C. Karan & W. I. Gardner (Eds.), *Habilitation practices with the developmentally disabled who present behavioral and emotional disorders* (pp. 77–91). Madison, WI: Rehabilitation Research and Training Center in Mental Retardation.

Kauffman, J. M. (1981). *Characteristics of children's behavior disorders* (2nd ed.). Columbus, OH: Charles E. Merrill.

Kiernan, W. E., & Stark, J. A. (Eds.). (1986). *Pathways to employment for adults with developmental disabilities.* Baltimore: Paul H. Brookes Publishing Co.

Landesman-Dwyer, S., & Berkson, G. (in press). Friendships and social behavior. In J. Wortis (Ed.), *Mental retardation and developmental disabilities: An annual review* (Vol. 13). New York: Plenum.

Mank, D. M., & Rhodes, L. E., & Bellamy, G. T. (1986). Four supported employment alternatives. In W. E. Kiernan & J. A. Stark (Eds.), *Pathways to employment for adults with developmental disabilities* (pp. 139–153). Baltimore: Paul H. Brookes Publishing Co.

Matson, J. (1984). Psychotherapy with persons who are mentally retarded. *Mental Retardation, 22,* 170–175.

Maurer, S., Teas, S., & Bates, P. (1981). *Project AMES:* Vol. I. 1979–1980. Des Moines: Iowa Department of Public Instruction.

Mayeda, T., Pelzer, I., & Magni, T. (1979). *Performance measures of skill and adaptive competencies of mentally retarded and developmentally disabled persons.* Los Angeles: University of California.

Melstrom, M. A. (1982). Social ecology of supervised communal facilities for mentally retarded adults: VII. Productivity and turnover rate in sheltered workshops. *American Journal of Mental Deficiency, 87,* 40–47.

Menolascino, F. J., & Stark, J. A. (Eds.). (1984). *Handbook of mental illness in the mentally retarded.* New York: Plenum.

Mitchell, R. E., Billings, A. G., & Moos, R. H. (1982). Social support and well-being: Implications for prevention programs. *Journal of Primary Prevention, 3,* 77–98.

Mithaug, D. E. (1981). *Prevocational training for retarded students.* Springfield, IL: Charles C Thomas.

Moss, J. W. (1979). *Post secondary vocational education for mentally retarded adults* (Final report to the Division of Developmental Disabilities, Rehabilitation Services Administration, U.S. Department of Health, Education, and Welfare, Grant No. 56P 50281/0).

National Association of Developmental Disabilities Councils, Employment Initiative Project. (1985). *Guidelines for evaluating, reviewing and enhancing employment-related services for people with developmental disabilities.* Washington, DC: Author.

Niziol, O. M., & DeBlassie, R. R. (1972). Work adjustment and the educable mentally retarded adolescent. *Journal of Employment and Counseling, 9,* 158–166.

O'Connor, G. (1983). Presidential address 1983: Social support of mentally retarded persons. *Mental Retardation, 21,* 187–196.

Pelzer, I., & Mayeda, T. (1980). *Item contents of performance measurement instrument for the developmentally disabled.* Los Angeles: University of California.

Peterson, R. O., & Jones, E. M. (1964). *Guide to jobs for the mentally retarded.* Pittsburgh: Marathon Institute for Research.

President's Committee on Employment of the Handicapped. (1984). *Avenues to employment: A guide.* Washington, DC: Author.

Reiss, S., & Trenn, E. (1984). Consumer demand for outpatient mental health services for people with mental retardation. *Mental Retardation, 22,* 112–116.

Richardson, S. A. (1978). Careers of mentally retarded young persons: Services, jobs, and interpersonal relations. *American Journal of Mental Deficiency, 82,* 349–358.

Romer, D., & Heller, T. (1983). Social adaptation of mentally retarded adults in community settings: A social-ecological approach. *Applied Research in Mental Retardation, 4,* 303–314.

Rosen, M., Clark, G. R., & Kivitz, M. S. (1977). *Habilitation of the handicapped: New dimensions in programs for the developmentally disabled.* Baltimore: University Park Press.

Rudrud, E. H., Ziarnik, J. P., Bernstein, G. S., & Ferrara, J. M. (1984). *Proactive vocational habilitation.* Baltimore: Paul H. Brookes Publishing Co.

Rusch, F. R. (1979). Toward the validation of social/vocational survival skills. *Mental Retardation, 17,* 143–145.

Rusch, F. R. (Ed.). (1986). *Competitive employment issues and strategies.* Baltimore: Paul H. Brookes Publishing Co.

Rusch, F., & Mithaug, D. (1980). *Vocational training for mentally retarded adults: A behavior analytic approach.* Champaign, IL: Research Press.

Schalock, R. L. (1986). Service delivery coordination. In F. R. Rusch (Ed.), *Competitive employment issues and strategies.* Baltimore: Paul H. Brookes Publishing Co.

Schalock, R. L., & Harper, R. S. (1978). Placement from community-based mental retardation programs: How well do clients do? *American Journal of Mental Deficiency, 83,* 240–247.

Schalock, R. L., & Karan, O. C. (1979). Relevant assessment: The interaction between evaluation and training. In G. T. Bellamy,, G. O'Connor, & O. C. Karan

(Eds.), *Vocational rehabilitation of severely handicapped persons: Contemporary service startegies*. Baltimore: University Park Press.

Schneider, K., Rusch, F. R., Henderson, R., & Geske, T. (1981). *Competitive employment for mentally retarded persons: Costs versus benefits*. Unpublished manuscript, University of Illinois, Department of Special Education, Champaign.

Schutz, R. P., & Rusch, F. R. (1982). Competitive employment: Toward employment integration for mentally retarded persons. In K. P. Lynch, W. E. Kiernan, & J. A. Stark (Eds.), *Prevocational and vocational education for special needs youth: A blueprint for the 1980's* (pp. 133–159). Baltimore: Paul H. Brookes Publishing Co.

Sowers, J., Thompson, L., & Connis, R. (1979). The food service vocational training program: A model for training and placement of the mentally retarded. In T. Bellamy, G. O'Connor, & O. Karan (Eds.), *Vocational rehabilitation of severely handicapped persons: Contemporary service strategies* (pp. 181–205). Baltimore: University Park Press.

Stark, J. A., Baker, D. H., Menousek, P. E., & McGee, J. J. (1982). Behavioral programming for severely mentally retarded/behaviorally impaired youth. In K. P. Lynch, W. E. Kiernan, & J. A. Stark (Eds.), *Prevocational and vocational education for special needs youth: A blueprint for the 1980s* (pp. 213–227). Baltimore: Paul H. Brookes Publishing Co.

Szymanski, L., & Grossman, H. (1984). Guest editorial: Dual implications of "dual diagnosis." *Mental Retardation, 22*, 155–156.

U.S. Department of Education, Office of Special Education and Rehabilitative Services. (1984). *Supported employment for adults with severe disabilities: An OSERS program initiative*. Unpublished manuscript.

U.S. Department of Health, Education, and Welfare. (1978). *Development of formal cooperative agreements between special education, vocational rehabilitation, and vocational education programs to maximize services to handicapped individuals* (Commissioner of Education and Commissioner of Rehabilitation Services [Memorandum]). Washington, DC.

U.S. Department of Health and Human Services. (1981). *Final report: Training and employment services for handicapped individuals*. Washington, DC: Office of the Assistant Secretary for Planning and Evaluation.

U.S. Department of Labor. (1977). *Sheltered workshop study: Workshop survey* (Vol. 1). Washington, DC: Author.

U.S. Department of Labor. (1979). *Sheltered workshop study: Study of handicapped clients in sheltered workshops* (Vol. 2). Washington, DC: Author.

Valera, R. (1982). Self advocacy and changing attitudes. *A public awareness viewpoint*. Washington, DC: American Coalition for Citizens with Disabilities.

Wehman, P. (1981). *Competitive employment: New horizons for severely disabled individuals*. Baltimore: Paul H. Brookes Publishing Co.

Wehman, P., & Hill, M. (1982). *Vocational training and placement of severely disabled persons: Volume 3. Project employability*. Richmond: Virginia Commonwealth University.

Wehman, P., Hill, M., Goodall, P., Cleveland, P., Brookes, V., & Pentecost, J. H. (1982). Job placement and follow-up of moderately and severely handicapped individuals after three years. *The Journal of the Association for the Severely Handicapped, 7*, 5–16.

Wehman, P., & Kregel, J. (1985). A supported work approach to competitive employment of individuals with moderate and severe handicaps. *Journal of Association for Persons with Severe Handicaps, 10*(1), 3–11.

Weiss, R. S. (1974). The provisions of social relationships. In Z. Rubin (Ed.), *Doing unto others: Joining, molding, conforming, helping, & loving* (pp. 17–26). Englewood Cliffs, NJ: Prentice-Hall.

Whitehead, C. (1979). Sheltered workshops in the decade ahead: Work and wages, or welfare. In G. T. Bellamy, G. O'Connor, & O. C. Karan (Eds.), *Vocational rehabilitation of severely handicapped persons: Contemporary service strategies* (pp. 71–84). Baltimore: University Park Press.

Will, M. (1984). *OSERS programming for the transition of youth with disabilities: Bridges from school to working life.* Washington, DC: Office of Special Education and Rehabilitative Services.

Themes for Consideration

Douglas Fenderson

There are a few themes that emerge consistently in this book. Madeleine Will began her foreword by speaking of fragmentation of services. That theme was reiterated in several of the chapters and responses. In fact, if one were to do a content analysis of the authors' deliberations, the concern about fragmentation of services, whether at the federal, state, or local level, would certainly be a major one.

The second theme reiterated in several discussions is that vocational and related personal skills should be learned in a natural community environment and not in artifically contrived ones. The "predictive validity" of various tests and of prevocational training is simply too low to be of practical value. There is increasing evidence that by approaching "criterion behavior" in the environments in which persons are to function, the outcomes are generally more satisfactory. In fact, this emphasis is so important that Will, Assistant Secretary of the Office of Special Education and Rehabilitative Services, has secured an additional appropriation of $5 million for replication and demonstration projects to extend and generalize this concept. Related ideas include task analysis, behavior management, and socialization skills. These are all part of an overall approach to the "transition from school to work."

Another major theme of this book raised initially by Will has to do with expectations. She said, in effect, that all too often one expects very little from persons with Down syndrome—and one tends to get what one expects. Expectations need to be raised not only by the families of individuals with Down syndrome, but by the schools, community service providers, and the whole array of rehabilitation and related professionals as well.

The importance of early work and community experience was emphasized. Paige Calvin is certainly a prime example of an accomplished person with Down syndrome who has been able to achieve because of opportunities afforded her within the home, the school, and the community. Achievements like Paige's have been shown to be predictive of ongoing success.

Ted Tjossem's efforts at the National Institute of Child Health and Human Development, Mental Retardation/Developmental Disabilities Branch has helped to define the major biomedical domains and topics for investigation in this subject area. There are new tools and techniques that are becoming increasingly productive, particularly in the area of molecular biology.

With regard to epidemiology, it was pointed out that population trend data may be useful for planning of community service programs but that there are limitations. They are subject to interpretation and are based on several assumptions as, indeed, are various Census Bureau projections. But, in any event, they provide rough approximations for purposes of service system planning. However, the subdomains of epidemiological data are not as accurate as they need to be. There are major problems with the validity of data from birth and other public records. This represents a major research need.

On the subject of early intervention, a dilemma is perceived. Not nearly enough is known, but there is a great deal that is known yet not consistently applied. Further study, as well as consistent application of current information, must be a major emphasis.

It was somewhat sobering to read the discussion of early intervention and to realize how much well-designed studies are needed. The practical problems of doing such studies are enormous; one problem is the infinity of variables and their interactions, ranging from the levels of cellular biology and organ characteristics to personal, family, and community aspects. Again, there is great need and potential for understanding this early fundamental process within the social environment as it contributes to developing building blocks for subsequent growth, development, and successful adaptation. This represents an important area for additional research.

"Diffusion of knowledge" or "information dissemination" is an area of study and application within several federal agencies. One of the recurring themes of this volume is that, in a number of areas, communication is not as effective as it could be. This fact provides a target at the national, state, and local levels with regard to application of these communication techniques.

Regarding "power bases," historically, there are programs associated with state departments of public welfare, education, and health; private medical practice; and community-based services. Several of this book's authors took aim at this fragmentation and the special restrictive eligibility rules. Again, there seems to be a need for leadership at all levels. It was suggested that a revolutionary concept, one that visualizes the individual with Down syndrome and the family to be at the center of concern and all the service programs revolving around them and their needs, is appropriate. It would be a more functional way of centralizing the relation between the needs of individuals, the flow of dollars, and the needs of families. This theme was reiterated repeatedly in the chapters and responses on living arrangements, federal funding, and public policy initiatives.

As a group, scientists are characterized by two "paradoxical" qualities. They tend to be very enthusiastic and at the same time quite skeptical. As applied to particular problems regarding alternative services, there is a need for those with the opportunity to provide leadership to be enthusiastic about what is happening and the potential for things to happen, but also to be realistic and somewhat skeptical about the things that are not happening. Let all scientists rededicate themselves to continue to be diligent both in enthusiasm and skepticism.

With regard to the elementary school years, there are very few data relevant to the effects of integration, let alone to the effects of certain skill-building elements. Most of the data reported are sketchy, descriptive, anecdotal, and they do not provide a tough-minded technology of approaches that can be readily applied to the understanding of what constitutes a strong educational base. Although for years there have been university affiliated facilities (UAFs), research through special education programs (SEP), and various studies through the National Institute of Handicapped Research (NIHR) and the National Institute of Health (NIH), the amount that is known about some of those very crucial issues in an applied sense is very limited. Certainly there is a whole research agenda needed for these issues.

Furthermore, the following questions must be answered: What is the basis for the curriculum for persons with Down syndrome? How is school time best used? Is this simply an approximation to some vision of "normal" adult roles or is it something that is altogether different and requires a new conceptualization of curriculum? These questions about the conceptual basis for curriculum were raised both in the elementary and secondary level discussions. Transition bridges from school to adult roles with special emphasis on work have been identified by Will as one of the most important areas to which the "transition" strategy should be directed. To achieve a successful employment goal usually implies resolution of other problems such as transportation and community living.

Speech and language development were also discussed. In regard to language development, language environment, and the indications of success in intervention, again, the question of diffusion of knowledge and stimulation of best practices around the country was raised. Novel investigations in the field of communication are absolutely essential. This is because of the large number of medical, neurological, cognitive, social, and environmental variables related to the development of communication skills. Longitudinal research is necessary in order to answer these questions. Investigators who must commit long periods of time—10 or 20 years in order to achieve conclusive results—require greater continuity in federal support. The use of observational and qualitative analysis may be more appropriate in handling some of these problems than more conventional quantitative approaches. Regarding speech, there was emphasis on the question of intelligibility and the need for additional clinical research to examine much more carefully the effectiveness of interventions.

In the discussion of the secondary curriculum, it was felt that what is needed is to start at the level of values. Values are basic and there must be some clear vision of adult roles. Nevertheless, without a sense of commitment or values, and a clear vision of adult roles, including work in the local community, it is very difficult to develop effective programs. It is like the introductory statement by Mager (1962) on educational objectives—"If you're not sure where you're going, you're liable to end up some place else" (p. ix).

Another recurring theme has to do with professional bias. Education is the usual prescription; educational materials should be developed to update them. As important as that undertaking may be, it should be remembered that the American Academy of Pediatrics tried a national continuing education program based on very well-developed materials regarding disabled children, including those with Down syndrome. Participation was very meager. One may not be able to teach physicians all of the nuances that they "need" to know in order to manage long-term medical care adequately for many children and adults with Down syndrome. This represents another area of unsolved problems.

Paradigm shifts suggest that textbooks need to be rewritten. This book will, in some sense, stimulate the development of programs and thinking on this entire subject.

Regarding independent living arrangements, various methods were discussed, with the key being the specific way in which the dollars flow. This seems to be another major target requiring emphasis by and collaboration of the private and public sectors.

The consensus of the authors of this book indicates that it is necessary to continue efforts to assure that all persons with Down syndrome are included in all aspects of society. This goal has not yet been achieved, and is the ultimate toward which all must strive.

REFERENCES

Mager, R. F. (1962). *Preparing instructional objectives.* Palo Alto, CA: Fearon.

Epilogue

Diane M. Crutcher

✦✦✦

Several points became apparent during the writing of this book. They are the cornerstone from which we all must work in order to ascertain the ultimate of services and rights for persons with Down syndrome.

Most important, the individual with Down syndrome is exactly that—an individual first, and an individual with a disability second. The right to live once born and the right to a reasonable quality of life should no longer be in doubt for persons with Down syndrome. In tandem with these statements, then, is the measuring of improvement and progress in terms of satisfaction in life on the part of persons with Down syndrome.

Persons with Down syndrome today are being raised in family homes to live and work in the community. Because of current interdisciplinary commitment, promise of yet further personal opportunities for persons with Down syndrome is evident. There is a profound positive impact on society from the shared existence between individuals with and without mental retardation. The community must become more accepting of family-scale residences and adult living arrangements that will encourage appropriate, realistic interactions for all.

The lessons learned from attention to the needs of persons with Down syndrome can be generalized. It is appropriate that people concerned with Down syndrome join in advocacy efforts directed toward support for individuals with a broad range of disabilities. Political progress in support of handicapped persons directly affects personal gains for individuals with Down syndrome, and this, in turn, has a reciprocal effect on the potential for political progress. Renewed promotion is needed for support of research and design of new human services relating to persons with special needs.

At this time, we have only cursory knowledge of the feelings and emotional elements in the lives of persons with Down syndrome and their families. As we attempt to serve this population, we must keep in mind what we do not know, and we must also remember that the parent/professional partnership is the best way for the child with Down syndrome to receive and benefit from the services he or she needs and deserves.

We do not currently have a cure for Down syndrome, although supportive therapies offer much assistance. Many other questions persist regarding a basic understanding of the special features of Down syndrome. There are important new approaches at the molecular and cellular level that give promise of obtaining fresh understanding of some specific biological problems. Major improvements in health care are now being applied to persons with Down syndrome, greatly enhancing their lives and life-span. There exist now many proven service delivery models and instructional techniques that have not yet been made available to serve all persons with Down syndrome, but should be.

The ultimate method for coordinating all facets of Down syndrome as it touches the child, the family, friends, and professionals is a National Down Syndrome Center to collect and disseminate information. It is vital to all who read this book and care about those with Down syndrome that it is understood where we are, what the "givens" are, where we need to go, and how we are going to get there—*together*.

Appendix

✛✛✛

The following individuals were involved in various aspects of the Down Syndrome State-of-the-Art Conference held April 23–25, 1985, in Boston, Massachusetts. The conference was made possible through Grant #300-85-0071, 1984, funded by the National Institute of Handicapped Research. The National Down Syndrome Congress served as the conference sponsor.

PRESENTERS/REACTORS

G. Thomas Bellamy, Ph.D.
Diane Bricker, Ph.D.
Paige Calvin
Claire Canning
Allen C. Crocker, M.D.
Michael Cummings, Ph.D.
Gunnar Dybwad, Ph.D.
Jean Elder, Ph.D.
Charles J. Epstein, M.D.
Douglas Fenderson, Ph.D.
H. D. Bud Fredricks, Ed.D.
Thomas Gilhool, Esq.
Marci Hanson, Ph.D.
Lewis Holmes, M.D.
DeAnna Horstmeier, Ph.D.
Carl Huether, Ph.D.
Georgiana Jagiello, M.D., D. Sc.
Orv C. Karan, Ph.D.
David Kurnit, M.D., Ph.D.
Ronald Melzer, Ph.D.
Jon F. Miller, Ph.D.
Ken Moses, Ph.D.
Thomas Nerney
Thomas J. O'Neill, A.C.S.W.
David Patterson, M.D.
Robert Perske
Siegfried M. Pueschel, M.D., Ph.D.,
    M.P.H.
John E. Rynders, Ph.D.
Miriam Schweber, Ph.D.
Sondra Spector, R.N.
Denis W. Stoddard, Ph.D.
Horace C. Thuline, M.D.
Carol Tingey, Ph.D., F.A.A.M.D.
Theodore Tjossem, Ph.D.
Ann P. Turnbull, Ed.D.
Madeleine Will
Jean M. Zadig, Ph.D.

PLANNING COMMITTEE

Allen C. Crocker, M.D.
Naomi Karp
Thomas J. O'Neill, A.C.S.W.
Diane M. Crutcher
DeAnna Horstmeier, Ph.D.
Thomas Nerney
Siegfried M. Pueschel, M.D., Ph.D.,
    M.P.H.
Theodore Tjossem, Ph.D.

CONFEREES

Alan Abeson, Ed.D.
Michael Begab, Ph.D.
Robert Crow, Ph.D.
Jo Ann Simons Derr, M.S.W.
Thomas E. Elkins, M.D., F.A.C.O.G.
Rebecca Fewell, Ph.D.
Professor Jesus Florez
Robert M. Greenstein, M.D.
Rudolf Hormuth, M.S.W.
Vince Hutchins, M.D.
Libby Kumin, Ph.D.
David J. Lang, M.D.
S. Michael Lawhon, M.D.
Ernest McCoy, M.D.
Ann Murphy, M.S.
JoAnne Putnam, Ph.D.
Alice Shea
Eunice Shishmanian
Mary Ann Smith, Ph.D.
Dr. Wolfgang Storm
Ludwik Szymanski, M.D.
Professor Conor Ward
Elizabeth Zausmer

Index

+++

Independence, *see* Residential options
Individuality, recognition of, 174–175, 383
  in residences, 340
  vocational rehabilitation and, 358–359
Individualized education program (IEP),
      196–197
  family involvement in, 302–303
  objectives of, 198
  Oregon high school, 206–207
  parental decision-making and, 291–293
Infants
  early intervention with, research on,
      155–158
  health concerns in, 114–119
    appropriate counseling and, 114–115
    cataracts, 117
    gastrointestinal anomalies, 115
    heart disease, 85–88, 115–117
    newborn and well-baby care, 118–119
  physical examination of, 118
  screening tests in, 118
  see also Children
Infection, 48
  middle ear, 122, 233
Infectious diseases, 120–121
Institutionalization movement, 3, 6–7
Instruction
  in Oregon High School model, 207
  see also Education
Instruction technology, Oregon High School
      program design versus, 228–229
Integration
  at elementary school level, 179–193,
      195–201
    Oregon survey of, 180–191
    settings for, 186–190
    see also Oregon survey of elementary
        education
  mainstreaming versus, 213
  at secondary school level, 213–215
    see also Education; Mainstreaming; Nor-
        malization
Intellectual development, early intervention
      and, 156–157
Intelligence tests, 320–321
Intelligibility, 242–243, 263–265
Intensive care homes, small, 345–346
Interferon receptor, 51
  increased dosage of, effects of, 71–73
  malformations and, 84
Intervention
  communication, 251–254, 263–267
  early, *see* Early intervention
  family transitions and, 302–303
  parents in, 293–294
Intraspindle apparatus, mutation of, 35
Ionizing radiation, 102
Irradiation hybrids

cytogenic analysis of, 57
production of, 54

Jobs Training Partnership Act (JTPA), 369

Karyotypes, 43–44

Language, oral versus sign, 242, 253–254
Language acquisition, 234–237
  deficits in, 237–238
Language development, 233–256, 381
  comprehension and, 246–248
  discourse in, 243–245
  early intervention and, 156–157
  environment and, 249–251
  future research questions about, 254–256
  language intervention and, 251–253
  phonology in, 242–243
    intervention in, 263–265
  semantics in, 241–242
  sign language training and, 253–254
  social maturity and, 319
  syntax in, 238–241
  vocabulary in, 245–246
Learning
  development and, 152–155, 172
  functional
    early intervention goals for, 160–161
    elementary, 196–197
  structuring environment for, 164–165
  see also Education
Learning process, early intervention and,
      162–163
Legislation
  Community and Family Living Amend-
      ments, 282
  history of, 10–13
  state zoning laws, 282
Lejeune, Jerome, 278
Leukemia, 48, 50–51
Linguistic abilities, *see* Language develop-
      ment
Linguistic environment, 265–267
Literacy, 187, 190, 199–201
Living options, 337–353
  see also Residential options
Looking behavior, 245–246

Mainstreaming
  early intervention and, 161–162, 175–176
  history of, 11–12
  integration versus, 213
  see also Integration; Normalization